CLINICAL CHALLENGES IN COPD

CLINICAL CHALLENGES IN COPD

Edited by

C. F. Donner and M. Carone

CLINICAL PUBLISHING

OXFORD

Clinical Publishing
an imprint of Atlas Medical Publishing Ltd

Oxford Centre for Innovation
Mill Street, Oxford OX2 0JX, UK

Tel: +44 1865 811116
Fax: +44 1865 251550
Web: www.clinicalpublishing.co.uk

Distributed in USA and Canada by:
Clinical Publishing
30 Amberwood Parkway
Ashland OH 44805, USA

Tel: 800-247-6553 (toll free within U.S. and Canada)
Fax: 419-281-6883
E-mail: order@bookmasters.com

Distributed in UK and Rest of World by:
Marston Book Services Ltd
PO Box 269
Abingdon
Oxon OX14 4YN, UK

Tel: +44 1235 465500
Fax: +44 1235 465555
E-mail: trade.orders@marston.co.uk

© Atlas Medical Publishing Ltd 2007

First published 2007

All rights reserved. No part of this publication may be reproduced, stored in a retrieval system, or transmitted, in any form or by any means, without the prior permission in writing of Clinical Publishing or Atlas Medical Publishing Ltd.

Although every effort has been made to ensure that all owners of copyright material have been acknowledged in this publication, we would be glad to acknowledge in subsequent reprints or editions any omissions brought to our attention.

A catalogue record for this book is available from the British Library

ISBN-10 1 904392 91 1
ISBN-13 978 1 904392 91 0

The publisher makes no representation, express or implied, that the dosages in this book are correct. Readers must therefore always check the product information and clinical procedures with the most up-to-date published product information and data sheets provided by the manufacturers and the most recent codes of conduct and safety regulations. The authors and the publisher do not accept any liability for any errors in the text or for the misuse or misapplication of material in this work.

Project manager: Gavin Smith, GPS Publishing Solutions, Hertfordshire, UK
Typeset by Mizpah Publishing Services Private Limited, Chennai, India
Printed in Spain by T G Hostench s.a., Barcelona, Spain

Contents

Editors vii

Contributors vii

Preface xi

1 Improvement of symptoms in a 62-year-old COPD patient after lung volume reduction surgery 1
   R. J. McKenna, Jr.

2 Patients with very frequent exacerbations of COPD: clinical stabilization after the prescription of inhaled corticosteroids 7
   P. M. A. Calverley, M. Cazzola

3 Reduction in the level of dyspnoea near the end of life 19
   D. A. Mahler, G. L. Scano

4 A COPD patient with bronchospasm episodes after the inhalation of tobacco smoke 29
   S. Nardini, G. Invernizzi

5 Improvement in exercise capacity after correcting calorie uptake in a patient with severe emphysema 37
   A. Del Ponte, S. Marinari

6 A 36-year-old patient with stage I – GOLD misdiagnosed as asthma 43
   I. Cerveri, R. Nimiano, J. Vestbo

7 A 68-year-old patient with COPD 49
   T. Troosters, R. Casaburi

8 Clinical approach to a COPD patient with muscle hypotrophy 65
   F. De Benedetto, S. Marinari, E. F. M. Wouters

9 Improvement of function and health status in a severely disabled patient with COPD 75
   P. W. Jones, M. Rosa Güell Rous

10 COPD caused by occupational exposure 85
   J. R. Balmes, D. Nowak

11	Body mass index as a prognostic factor in COPD B. R. Celli	97
12	Multiple vertebral fractures in a COPD patient on long-term inhaled corticosteroids F. De Benedetto, A. Spacone	105
13	Managing acute respiratory failure during exacerbation of COPD A. Torres, M. Ferrer, S. Nava	115
14	Difficult weaning in a COPD patient with acute respiratory failure after use of benzodiazepines C. Girault, N. Ambrosino	125
15	Suspected exacerbation of COPD in a 56-year-old woman with atrial fibrillation S. Ramanuja, M. D. L. Morgan	135
16	Antibiotic allergy in a COPD patient with frequent bacterial exacerbations S. Sethi, F. Blasi	143
17	Tuberculosis re-exacerbation in an older smoker with COPD L. Casali, J.-P. Zellweger	155
18	A 58-year-old woman with COPD and acute fever after visiting relatives in the countryside – farmer's lung M. Iversen, G. Moscato	161
19	Higher than expected rest hypoxaemia in a 74-year-old COPD patient with only mild airway obstruction E. M. Clini, A. M. D'Armini, I. Sampablo	169
20	A 52-year-old woman with mild COPD and significant oxygen desaturation during exertion J. Zieliński, T. J. Ringbaek	179
21	Hemidiaphragmatic paralysis after cardiac surgery in a 62-year-old COPD patient S. Zanaboni, L. Appendini, B. Schönhofer	191

Abbreviations   199

Index   203

Editors

Claudio F. Donner, MD, Medical Director, Mondo Medico, Multidisciplinary and Rehabilitation Outpatient Clinic, Borgomanero (NO), Italy

Mauro Carone, MD, 'Salvatore Maugeri' Foundation IRCCS, Scientific Institute of Veruno (NO), Italy

Contributors

Nicolino Ambrosino, MD, Pulmonologist, Pulmonary Unit, Cardiothoracic Department, University Hospital Pisa, Pisa, Italy

Lorenzo Appendini, MD, Consultant in Pneumology and Critical Care Medicine, Division of Pneumology, 'Salvatore Maugeri' Foundation IRCCS, Institute of Care and Research, Scientific Institute of Veruno, Veruno (NO), Italy

John R. Balmes, MD, Professor, University of California San Francisco, Division of Occupational and Environmental Medicine, San Francisco General Hospital, San Francisco, California, USA

Francesco Blasi, MD, PhD, Professor of Respiratory Medicine, Institute of Respiratory Diseases, University of Milan, Milan, Italy

Peter M. A. Calverley, MD, FRCP, FRCPE, Professor of Respiratory Medicine; Honorary Consultant Physician, University Department of Medicine, University Hospital Aintree, Liverpool, UK

Richard Casaburi, MD, PhD, Rehabilitation Clinical Trials Center, Los Angeles Biomedical Research Institute at Harbor-UCLA Medical Center, Torrance, California, USA

Lucio Casali, MD, PhD, Chair of Respiratory Diseases, Faculty of Medicine and Surgery, University of Perugia, Sede di Terni, Italy

Mario Cazzola, MD, Associate Professor of Respiratory Medicine, Unit of Respiratory Diseases, Department of Internal Medicine, University of Rome 'Tor Vergata', Rome, Italy

BARTOLOME R. CELLI, MD, Professor of Medicine, Tufts University, Chief Pulmonary, Critical Care and Sleep Medicine, Caritas St Elizabeth's Medical Center Boston, Massachusetts, USA

ISA CERVERI, MD, Consultant Pulmonologist, Department of Respiratory Diseases, IRCCS Policlinico San Matteo, University of Pavia, Pavia, Italy

ENRICO M. CLINI, MD, Associate Professor of Respiratory Medicine, University of Modena, Institute of Respiratory Diseases, Ospedale Policlinico, Modena, Italy

ANDREA M. D'ARMINI, MD, Associate Professor of Cardiac Surgery, University of Pavia, Division of Cardiac Surgery, IRCCS Policlinico San Matteo, Pavia, Italy

FERNANDO DE BENEDETTO, MD, Director, Department of Pneumology, San Camillo De Lellis Hospital, Chieti, Italy

ADRIANA DEL PONTE, MD, Department of Internal Medicine and Aging, Chieti Hospital, Chieti, Italy

MIGUEL FERRER, MD, PhD, Pneumology Service, Institute and Clinic of the Thorax, IDIBAPS, Faculty of Medicine, University of Barcelona, Barcelona, Spain

CHRISTOPHE GIRAULT, MD, Medical Intensive Care Physician, Medical Intensive Care Department and GRHV Research Group, Rouen University Hospital Charles Nicolle, Rouen, France

M. ROSA GÜELL ROUS, MD, Department of Pneumology, Hospital de la Santa Creu i de Sant Pau, Barcelona, Spain

GIOVANNI INVERNIZZI, MD, Allergologist, Tobacco Control Unit, National Tumour Institute and SIMG-Italian College of General Practitioners, Milan, Italy

MARTIN IVERSEN, Dr Med Sci, Consultant Pulmonologist, Medical Department, Lung Transplantation Unit, Copenhagen University Hospital, Copenhagen, Denmark

PAUL W. JONES, PhD, FRCP, Department of Respiratory Medicine, St George's Hospital Medical School, London, UK

DONALD A. MAHLER, MD, Professor of Medicine, Dartmouth Medical School, Hanover, New Hampshire, USA

STEFANO MARINARI, MD, Department of Pneumology, San Camillo De Lellis Hospital, Chieti, Italy

ROBERT J. MCKENNA JR, MD, Surgical Director, Cedars-Sinai Center for Chest Diseases, Thoracic Surgery and Trauma, Los Angeles, California, USA

MICHAEL D. L. MORGAN, MD, FRCP, Consultant Respiratory Physician, Department of Respiratory Medicine, University Hospitals of Leicester, Glenfield Hospital, Leicester, UK

GIANNA MOSCATO, MD, Head, Allergy and Immunology Unit, 'Salvatore Maugeri' Foundation IRCCS, Institute of Care and Research, Scientific Institute of Pavia, Pavia, Italy

STEFANO NARDINI, MD, Pneumologist, U.O. di Pneumologia, Regione Veneto, Sinistra Piave, Vittorio Veneto, Italy

Contributors

STEFANO NAVA, MD, Respiratory Intensive Care Unit, 'Salvatore Maugeri' Foundation IRCCS, Institute of Care and Research, Scientific Institute of Pavia, Pavia, Italy

ROSANNA NIMIANO, MD, Consultant Pneumologist, Department of Respiratory Diseases, Fondazione IRCSS Policlinico S. Matteo, Universita de Pavia, Pavia, Italy

DENNIS NOWAK, MD, Director, Institute and Outpatient Clinics for Occupational and Environmental Medicine, Ludwig-Maximilians-University, Munich, Germany

SRINIVASAN RAMANUJA, MD, Allergy/Immunology Fellow-in-Training, Allergy/Immunology Fellowship Training program, Department of Medicine, Division of Basic and Clinical Immunology, University of California-Irvine, California, USA

THOMAS J. RINGBAEK, MD, DMSc, Consultant in Respiratory Medicine, Department of Cardiology and Respiratory Medicine, University Hospital, Hvidovre, Denmark

ITALO SAMPABLO, MD, Associate Professor of Respiratory Medicine, Universitari Dexeus, Pneumology Service Institute, Barcelona, Spain

GIORGIO L. SCANO, MD, Associate Professor in Respiratory Medicine, Department of Internal Medicine, Section of Immunology and Respiratory Medicine, University of Florence, Careggi General Hospital, Florence, Italy

BERND SCHÖNHOFER, MD, PhD, Department for Pneumology and Intensive Care Medicine, Hospital Oststadt-Heidehaus, Klinikum Region Hannover, Hannover, Germany

SANJAY SETHI, MD, Associate Professor of Medicine, Division of Pulmonary, Critical Care and Sleep Medicine, State University of New York at Buffalo, Attending Physician, VA Western New York Healthcare System, New York, USA

ANTONELLA SPACONE, MD, Department of Pneumology, San Camillo De Lellis Hospital, Chieti, Italy

ANTONI TORRES, MD, PhD, Pneumology Service, Institute and Clinic of the Thorax, IDIBAPS, Faculty of Medicine, University of Barcelona, Barcelona, Spain

THIERRY TROOSTERS, PT, PhD, Associate Professor, Rehabilitation Sciences, Faculty of Kinesiology and Rehabilitation Sciences, Respiratory Division, Katholieke Universiteit Leuven, Leuven, Belgium

JØRGEN VESTBO, MD, PhD, Professor of Respiratory Medicine, University of Manchester, North West Lung Centre, Wythenshawe Hospital, Manchester, UK

EMIEL F. M. WOUTERS, MD, PhD, Professor of Medicine, University Hospital Maastricht, Department of Respiratory Medicine, Maastricht, The Netherlands

SILVIO ZANABONI, MD, Chair of Anaesthesia and Rescuscitation, 'Maggiore della Carità' Hospital, University of Eastern Piedmont, Novara, Italy

JEAN-PIERRE ZELLWEGER, MD, Senior Consultant, University Medical Policlinic, Lausanne, Switzerland

JAN ZIELIŃSKI, MD, PhD, FCCP, Professor of Medicine, Department of Respiratory Medicine, Institute of Tuberculosis and Lung Disease, Warsaw, Poland

Preface

When we first discussed *Clinical Challenges in COPD* with the publishers, we both agreed to produce something quite different from the usual textbook format of publications in respiratory medicine. The majority of books on the subject of COPD have largely the same characteristics, with differences only in the depth and type of information provided, depending on whether the specific target readership is the general practitioner, pulmonary clinician or academic clinician. With this new venture, we hoped and planned to produce a publication on COPD that addressed *all* clinicians dealing with pulmonary patients in an innovative format. We wanted to break away from the traditional idea of expounding a list of diseases or therapeutic approaches: even if these were well described in terms of their aetiology, pathogenesis, diagnosis and treatment, we felt that we would not be adding anything new to the stock of literature already published in this field. We also did not want simply to provide a list of clinical cases.

In this book, we have tried to integrate all of these aspects and present them from a novel viewpoint: starting from the description of a *real* clinical case – such as the clinician typically encounters in everyday clinical practice – the idea was to open up a panel discussion, as it were, on all aspects related to the diagnosis and treatment of the case that would be of interest to the clinical specialist. In this way, we hoped to give the reader an update on the state-of-the-art on specific aspects of respiratory medicine relevant to clinical practice, presented in a novel, easy-to-read manner.

We selected 21 topics, which, while they do not represent all aspects of COPD, cover all of the *real* cases that a clinician may encounter in everyday clinical practice.

All chapters have a similar structure, providing:

- a background, to set the scene and give the general picture of the specific clinical problem;
- a case report, including history, basic diagnostic assessment, differential diagnosis, and treatment (pharmacological, rehabilitation and follow-up);
- a discussion, examining the different possible scenarios arising from the different assessment approaches;
- a conclusion, summing up what has emerged from the discussion and giving clear options for diagnosis, management and follow-up of the specific patient/disease.

The discussion section, in particular, follows the style of a panel discussion: it examines the four or five questions most likely to come from the floor, debating these from the different angles possible. For this reason, where there were debatable perspectives, we sought to have two or more co-authors to enable interaction as though they were part of a panel of experts.

The authors are outstanding authorities in their specific field, each with many high-level publications to their name. Notwithstanding their expert status, we asked them to write in a colloquial manner, as if they were talking from the floor. As such, we hope to offer here a distillation of the best knowledge available in the field, to provide clinicians with a useful tool to keep on their desk for rapid consultation in daily practice. We would like to thank all of the authors for the time and effort they have devoted to the task despite their heavy clinical and scientific commitments and for their goodwill in following the editors' guidance to produce an innovative book. We hope that this publication will not only be useful reading, but also a 'companion' for all clinicians who, we are confident, will appreciate this new format.

Claudio F. Donner
Mauro Carone
Italy, December 2006

1

Improvement of symptoms in a 62-year-old COPD patient after lung volume reduction surgery

R. J. McKenna Jr.

BACKGROUND

Emphysema is a disease that causes great morbidity and mortality worldwide and for which the medical treatment has had little impact upon quality of life or survival. Therefore, a variety of operations have been tried over the years in an attempt to help patients suffering from severe emphysema. This chapter will use a case report to present the current status of lung volume reduction surgery (LVRS) in the treatment of severe emphysema.

In the US, there are approximately 14 million people who suffer from chronic obstructive pulmonary disease (COPD) and about 2 million of these have primarily emphysema. This is the third most common overall cause of death in the country.

Unfortunately, medical management has had little impact on the morbidity and mortality of emphysema. Pulmonary rehabilitation has slightly improved quality of life and has reduced the number of hospitalizations, but has failed to improve pulmonary function or to improve survival [1]. Oxygen therapy for patients with hypoxaemia (oxygen saturations < 90%) has been shown to improve survival.

Otto Brantigan first performed what we now call LVRS in the 1950s at the University of Maryland. Through unilateral thoracotomy incisions, he performed wedge resections of the lung in areas of severe emphysema. This procedure did produce significant clinical improvement in patients, but there was an 18% hospital mortality rate and there was no good scientific documentation of the benefit. Wakabayashi [2] used unilateral thoracoscopy and the Nd:YAG laser to reduce lung volume, but there was little scientific documentation of the benefit and again there was significant morbidity and mortality, so this did not become popular. Cooper et al. [3] introduced modern LVRS as bilateral wedge resections of the lung through a median sternotomy with bovine pericardium to buttress the staple lines on the lung. McKenna et al. [4] performed a randomized, prospective trial to confirm that the staple procedure produced better improvement in pulmonary function than the laser procedure. Subsequent studies established a bilateral staple operation as the standard procedure [5].

The basic concept of LVRS was to identify patients with a heterogeneous pattern of emphysema (usually in the upper lobes). The operation removed approximately 30% of each lung. Removal of areas of lung parenchyma that were not essentially a functional tissue allowed the remaining lung to function more effectively. This resulted in improved elastic recoil of the lung [6].

Robert J. McKenna Jr, MD, Surgical Director, Cedars-Sinai Center for Chest Diseases, Thoracic Surgery and Trauma, Los Angeles, California, USA

The National Emphysema Treatment Trial (NETT) was a randomized, prospective trial comparing best medical management with or without LVRS [7]. Of the 1210 patients in the trial, 608 underwent LVRS and 610 underwent medical management alone. The first NETT publication of results confirmed that older patients with the most severe emphysema (FEV_1 < 20% and diffusion capacity of the lung for carbon monoxide [DLCO] < 20%) and homogeneous emphysema were at risk for greatest morbidity and mortality, with little chance of benefit [8]. The overall results of the NETT showed that, for patients with upper lobe emphysema and poor exercise tolerance, LVRS provided better pulmonary function, exercise tolerance, quality of life, and survival than medical management. For patients with upper lobe emphysema and better exercise tolerance, LVRS provided better pulmonary function, exercise tolerance, and quality of life, but no survival benefit, compared to medical management [9]. For patients with non-upper lobe emphysema and poor exercise tolerance, LVRS provided better pulmonary function, exercise tolerance, and quality of life, but no survival benefit, compared to medical management. A substudy in the NETT showed that bilateral staple LVRS *via* a median sternotomy or video assisted thoracoscopic surgery (VATS) had the same morbidity, mortality and benefit, although the VATS approach had a shorter length of stay and cost [10]. Other randomized trials have confirmed these results [11–13].

This chapter will illustrate the basic workup and procedure for LVRS and then discuss the different possible scenarios arising from the diverse possible assessment and approaches.

CASE REPORT

A 62-year-old male complained of significant limitation in activities of daily living. He had severe dyspnoea with taking a shower, bending over, carrying anything, and activities around the house. He could walk approximately 15 m without stopping. He had smoked two packs of cigarettes per day for 30 years before dyspnoea, which led him to stop smoking 10 years ago. He had 2–5 episodes of bronchitis per year and had been hospitalized three times for acute exacerbations of his emphysema.

Tests confirmed that he had severe emphysema. His computed tomography (CT) scan showed severe emphysema in the upper lobes bilaterally and much better parenchyma in the lower lobes. A lung perfusion scan confirmed the heterogeneity. In some patients the CT scan does not show heterogeneity, while the perfusion scan (particularly in the oblique and lateral views) shows significant heterogeneity. His pulmonary function tests (PFTs) showed an FEV_1 of 910 ml (32% predicted), total lung capacity (TLC) of 7.11 (141% of predicted), a residual volume (RV) of 5.91 (267% of predicted), and DLCO of 34%. His 6-min walk was 120 m.

He had received maximal medical management that included inhalers, oxygen at night, and prednisone for episodes of acute bronchitis. He completed a pulmonary rehabilitation program that included education, upper body conditioning, and exercise on the treadmill. He exercised daily on the treadmill for 30 min at 1 mile/h. The rehabilitation coordinator confirmed that he was compliant and showed good effort. This is critical because non-compliant patients have greater morbidity and mortality for LVRS, so they are turned down for the procedure. PFTs after rehabilitation showed no change, while his 6-min walk test increased to 132 m.

Because the patient was still severely limited after maximal medical management, he underwent LVRS. The bilateral VATS procedure took 60 min. There were no adhesions on either side and approximately 70% of the right upper lobe was resected and 60% of the upper division was resected. He was extubated in the operating room. The patient had no air leaks noted in the operating room, but the right side developed a small leak in the recovery room and the left side developed a moderate sized leak. He was followed for 2 days in the intensive care unit, where he received nebulizer treatment and was ambulated three times per day.

Table 1.1 Typical PFTs for a candidates for LVRS

PFT	Predicted value (%)
FEV_1	<45
TLC	>100 (mean = 143)
RV	>200 (mean = 270)

FEV_1 = forced expiratory volume in the first second; PFT = pulmonary function test; RV = residual volume; TLC = total lung capacity.

He was transferred to the ward on the third postoperative day. His right-sided air leak resolved so the chest tubes on the right were removed on the fourth postoperative day. Because he still had an air leak on the left, his chest tubes were disconnected from the chest drainage system and connected to Heimlich valves. His postoperative course was otherwise uneventful and he was discharged on the seventh postoperative day with a left chest tube and Heimlich valve for a persistent air leak. The tube was removed when the patient returned to the office 3 days later and was found to have no air leak. He continued in pulmonary rehabilitation for the next month. His quality of life improved significantly. His postoperative PFTs showed an FEV_1 of 1350 ml (47% predicted), TLC of 5.59 l (111% of predicted), an RV of 3.91 l (177% of predicted), and DLCO of 39%. His 6-min walk was 149 m.

DISCUSSION

Patient selection is the key to a successful result after LVRS. Only 10–20% of patients with severe emphysema are potential candidates for LVRS. It is a palliative procedure, so the patients must have symptoms that warrant the procedure. Table 1.1 shows the typical pulmonary function for patients who undergo LVRS.

What is the importance of the preoperative pulmonary rehabilitation?

Rehabilitation provides only a small impact on quality of life and does not improve pulmonary function, however it is important for patient selection and preparing the patient for LVRS [14]. In the hospital after LVRS, the patient must work very hard at pulmonary toilet and ambulation to minimize complications. This is important for patient selection because patients who show a strong effort in preoperative rehabilitation demonstrate that they are adequately motivated to do well after LVRS. Achieving certain goals, such as the ability to walk for 30 min without stopping on the treadmill also conditions patients to minimize complications after LVRS.

Can the lung function be too bad for LVRS?

Patients with an $FEV_1 < 20\%$ or a DLCO < 20% predicted value have an increased risk of mortality and a low chance of benefit from emphysema [8]. However, some patients with those PFTs can still benefit from LVRS, especially if they have a strongly heterogeneous pattern of emphysema [9].

Must patients have a heterogeneous pattern of emphysema?

The basic concept of LVRS is to resect areas of non-functioning lung to allow other areas to function more effectively. By definition, that means a heterogeneous pattern of emphysema.

The NETT identified the best patients for LVRS as those with a bilateral upper lobe pattern of emphysema and poor exercise tolerance. They had improvement in exercise tolerance, lung function, quality of life, and survival. Patients with either bilateral upper lobe emphysema and better exercise tolerance or patients with poor exercise tolerance and no upper lobe emphysema achieve better exercise tolerance, lung function, and quality of life, but not longer survival. PFTs confirm that the patients have severe emphysema, but do not predict heterogeneity, which is the most important selection factor. Gelb et al. [15] showed that only 30% of patients with $FEV_1 < 50\%$ have severe emphysema scores on thin cut CT scans. Even fewer patients have significant heterogeneity on thin slice CT scans. A complete evaluation of the radiological pattern of emphysema requires a chest X-ray, CT scan and lung perfusion scan. For an experienced observer, the chest X-ray shows the pattern of emphysema in most patients [16]. The CT confirms this. There are a few patients with a strongly heterogeneous pattern of emphysema that is apparent only on the perfusion scan, so this is an important test [17].

What are other contraindications to LVRS?
Patients with conditions that would increase the risk for LVRS or would significantly shorten the life expectancy of the patient have a relative contraindication for the procedure. The NETT showed that older patients (>70 years), patients with $FEV_1 < 20\%$, DLCO < 20% predicted value, and homogeneous disease have increased risk of mortality with little chance of benefit. Some studies have reported that patients with poor lung function tests, but with good target areas for LVRS had good results. Patients with shortened life expectancies due to medical illnesses, such as cancer or heart disease, are not candidates. Depression and anxiety interfere with postoperative compliance so those conditions must be assessed preoperatively.

Is there a role for unilateral LVRS?
The intent of the operation is a bilateral staple procedure through either a median sternotomy or VATS. Occasionally, patients are only candidates for unilateral VATS because they have had a resection on one side, pleural symphysis on one side, heterogeneous emphysema on only one side, or if they develop a large air leak on the first side of an operation where a bilateral procedure was intended. If a large leak occurs on both sides, the patients often have respiratory failure, require ventilation, and have a high mortality rate. In general, a bilateral operation can be performed with the same morbidity, mortality, and length of stay as a unilateral operation, but the improvement is considerably better after the bilateral operation [5].

Are patients with α_1 anti-trypsin deficiency candidates for LVRS?
Patients with α_1 anti-trypsin deficiency can benefit from LVRS. Series have shown that the improvement in FEV_1 may not be as great, but the improvement in quality of life may be significant [18]. It also appears that the duration of the benefit may not be as long as the benefit for LVRS in smoking-related emphysema.

What is the postoperative course after LVRS?
The care of patients after LVRS can be challenging. There is a 5% hospital mortality rate. Patients are usually extubated in the operating room. They are followed initially in the intensive care unit. Aggressive pulmonary toilet with nebulizer treatments and chest physical therapy is critical. Broad-spectrum antibiotics are added if the patients show any signs of increasing hypoxia or fever. Ninety percent of patients develop an air leak after LVRS. Other complications are seen in Table 1.2 [10].

Table 1.2 Typical complications after LVRS

Complication	Incidence (%)
None	–
Air leak	90
Atrial fibrillation	3
Other arrhythmias	22
Tracheostomy	10
Pneumonia	20
Re-admission to intensive care	10

What about bronchoscopic LVRS?
Recently, in an effort to reduce the morbidity and mortality of LVRS, a variety of different bronchoscopic procedures have been experimented to provide volume reduction [19, 20]. The hope is to develop a bronchoscopic procedure to induce atelectasis. The techniques have included bronchial valves, bronchial blockers, and biologic glue to maintain atelectasis. The preliminary data with these procedures show some benefit, although the improvement has not been as much as with LVRS. Another novel approach has been the placement of a stent through fistulae created between the bronchus and areas of emphysema. This bypasses the collapsed small airways and allows better air movement. Unfortunately, while these stents initially work well, mucus and scars quickly close the stents and make them non-functional. The future of LVRS may be with endobronchial approaches, but the current prototypes do not work well enough to replace LVRS.

SUMMARY

LVRS is an exciting new treatment for patients with emphysema who are symptomatic despite maximal medical management. The key to success after LVRS is proper patient selection. The most important factor is a heterogeneous pattern of emphysema, usually in the upper lobes. The NETT showed that LVRS, compared to medical management, provides better quality of life, pulmonary function, exercise tolerance, and survival for patients with upper lobe emphysema and poor exercise tolerance.

REFERENCES

1. Decramer M. Treatment of chronic respiratory failure: lung volume reduction surgery versus rehabilitation. *Eur Respir J* 2003; 22:47S–56S.
2. Wakabayashi A. Unilateral thorascopic laser pneumoplasty of diffuse bullous emphysema. *Chest Surg Clin N Am* 1995; 5:833–850
3. Cooper JD, Trulock EP, Triantafillou AN et al. Bilateral pneumectomy (volume reduction) for chronic obstructive pulmonary disease. *J Thorac Cardiovasc Surg* 1995; 109:106–116.
4. McKenna R, Brenner M, Gelb AF et al. A randomized, prospective trial of stapled lung reduction versus laser bullectomy for diffuse emphysema. *J Thorac Cardiovasc Surg* 1996; 111:310–322.
5. McKenna RJ Jr, Brenner M, Fischel RJ, Gelb AF. Should lung reduction surgery for emphysema be unilateral or bilateral? *J Thorac Cardiovasc Surg* 1996; 112:1331–1339.
6. Gelb AF, Zamel N, McKenna RJ Jr, Brenner M. Mechanism for short-term improvement in lung function after emphysema resection. *Am J Respir Crit Care Med* 1996; 154:945–951.
7. The National Emphysema Treatment Trial Research Group. Rationale and Design of the National Emphysema Treatment Trial (NETT): A prospective randomized trial of lung volume reduction surgery. *J Cardiopulm Rehabil* 2000; 20:24–36.
8. The National Emphysema Treatment Trial Research Group. Patients at high risk of mortality from lung volume reduction surgery. *New Engl J Med* 2001; 345:1075–1083.

9. National Emphysema Treatment Trial Research Group. A randomized trial comparing lung-volume-reduction surgery with medical therapy for severe emphysema. *N Engl J Med* 2003; 348:2059–2073.
10. McKenna RJ Jr, Benditt JO, DeCamp M *et al.*; for the National Emphysema Treatment Trial (NETT) Research Group. National Emphysema Treatment Trial: A comparison of median sternotomy versus VATS for lung volume reduction surgery. *J Thorac Cardiovasc Surg* 2004; 127:1350–1360.
11. Criner GJ, Cordova FC, Furukawa S *et al.* Prospective randomized trial comparing bilateral lung volume reduction surgery to pulmonary rehabilitation in severe chronic obstructive pulmonary disease. *Am J Respir Crit Care Med* 1999; 160:2018–2027.
12. Geddes D, Davis M, Koyoma H *et al.* Effect of lung volume reduction surgery in patients with emphysema. *N Engl J Med* 2000; 343:239–245.
13. Pompeo E, Marino M, Nofroni I *et al.* Reduction pneumoplasty versus respiratory rehabilitation in severe emphysema: a randomized study. *Ann Thorac Surg* 2000; 70:948–953.
14. McKenna RJ Jr, Brenner M, Singh N *et al.* Patient selection for lung volume reduction surgery. *J Thorac Cardiovasc Surg* 1997; 114:957–967.
15. Gelb AF, Hogg JC, Muller NL *et al.* Contribution of emphysema and small airways in COPD. *Chest* 1996; 109:353–359.
16. Maki DD, Miller WT Jr, Aronchick JM *et al.* Advanced emphysema: preoperative chest radiographic findings as predictors of outcome following lung volume reduction surgery. *Radiology* 1999; 212:49–55.
17. Jamadar DA, Kazerooni EA, Martinez FJ *et al.* Semi-quantitative ventilation/perfusion scintigraphy and single-photon emission tomography for evaluation of lung volume reduction surgery candidates: description and prediction of clinical outcome. *Eur J Nucl Med* 1999; 26:734–742.
18. Gelb AF, McKenna RJ Jr, Brenner M *et al.* Lung function after bilateral lower lobe lung volume reduction surgery for alpha1-antitrypsin emphysema. *Eur Respir J* 1999; 14:928–933.
19. McKenna RJ Jr. Bronchial blockers for LVRS. *J Bronchology* (in press).
20. Wood D, McKenna RJ Jr. A pilot multi-center trial of the intrabronchial valve for treatment of severe emphysema. *Ann Thorac Surg* (in press).

2

Patients with very frequent exacerbations of COPD: clinical stabilization after the prescription of inhaled corticosteroids

P. M. A. Calverley, M. Cazzola

BACKGROUND

Chronic obstructive pulmonary disease (COPD) is characterized by airflow limitation that is persistent, progressive and associated with an abnormal inflammatory response to inhaled toxic particulates, especially tobacco [1]. One further feature which is not present in every case but which certainly becomes more important as the disease progresses clinically is the tendency to experience periodic worsening of symptom intensity that are defined as exacerbations of COPD [2]. These episodes can be difficult to define in clinical trials, but patients seldom have problems identifying when they occur. An exacerbation represents a deterioration in the patient's clinical condition which is beyond the normal day-to-day variation and is sustained for at least 48 h [3]. The impact of these exacerbations varies depending upon disease severity. Thus, a period of 'winter bronchitis' in a patient with relatively mild airflow obstruction appears to produce less systemic upset and to impair the patient's performance less than an apparently similar bronchial infection in a patient with a much lower FEV_1 where hospitalization may occur. Thus, episodes in patients with more severe disease are certainly more dangerous to the patient and more expensive to the healthcare provider.

Exacerbations are related to many aspects of the definition of COPD developed above. They are clearly related to the degree of airflow obstruction [4] and are more frequently recognized as clinically significant events when the mean FEV_1 falls below 50% of predicted. They have been characterized physiologically with qualitatively similar changes in lung function irrespective of whether the patient was breathing spontaneously or requiring assisted ventilation [5, 6]. Although airflow obstruction worsens when patients exacerbate the absolute change in indices of expiratory flow is relatively small (of the order of 100–300 ml FEV_1) [5, 7] and is easily missed given the known day-to-day variability in lung function testing [8]. More impressive are the changes in operating lung volumes. Two recent studies have shown that patients recovering from exacerbations that required hospitalizations exhibit increases in end-expiratory lung volume, principally due to a rise in residual volume and these changes diminish in the days and weeks after hospital attendance [5, 9]. These changes are accompanied by an increase in respiratory frequency, but the most important change during resolution of the exacerbation is a change in the operating lung

---

Peter M. A. Calverley, MD, FRCP, FRCPE, Professor of Respiratory Medicine; Honorary Consultant Physician, University Department of Medicine, University Hospital Aintree, Liverpool, UK

Mario Cazzola, MD, Associate Professor of Respiratory Medicine, Unit of Respiratory Diseases, Department of Internal Medicine, University of Rome 'Tor Vergata', Rome, Italy

© Atlas Medical Publishing Ltd 2007

volume rather than the rate at which the patient is breathing. These changes in lung volume are also accompanied by more subtle changes in lung mechanics and in particular an increase in the inspiratory threshold load (intrinsic positive end-expiratory pressure), which is a feature of many patients with COPD and is associated with dynamic regulation of lung volumes at rest [10]. Changes in both the work done to overcome the intrinsic load of breathing and a combination of an increased elastic and resisted work of breathing go a long way to account for the increased breathlessness which accompanies exacerbations that is a striking feature of these episodes [11]. In contrast, changes in ventilation and perfusion matching are the main reason for the hypoxaemia, which commonly accompanies exacerbations of COPD [12]. Lung ventilation perfusion changes are particularly marked and there is an increase in the physiological dead space, which can lead to hypercapnia. This is a major determinant of prognosis since worsening hypercapnia is associated with respiratory acidosis, which is a poor prognostic marker.

If the physiological dysfunction that characterizes COPD explains the pattern of exacerbations, the worsening of airway inflammation is a principal reason why these physiological changes occur. Only limited data are available from endobronchial biopsy studies in intensive care but these data support that an increase in CD8+ T cells and increased neutrophil traffic through the airway wall is seen in more severe COPD exacerbations [13]. Using protected brush bronchoscopy it has been possible to demonstrate that lower respiratory tract colonization occurs with *Haemophilus influenza* and, to a lesser degree, *Streptococcus* [14]. The presence of this finding significantly increases the risk of exacerbation although subtle changes in the strain type of a colonizing micro-organism may occur without obvious changes in the total microbiological load and a change to a new strain of *Haemophilus* can precipitate clinical deterioration [15]. A wide range of aetiological factors, both bacterial and viral, have been established in COPD [16, 17]. Many useful data have come from the careful follow-up of COPD patients who completed a daily exacerbation diary card scoring their perceived symptomatology relative to the previous day [18]. Using polymerase chain reaction (PCR) analysis of specimens from patients, when stable and during exacerbations, it has been possible to show that viruses such as rhinovirus and respiratory syncytial virus account for a significant number of exacerbations and are often present together with bacterial pathogens [19]. Patients who have a higher residual bacterial load may also show exacerbations with purulent sputum [20] although the significance of bronchiectasis defined on computed tomography (CT) scanning in COPD patients is debatable [21, 22].

Exacerbations contribute to general patient ill-health, have an extended impact on the patient's health status [23] and are accompanied by weight loss, which can cumulate and contribute to the systemic impact of COPD [24]. Studies have reported a relationship between the number of exacerbations and the rate of decline of lung function, which appears to explain up to 25% of the variability in decline between COPD subjects [25]. Studies over a longer period in the east London cohort have supported this finding [26]. More recently, in patients who were hospitalized, exacerbations have been shown to be an independent predictor of mortality, which is something that clinicians have recognized for a long time but which has been hard to demonstrate statistically until now [27].

The management of a COPD exacerbation usually involves an increase in the dose and frequency of inhaled bronchodilators and commonly requires high-dose combined bronchodilator therapy given by nebulization in patients admitted to hospital. There has been some uncertainty about whether adding anticholinergics and β-agonists in high dose is necessary and one clinical study based on the recovery of FEV_1 found that there was no advantage in doing so [28]. However, this study is probably statistically underpowered to detect an effect which has been seen when more rigorous studies in stable patients were conducted [29]. Moreover, high-dose nebulized bronchodilators do affect operating lung volumes to a greater degree than FEV_1 and the changes in FEV_1 are really extremely small during the early stages of the disease when important volume changes can be detected [5]. In these circumstances, it would be prudent to combine treatment in the sickest patients until better data showing that this is unnecessary become available.

After some years of debate, there is now clear evidence that using oral corticosteroids is beneficial in a range of patients with COPD who present with exacerbations. Oral corticosteroids increase the rate of improvement of post-bronchodilator FEV_1, shorten hospital stay and reduce the chances of relapse when compared with conventional therapy without corticosteroids [30–32]. The optimal dose has not been defined but clinical practice suggests that not more than 30 ml of prednisolone given orally for 5–7 days is required. Certainly, there is a measurable incidence of hyperglycaemia in patients exposed to corticosteroids and the temptation to extend this treatment for longer periods should be resisted. There appears to be no particular advantage in giving large doses of corticosteroids by injection or doses by nebulization, the latter being not more effective than oral therapy [33].

The role of antibiotics in exacerbations remains contentious although these drugs are widely used and their use in this way contributes significantly to the development of multiply resistant micro-organisms. The best studies conducted in this field are now over 25 years old [34] but the guidance they suggest, namely, that patients who have clear evidence of infection with an increase in symptoms together with an increase in the volume and a changing colour of the sputum to green constitute the group of patients where antibiotics can be most clearly seen to be effective [35]. The use of broad-spectrum antibiotics routinely is not recommended although one interesting study from North Africa has suggested that using ofloxacin reduced the incidence of pneumonia in an intensive care unit [36]. Hospitalized patients benefit from control oxygen therapy although, unsurprisingly, there are no good clinical trials to confirm this. Nonetheless, although the known effects of oxygen in decreasing ventilatory demand are likely to be valuable in the setting of an acute exacerbation that requires hospitalization, care needs to be taken to prevent oxygen-induced hypercapnia [37], which appears to be mainly due to ventilatory depression in milder cases although high concentrations of oxygen can affect ventilation perfusion matching in more severe disease. These problems can worsen the tendency to respiratory acidosis, which may already be present, and there are now excellent data to support the use of non-invasive ventilation in managing such patients [38].

The principles of hospital management are generally applicable – but to a lesser degree – in the community where increased doses of bronchodilators and the use of oral corticosteroids are usually all that is required. Nonetheless, exacerbations in this setting can be distressing and contribute to the decline in health status which is typical of more advanced COPD [39], so that exacerbation prevention remains an important therapeutic goal. It would be reasonable to assume that smoking cessation would prevent exacerbations of COPD, and over the long-term this is clearly true as ex-smokers are less likely to be hospitalized as a result of COPD exacerbation [40]. Trials on the outcome of smoking cessation and exacerbation risk in patients with more severe disease are currently lacking. Influenza vaccination clearly reduces the number of exacerbations associated with influenza [41], but the evidence in favour of pneumococcal vaccination is rather less firm although it has been widely advocated [27]. Pulmonary rehabilitation and treatment with domiciliary oxygen, where appropriate, may also impact on exacerbation frequency although the data on this are somewhat inconsistent [42]. The use of long-acting inhaled bronchodilators appears to reduce exacerbation frequency with evidence of an impact with β-agonists [43] and even more clearly with long-acting inhaled anticholinergic drugs like tiotropium. A recent large study from the Veterans' Administration in the USA showed a clear reduction in hospitalization due to exacerbation in patients randomized to receive tiotropium. The role of inhaled corticosteroids (ICS) in exacerbation prevention has been much more controversial but the majority of studies, whatever the design, suggest that some effect is present, at least in patients with severe but not necessarily very severe COPD [44]. In the latter setting, patients who have ICS combined with long-acting β-agonist (LABA) appear to do better than those in whom ICS are used for preventative reasons alone [45].

Thus, a range of treatment options both to actively manage the episode and prevent its occurrence is available. Despite this, exacerbations become a progressively more intrusive part of the patient's disease as their illness progresses.

CASE REPORT

C.P., a 58-year-old retired female shop assistant was first seen as an out-patient in mid-June 2002. She complained of worsening exertional breathlessness, which prevented her taking as much exercise as she would like and this had been slowly worsening over the preceding 3 years. She was no longer able to walk to the shops, which were some 200 m from her home, without having to stop to get her breath. She found it difficult to manage the steep flight of stairs in her house and had to restrict the amount and duration of cleaning she could undertake at home. She slept with two pillows, which was her usual habit, and denied ankle swelling, chest pain or palpitations. She was troubled by a 'smoker's cough' that had been present for many years and that was productive of approximately an egg-cup full of sputum each day. This material was usually pale green in colour but became a darker green intermittently, usually when she was having symptoms of sneezing and upper respiratory tract discomfort. When this occurred her breathing became more laboured and she used many puffs of the blue inhaler (salbutamol), which her family doctor had given her the previous year. These episodes developed over 48–72 h and she usually had to go to her bed for a day or two until she was well enough to recover, a process that took 1–2 weeks in her view.

The first of these troublesome episodes had occurred some 2.5 years previously and 9 months had passed before a second more severe episode had been noted in the winter of 2001. She attended her physician who prescribed broad-spectrum antibiotics and the 'as needed' β-agonist inhaler she still used. This initially improved her condition, but 2 weeks after stopping treatment her symptoms returned and a further course of antibiotics was prescribed. This pattern of relapse and recurrences, which were partially responsive to treatment, continued until the summer of 2001 when she improved more substantially after her first course of oral corticosteroids. She was well until late November of that year but after a 'flu-like' illness became very breathless with accompanying wheeziness and was thought to be febrile. Further antibiotic and oral corticosteroid treatments were less successful in controlling these symptoms and a chest X-ray performed at the hospital revealed no focal pathology but was reported as 'changes of chronic bronchitis only'. Over this period she lost weight and became depressed, waking early in the morning feeling quite despondent. She gave up her work on the grounds of ill health and her ability to cope at home was significantly reduced.

Finally, in late March 2002 she was hospitalized with severe breathlessness at rest, which had developed over a few days on top of her already impaired physical state. She was treated with high doses of oral corticosteroids, nebulized bronchodilators and oxygen given for Type 1 respiratory failure. After 5 days, she was discharged home with support from the community outreach COPD team.

C.P. has smoked from her teenage years and despite advice from her doctors continued to smoke 20 cigarettes per day, although claiming that she had 'cut down' from her usual 30 per day. Altogether she had a 50 pack-year smoking history. Past medical history was unremarkable apart from a period during her early childhood when she wheezed and coughed and lost some time from school. Her mother had been treated for tuberculosis and the other family members screened but had not received additional chemotherapy. She drank socially but never excessively, at least not since divorcing from her husband of 15 years, an event that had occurred 10 years previously. Her two daughters both lived locally and called in to ensure that she was well and she continued to be self-caring, which was her normal habit.

When she was seen she was thin (body mass index = 19 kg/m^2), but not cyanosed or tachypnoeic at rest. She was not anaemic or using her accessory muscles of respiration while resting although she did appear to become breathless when she got undressed to lie down on the examination couch. Cardiovascular examination was unremarkable with rather distant heart sounds and it was hard to locate her apex beat. Respiratory examination confirmed that she had a hyper-inflated chest with a short trachea palpable above the sternal angle, pulmonary over-inflation and some in-drawing of the lower ribs on inspiration. Occasional wheezes were heard on auscultation but in general her breath sounds were reduced; there was no evidence of right-heart failure.

Her haemoglobin was at the upper limit of the laboratory normal range for women, being 16.2 g/dl with a normal white count and platelet count. Her packed cell volume was 48%. Her ECG showed that she was in sinus rhythm with right-axis deviation and a minor intra-ventricular conduction defect whilst her chest X-ray showed large lung fields with flat hemi-diaphragms and a narrow cardiac contour. There were decreased vessel markings in both upper lobes but the airway walls appeared to be visible in some parts of the left lower lobe, where there had also been some blunting of the left costophrenic angle.

On pulmonary function testing her FEV_1 was 0.92 l compared with the predicted value of 3.1 l and her forced vital capacity (FVC) was 2.8 l compared with predicted value of 4.0 l. These results did not change significantly after high-dose nebulized bronchodilators, her FEV_1 only rising to 1.24 l. Measurements of her lung volume in a body plethysmograph showed her total lung capacity to be 110% of predicted with a residual volume of 180% predicted. The maximum expiratory flow volume loop showed a 'collapse' pattern with a reduced peak flow, but a marked reduction in the mid and late expiratory flows. Her gas transfer factor was 63% of predicted and when corrected for alveolar volume her KCO was 70% predicted.

A CT scan confirmed the presence of mixed centri- and pan-acinar emphysema in both upper lobes, more marked on the left than the right. There was less severe emphysematous change throughout the lower zones. There was evidence of some tubular bronchiectasis in the left lower lobe with a positive signet ring sign in which the airways were larger than the adjacent pulmonary vessels.

She was unable to produce any sputum for microbiology at the clinic although a previous record had shown that she had grown *Moraxella catarrhalis* on one occasion and *Haemophilus influenzae* on two previous occasions when her sputum had been cultured.

PROBLEMS AND POSSIBLE CLINICAL RESOLUTION TO THE SCENARIO

This case describes a typical patient suffering from severe COPD with frequent exacerbations. It raises two major criticisms of the management of the disease as prescribed by the patient's primary care physician and, partially, as perceived by the patient.

The patient suffered from several exacerbations before she started with an oral corticosteroid course. Although the management of COPD exacerbations involves increasing the dose and/or frequency of existing bronchodilator therapy [1], GOLD guidelines advise that oral corticosteroids should be considered in addition to bronchodilators if the patient's baseline FEV_1 is less than 50% predicted [46]. In particular, as we have highlighted before, out-patient treatment of acute COPD exacerbation with an oral corticosteroid accelerates recovery of lung function, reduces the treatment failure rate, improves subjective dyspnoea [47] and may reduce the risk of early relapse [32]. In any case, it is likely that, since her first episodes of acute exacerbation were milder and less symptomatic, the patient sought her physician only when symptoms became more pronounced. We cannot omit to underline that the factors affecting how patients with COPD interpret changes in their symptoms are likely to be complex, including their understanding of COPD, which is often poor [48], the relationship with disease severity, and psychological overlay in patients with high levels of anxiety and depression [49].

The second criticism, which is even more important, is linked to the management of the disease during the stable phases. COPD exacerbations are morbid and costly events, and treatment of an established exacerbation has only a modest effect in shortening its duration [50]. Reducing the number of exacerbations of COPD is an important goal of treatment and this concept has been stressed in several treatment guidelines or position papers [1, 46, 51]. In fact, strategies that reduce the frequency of acute exacerbations and their severity have clinical, public health, and economic implications. Smoking cessation, and vaccination against influenza and pneumococcal pneumonia are the most important strategies to prevent and control exacerbations [1, 46, 51]. Potentially interesting alternative strategies for an improved control of symptoms and exacerbations in COPD include the use of mucolytic, anti-oxidant, and immunomodulator agents [1, 46, 51]. Apparently, none of these actions was undertaken.

The proven effectiveness of ICS in treating asthma suggested a potential role in the long-term management of patients with COPD. Inflammation is thought to play a pivotal role in the pathogenesis of COPD, and a potent anti-inflammatory agent might therefore have a disease-modifying effect. However, compared with the case of asthma, there is much more controversy about the role of ICS in preventing exacerbations of COPD [52, 53]. A systematic review of nine randomized trials, which evaluated the long-term effects (≥ 6 months) of ICS for stable COPD and involved a total of 3976 patients with COPD, has demonstrated that, although these agents had no important effect on the yearly decline in FEV_1, regular use of ICS in the doses employed in these trials reduced the chance of an exacerbation, and the total exacerbation rate, by almost one-third [54]. The risk ratio was 0.70, with similar benefits in those who were and were not pre-treated with systemic steroids.

Three further large multicentre studies have been reported in which exacerbations were evaluated using a similar definition in a large number of patients followed up for 1 year. Rather surprisingly, in all three studies no relation was seen between self-reported smoking status and response to therapy. In the TRISTAN (TRial of Inhaled STeroids ANd long-acting β_2-agonists) investigation, ICS therapy was associated with an approximate 20% reduction in the overall number of exacerbations compared with placebo, although patients in the placebo limb were again more likely to be withdrawn [43]. The effect was similar for exacerbations treated with oral corticosteroids, which have conventionally been thought to be more severe episodes.

Two studies of inhaled budesonide for COPD exacerbations in almost identical patient populations have now been reported, both examining patients with a significantly lower pre-bronchodilator FEV_1 than in the TRISTAN study (36 vs. 43% predicted, respectively). The first of them, by Szafranski *et al.* [55], used a design similar to that of the TRISTAN study but included patients with an FEV_1 below 50% predicted. The exacerbation rate while receiving placebo was 1.8 episodes per year, almost 50% greater than in the placebo limb of the TRISTAN study, where it was 1.3 episodes per year. There was a small reduction in the exacerbation rate among individuals treated with inhaled budesonide, a finding confirmed in a subsequent study by Calverley *et al.* [45], which adopted a design modelled on the FACET investigation in asthma. In the latter study there was an effect of budesonide on the number of courses of oral prednisolone, but in neither of these investigations, in which budesonide was given at a dose of 400 µg twice daily, did ICS treatment produce a statistically significant reduction in the number of exacerbations.

It is not a surprise, therefore, that the present GOLD recommendation [46] is to treat symptomatic COPD patients with an $FEV_1 < 50\%$ predicted and repeated exacerbations using regular ICS treatment.

Our patient, however, only received oral corticosteroid courses. Although oral corticosteroids are given to a substantial number of patients with COPD, the improvement in FEV_1 with these agents in stable COPD is inconsistent and at best modest, and the benefits do not outweigh the increase in side-effects [56]. A Cochrane research study has documented that it would be necessary to treat seven patients with oral corticosteroids to achieve one extra case of increasing FEV_1 by more than 20%, with a placebo group risk of 0.13 [57]. Moreover, there are small statistically significant advantages for functional capacity and respiratory symptom of wheeze with oral steroid treatment compared to placebo but, and this is very important for our patient, no significant difference in risk of suffering from an exacerbation or rate of serious exacerbations over 2 years with low-dose oral steroid treatment.

It is noteworthy that use of oral corticosteroids in patients with COPD may also result in weight loss and muscle catabolism [58]. Anorexia is one of the side-effects of corticosteroid treatment and increased corticosteroid plasma levels [59]. However, corticosteroids induce a greater weight loss than can be explained by anorexia only. Weight loss itself also induces changes in protein and amino acid metabolism of muscle [60]. This must be considered a problem for a patient such as we have described, who was also losing weight. Really, unexplained weight loss occurs in about 50% of patients with severe COPD and chronic respiratory failure, but it can also be seen in about 10–15% of patients with mild-to-moderate disease [61]. Loss of skeletal muscle mass is the main cause of weight loss in COPD, with loss of fat mass contributing to a lesser extent [62]. Several studies have provided clear evidence for involvement of tumour necrosis factor alpha (TNFα) in the pathogenesis of tissue depletion in patients with COPD. Increased plasma levels of TNFα and soluble TNF receptors were found in patients with COPD, particularly those suffering from weight loss [63, 64]. This increase in plasma levels of TNFα and soluble TNF receptors indicates the presence of a systemic inflammation. During acute exacerbations, levels of TNFα [65] increase markedly in sputum, and TNF receptors increase in the systemic circulation [66]. Moreover, the rise in systemic inflammatory molecules during acute exacerbations correlates closely with the increase in sputum indices of inflammation, suggesting that there may be a link between lung and systemic inflammation [67]. There is evidence that fluticasone and budesonide inhibit TNFα release in human alveolar macrophages [68]. The documentation that 2 weeks of treatment with inhaled fluticasone reduced systemic inflammation by more than 50% and that these effects were maintained after an additional 8 weeks of inhaled fluticasone [69] seems to suggest that long-term treatment with an ICS could be beneficial even for the weight loss, but, unfortunately, solid evidence of this possibility is still lacking.

It must be highlighted that the patient was also suffering from tubular bronchiectasis. Twenty nine percent of patients with COPD who developed an exacerbation in primary care were found to have some bronchiectatic changes when evaluated by high-resolution computed tomography (HRCT) scanning [22]. The extent of bronchiectasis has been shown to be negatively correlated with FEV_1% predicted [70], suggesting that in patients with COPD bronchiectasis may develop in the presence of progressive airway obstruction. Interestingly, a relationship between the detection of radiological bronchiectasis on HRCT and more severe COPD exacerbations, as assessed by time to symptom recovery, has been documented [21]. Intense neutrophil infiltration into the tracheobronchial tree occurs in bronchiectasis [71], which aggravates the underlying tracheobronchial damage. Neutrophil-derived toxic products, such as elastase, cause ultrastructural and functional damage [72] and release of pro-inflammatory mediators in the tracheobronchial tree [73]. There is ample evidence to suggest that this neutrophil influx into the bronchiectatic airways is mediated by pro-inflammatory cytokines and leukotriene B_4 (LTB_4) [71]. It has been documented that low-dose inhaled steroid therapy (beclomethasone 0.4 mg/day) had no effects on sputum proteolytic or immune complex activities [74], but higher dosage (beclomethasone 1.5 mg/day or budesonide 1.6 mg/day) improved sputum volume [75], bronchial hyperreactivity, dyspnoea and cough [76], and spirometry [77]. Moreover, high-dose inhaled fluticasone (1 mg/day) therapy is effective in reducing the sputum inflammatory indices in severe bronchiectasis [78]. A 12-month study with inhaled fluticasone has documented that ICS treatment is beneficial to patients with bronchiectasis, particularly those with *Pseudomonas aerurginasa* infection [79].

All these findings tell us that the patient described here would have had to receive a regular course with an ICS in order to achieve a clinical stabilization and reduce the risk of suffering from frequent exacerbations. Nonetheless, it must be highlighted that she was a current smoker. It is highly likely that smoking cessation would reduce the number of exacerbations in our patient because an acknowledged effect is a reduction in cough and sputum production [80]. These variables are important predictors of the risk of frequent exacerbations at least in the London observational cohort [81]. In any case, the current opinion is that there is a link between smoking and resistance to the anti-inflammatory effects of corticosteroids due to an inhibitory effect of cigarette smoke on the histone deacetylases, which are nuclear enzymes required for corticosteroids to switch off inflammatory genes [82, 83]. Consequently, a strong cessation intervention in our patient should have been considered, even though it is well-known that some cigarette smokers are able to quit, but many are not, and standard medications to assist in smoking cessation (e.g. nicotine-replacement therapies and sustained-release bupropion) are ineffective in many remaining smokers [84]. Nonetheless, even in the event that she had been unable to stop smoking, the clear documentation that there is no relation between self-reported smoking status and response to therapy with an ICS [43, 45, 55] should have prompted her physician to prescribe a regular treatment with such a drug.

SUMMARY

Exacerbations are related to the degree of airflow obstruction, especially when the mean FEV_1 falls below 50% of predicted. In patients with frequent episodes of exacerbation, a regular course of ICS may determine clinical stabilization and reduce the risk of exacerbations. In such patients, the smoking habit needs to be discontinued, as it is highly likely that smoking cessation would reduce the number of exacerbations given the established link between smoking and resistance to the anti-inflammatory effects of corticosteroids. However, quite often smokers report to have just a 'smoker's cough', thus not perceiving this symptom as an expression of disease but merely as a 'harmless' side-effect of smoking. Consequently, especially in COPD patients with frequent exacerbations, a strong cessation intervention must be considered. In these circumstances, optimizing therapy can make a considerable difference to the patient.

However, drug treatment alone is seldom enough to achieve this goal. Pharmacological therapy should be seen as an integral part of a comprehensive patient management which includes diverse components such as pulmonary rehabilitation, smoking cessation and appropriate nutritional advice. With such a combined approach it may be possible to break the 'vicious spiral' of recurrent exacerbations, immobility, deteriorating health status and further exacerbation, and dramatically improve patients' well-being.

REFERENCES

1. Celli BR, MacNee W. Standards for the diagnosis and treatment of patients with COPD: a summary of the ATS/ERS position paper. *Eur Respir J* 2004; 23:932–946.
2. Burge S, Wedzicha JA. COPD exacerbations: definitions and classifications. *Eur Respir J Suppl* 2003; 41: 46s–53s.
3. Rodriguez-Roisin R. Toward a consensus definition for COPD exacerbations. *Chest* 2000; 117(suppl 2): 398S–401S.
4. Jones PW, Willits LR, Burge PS *et al*. Disease severity and the effect of fluticasone propionate on chronic obstructive pulmonary disease. *Eur Respir J* 2003; 21:68–73.
5. Stevenson NJ, Walker PP, Costello RW *et al*. Lung mechanics and dyspnea during exacerbations of chronic obstructive pulmonary disease. *Am J Respir Crit Care Med* 2005; 172:1510–1516.
6. Vitacca M, Porta R, Bianchi L *et al*. Differences in spontaneous breathing pattern and mechanics in patients with severe COPD recovering from acute exacerbation. *Eur Respir J* 1999; 13:365–370.
7. Seemungal TA, Donaldson GC, Bhowmik A *et al*. Time course and recovery of exacerbations in patients with chronic obstructive pulmonary disease. *Am J Respir Crit Care Med* 2000; 161:1608–1613.

8. Miller MR, Hankinson J, Brusasco V et al. Standardization of spirometry. *Eur Respir J* 2005; 26:319–338.
9. Parker CM, Voduc N, Aaron SD et al. Physiological changes during symptom recovery from moderate exacerbations of COPD. *Eur Respir J* 2005; 26:420–428.
10. Calverley PM, Koulouris NG. Flow limitation and dynamic hyperinflation: key concepts in modern respiratory physiology. *Eur Respir J* 2005; 25:186–199.
11. O'Donnell DE, Bertley JC, Chau LK et al. Qualitative aspects of exertional breathlessness in chronic airflow limitation: pathophysiologic mechanisms. *Am J Respir Crit Care Med* 1997; 155:109–115.
12. Rodriguez-Roisin R, Barbera JA, Roca J. Pulmonary gas exchange. In: Calverley PMA, MacNee W, Pride NB et al. (eds). *Chronic Obstructive Pulmonary Disease*. Arnold, London, 2003, pp 175–193.
13. Qiu Y, Zhu J, Bandi V et al. Biopsy neutrophilia, neutrophil chemokine and receptor gene expression in severe exacerbations of chronic obstructive pulmonary disease. *Am J Respir Crit Care Med* 2003; 168:968–975.
14. Sethi S, Murphy TF. Bacterial infection in chronic obstructive pulmonary disease in 2000: a state-of-the-art review. *Clin Microbiol Rev* 2001; 14:336–363.
15. Sethi S, Evans N, Grant BJ et al. New strains of bacteria and exacerbations of chronic obstructive pulmonary disease. *N Engl J Med* 2002; 347:465–471.
16. Seemungal T, Harper-Owen R, Bhowmik A et al. Respiratory viruses, symptoms, and inflammatory markers in acute exacerbations and stable chronic obstructive pulmonary disease. *Am J Respir Crit Care Med* 2001; 164:1618–1623.
17. Wedzicha JA. Exacerbations: etiology and pathophysiologic mechanisms. *Chest* 2002; 21(suppl): 136S–141S.
18. Seemungal TA, Donaldson GC, Paul EA et al. Effect of exacerbation on quality of life in patients with chronic obstructive pulmonary disease. *Am J Respir Crit Care Med* 1998; 157:1418–1422.
19. Rohde G, Wiethege A, Borg I et al. Respiratory viruses in exacerbations of chronic obstructive pulmonary disease requiring hospitalization: a case-control study. *Thorax* 2003; 58:37–42.
20. Wilkinson TM, Patel IS, Wilks M et al. Airway bacterial load and FEV_1 decline in patients with chronic obstructive pulmonary disease. *Am J Respir Crit Care Med* 2003; 167:1090–1095.
21. Patel IS, Vlahos I, Wilkinson TM et al. Bronchiectasis, exacerbation indices, and inflammation in chronic obstructive pulmonary disease. *Am J Respir Crit Care Med* 2004; 170:400–407.
22. O'Brien C, Guest PJ, Hill SL et al. Physiological and radiological characterization of patients diagnosed with chronic obstructive pulmonary disease in primary care. *Thorax* 2000; 55:635–642.
23. Spencer S, Jones PW. Time course of recovery of health status following an infective exacerbation of chronic bronchitis. *Thorax* 2003; 58:589–593.
24. Vermeeren MA, Wouters EF, Geraerts-Keeris AJ et al. Nutritional support in patients with chronic obstructive pulmonary disease during hospitalization for an acute exacerbation; a randomized controlled feasibility trial. *Clin Nutr* 2004; 23:1184–1192.
25. Kanner RE, Anthonisen NR, Connett JE. Lower respiratory illnesses promote FEV_1 decline in current smokers but not ex-smokers with mild chronic obstructive pulmonary disease: results from the lung health study. *Am J Respir Crit Care Med* 2001; 164:358–364.
26. Donaldson GC, Seemungal TA, Bhowmik A et al. Relationship between exacerbation frequency and lung function decline in chronic obstructive pulmonary disease. *Thorax* 2002; 57:847–852.
27. Soler-Cataluna JJ, Martinez-Garcia MA, Roman Sanchez P et al. Severe acute exacerbations and mortality in patients with Chronic Obstructive Pulmonary Disease. *Thorax* 2005; 60:925–931.
28. Moayyedi P, Congleton J, Page RL et al. Comparison of nebulised salbutamol and ipratropium bromide with salbutamol alone in the treatment of chronic obstructive pulmonary disease. *Thorax* 1995; 50:834–837.
29. Hadcroft J, Calverley PM. Alternative methods for assessing bronchodilator reversibility in chronic obstructive pulmonary disease. *Thorax* 2001; 56:713–720.
30. Davies L, Angus RM, Calverley PMA. Oral corticosteroids in patients admitted to hospital with exacerbations of chronic obstructive pulmonary disease: a prospective randomised controlled trial. *Lancet* 1999; 354:456–460.
31. Niewoehner DE, Erbland ML, Deupree RH et al. Effect of systemic glucocorticoids on exacerbations of chronic obstructive pulmonary disease. *N Engl J Med* 1999; 340:1941–1947.
32. Aaron SD, Vandemheen KL, Hebert P et al. Outpatient oral prednisone after emergency treatment of chronic obstructive pulmonary disease. *N Engl J Med* 2003; 348:2618–2625.
33. Maltais F, Ostinelli J, Bourbeau J et al. Comparison of nebulized budesonide and oral prednisolone with placebo in the treatment of acute exacerbations of chronic obstructive pulmonary disease: a randomized controlled trial. *Am J Respir Crit Care Med* 2002; 165:698–703.

34. Anthonisen NR, Manfreda J, Warren CP et al. Antibiotic therapy in exacerbations of chronic obstructive pulmonary disease. *Ann Intern Med* 1987; 106:196–204.
35. Stockley RA, O'Brien C, Pye A et al. Relationship of sputum color to nature and outpatient management of acute exacerbations of COPD. *Chest* 2000; 117:1638–1645.
36. Nouira S, Marghli S, Belghith M et al. Once daily oral ofloxacin in chronic obstructive pulmonary disease exacerbation requiring mechanical ventilation: a randomised placebo-controlled trial. *Lancet* 2001; 358:2020–2025.
37. Calverley PMA. Oxygen-induced hypercapnia revisited. *Lancet* 2000; 356:1538–1539.
38. Lightowler JV, Wedzicha JA, Elliott MW et al. Non-invasive positive pressure ventilation to treat respiratory failure resulting from exacerbations of chronic obstructive pulmonary disease: Cochrane systematic review and meta-analysis. *BMJ* 2003; 326:185–187.
39. Spencer S, Calverley PM, Burge PS et al. Impact of preventing exacerbations on deterioration of health status in COPD. *Eur Respir J* 2004; 23:698–702.
40. Godtfredsen NS, Vestbo J, Osler M et al. Risk of hospital admission for COPD following smoking cessation and reduction: a Danish population study. *Thorax* 2002; 57:967–972.
41. Wongsurakiat P, Maranetra KN, Wasi C et al. Acute respiratory illness in patients with COPD and the effectiveness of influenza vaccination: a randomized controlled study. *Chest* 2004; 125:2011–2020.
42. Troosters T, Casaburi R, Gosselink R et al. Pulmonary rehabilitation in chronic obstructive pulmonary disease. *Am J Respir Crit Care Med* 2005; 172:19–38.
43. Calverley P, Pauwels R, Vestbo J et al. Combined salmeterol and fluticasone in the treatment of chronic obstructive pulmonary disease: a randomised controlled trial. *Lancet* 2003; 361:449–456.
44. Calverley PM. The role of corticosteroids in chronic obstructive pulmonary disease. *Semin Respir Crit Care Med* 2005; 26:235–245.
45. Calverley PM, Boonsawat W, Cseke Z et al. Maintenance therapy with budesonide and formoterol in chronic obstructive pulmonary disease. *Eur Respir J* 2003; 22:912–919.
46. Global initiative for chronic obstructive lung disease. Global strategy for the diagnosis, management and prevention of Chronic Obstructive Pulmonary Disease. NHLBI/WHO workshop report. Bethesda, MD: National Heart, Lung and Blood Institute; April 2001; update of the management sections, GOLD website (www.goldcopd.com). Date updated: September 2005.
47. Thompson WH, Nielson CP, Carvalho P et al. Controlled trial of oral prednisone in outpatients with acute COPD exacerbation. *Am J Respir Crit Care Med* 1996; 154:407–412.
48. Rennard S, Decramer M, Calverley PMA et al. Impact of COPD in North America and Europe in 2000: subjects' perspective of confronting COPD international survey. *Eur Respir J* 2002; 20:799–805.
49. Okubadejo AA, Jones PW, Wedzicha JA. Quality of life in patients with chronic obstructive pulmonary disease and severe hypoxaemia. *Thorax* 1996; 51:44–47.
50. Niewoehner DE. Interventions to prevent chronic obstructive pulmonary disease exacerbations. *Am J Med* 2004; 117(suppl 12A):41S–48S.
51. Chronic obstructive pulmonary disease. National clinical guideline on management of chronic obstructive pulmonary disease in adults in primary and secondary care. *Thorax* 2004; 59(suppl 1):1–232.
52. Calverley PM. Effect of corticosteroids on exacerbations of asthma and chronic obstructive pulmonary disease. *Proc Am Thorac Soc* 2004; 1:161–166.
53. Cazzola M, Matera MG, Pauwels R. Corticosteroids in COPD. In: Celli BR (ed.). *Pharmacotherapy in Chronic Obstructive Pulmonary Disease*. Marcel Dekker, New York, 2004, pp 265–298.
54. Alsaeedi A, Sin DD, McAlister FA. The effects of inhaled corticosteroids in chronic obstructive pulmonary disease: a systematic review of randomized placebo-controlled trials. *Am J Med* 2002; 113:59–65.
55. Szafranski W, Cukier A, Ramirez A et al. Efficacy and safety of budesonide/formoterol in the management of chronic obstructive pulmonary disease. *Eur Respir J* 2003; 21:74–81.
56. Donohue JF, Ohar JA. Effects of corticosteroids on lung function in asthma and Chronic Obstructive Pulmonary Disease. *Proc Am Thorac Soc* 2004; 1:152–160.
57. Walters JA, Walters EH, Wood-Baker R. Oral corticosteroids for stable chronic obstructive pulmonary disease. *Cochrane Database Syst Rev* 2005; CD005374.
58. Wouters EF, Creutzberg EC, Schols AM. Systemic effects in COPD. *Chest* 2002; 121(suppl):127S–130S.
59. Koerts-de Lang E, Hesselink MK, Drost MR et al. Enzyme activity of rat tibialis anterior muscle differs between treatment with triamcinolone and prednisolone and nutritional deprivation. *Eur J Appl Physiol Occup Physiol* 1999; 79:274–279.
60. de Blaauw I, Schols AM, Koerts-deLang E et al. De novo glutamine synthesis induced by corticosteroids in vivo in rats is secondary to weight loss. *Clin Nutr* 2004; 23:1035–1042.

61. Creutzberg EC, Schols AM, Bothmer-Quaedvlieg FCM *et al*. Prevalence of an elevated resting energy expenditure in patients with chronic obstructive pulmonary disease in relation to body composition and lung function. *Eur J Clin Nutr* 1998; 52:396–401.
62. Schols AM. Nutrition in chronic obstructive pulmonary disease. *Curr Opin Pulm Med* 2000; 6:110–115.
63. Di Francia M, Barbier D, Mege JL *et al*. Tumor necrosis factor-α levels and weight loss in chronic obstructive pulmonary disease. *Am J Respir Crit Care Med* 1994; 150:1453–1455.
64. De Godoy I, Donahoe M, Calhoun WJ *et al*. Elevated TNF-α production by peripheral blood monocytes of weight-losing COPD patients. *Am J Respir Crit Care Med* 1996; 153:633–637.
65. Aaron SD, Angel JB, Lunau M *et al*. Granulocyte inflammatory markers and airway infection during acute exacerbation of chronic obstructive pulmonary disease. *Am J Respir Crit Care Med* 2001; 163: 349–355.
66. Dentener MA, Creutzberg EC, Schols AM *et al*. Systemic anti-inflammatory mediators in COPD: increase in soluble interleukin 1 receptor II during treatment of exacerbations. *Thorax* 2001; 56:721–726.
67. Roland M, Bhowmik A, Sapsford RJ *et al*. Sputum and plasma endothelin-1 levels in exacerbations of chronic obstructive pulmonary disease. *Thorax* 2001; 56:30–35.
68. Ek A, Larsson K, Siljerud S *et al*. Fluticasone and budesonide inhibit cytokine release in human lung epithelial cells and alveolar macrophages. *Allergy* 1999; 54:691–699.
69. Sin DD, Lacy P, York E *et al*. Effects of fluticasone on systemic markers of inflammation in chronic obstructive pulmonary disease. *Am J Respir Crit Care Med* 2004; 170:760–765.
70. Smith IE, Jurriaans E, Diederich S *et al*. Chronic sputum production: correlation between clinical features and findings on high resolution computed tomographic scanning of the chest. *Thorax* 1996; 51:914–918.
71. Eller J, de Silva JRL, Poulter LW *et al*. Cells and cytokines in chronic bronchial infection. *Ann N Y Acad Sci* 1994; 725:331–345.
72. Amitani R, Wilson R, Rutman A *et al*. Effects of human neutrophil elastase and bacterial proteinases on human respiratory epithelium. *Am J Respir Cell Mol Biol* 1991; 4:26–32.
73. Nakamura H, Yoshimura K, McElvaney NG *et al*. Neutrophil elastase in respiratory epithelial lining fluid of individuals with cystic fibrosis induces interleukin-8 gene expression in a human bronchial epithelial cell line. *J Clin Invest* 1992; 89:1478–1484.
74. Schiotz PO, Jorgensen M, Flensborg EW *et al*. Chronic *Pseudomonas aeruginosa* in lung infection in cystic fibrosis. A longitudinal study of immune complex activity and inflammatory response in sputum sol-phase of cystic fibrosis patients with chronic *Pseudomonas aeruginosa* lung infections: influence of local steroid treatment. *Acta Paediatr Scand* 1983; 72:283–287.
75. Elborn JS, Johnston B, Allen F *et al*. Inhaled steroids in patients with bronchiectasis. *Respir Med* 1992; 86:121–124.
76. Van Haren EHJ, Lammers JWJ, Festen J *et al*. The effects of inhaled corticosteroid budesonide on lung function and bronchial hyper-responsiveness in adult patients with cystic fibrosis. *Respir Med* 1995; 89:209–214.
77. Nikolaizik WH, Schoni MH. Pilot study to assess the effect of inhaled corticosteroids on lung function in patients with cystic fibrosis. *J Pediatr* 1996; 128:271–274.
78. Tsang KW, Ho PL, Lam WK *et al*. Inhaled fluticasone reduces sputum inflammatory indices in severe bronchiectasis. *Am J Respir Crit Care Med* 1998; 158:723–727.
79. Tsang KW, Tan KC, Ho PL *et al*. Inhaled fluticasone in bronchiectasis: a 12 month study. *Thorax* 2005; 60:239–243.
80. Calverley PM. Reducing the frequency and severity of exacerbations of chronic obstructive pulmonary disease. *Proc Am Thorac Soc* 2004; 1:121–124.
81. Patel IS, Seemungal TA, Wilks M *et al*. Relationship between bacterial colonization and the frequency, character, and severity of COPD exacerbations. *Thorax* 2002; 57:759–764.
82. Ito K, Lim S, Caramori G *et al*. Cigarette smoking reduces histone deacetylase 2 expression, enhances cytokine expression and inhibits glucocorticoid actions in alveolar macrophages. *FASEB J* 2001; 15: 1100–1102.
83. Barnes PJ, Ito K, Adcock IM. A mechanism of corticosteroid resistance in COPD: inactivation of histone deacetylase. *Lancet* 2004; 363:731–733.
84. George TP, O'Malley SS. Current pharmacological treatments for nicotine dependence. *Trends Pharmacol Sci* 2004; 25:42–48.

3

Reduction in the level of dyspnoea near the end of life

D. A. Mahler, G. L. Scano

BACKGROUND

Information about the impact of chronic obstructive pulmonary disease (COPD) on control of symptoms, health status, and activities of daily living is quite limited in the latter stages of the illness [1–4]. In 1996, Connors et al. [1] described the outcomes of 1016 patients with COPD following hospitalization in the US for an acute exacerbation. After 6 months, only 26% of the patients were both alive and able to report a good, very good, or excellent quality of life [1]. In comparing the course of illness and patterns of care of patients with non-small cell lung cancer and COPD, Claessens et al. [2] reported that 'severe dyspnoea' occurred in 32% of patients with lung cancer and in 56% of patients with COPD. The symptoms of dyspnoea and pain were considered problematic in both groups of patients [2]. In 2005, Elkington et al. [5] assessed the healthcare needs of 209 patients with COPD who had died. Based on reports from informants (those close to the deceased and involved in caring for them in the last months of life), 98% of patients were breathless all the time or sometimes in their last year; and breathlessness was partly relieved in over 50% of those treated [5].

These data illustrate the challenge faced by caregivers and healthcare systems in reducing the intensity of breathing discomfort experienced by nearly all patients with COPD as the disease advances and progresses near the end of their life. Dudgeon [6] has recently reviewed treatment strategies for relieving dyspnoea at the end of life, and there is considerable information available about the management of dyspnoea in patients with cancer [7–9].

CASE REPORT

HISTORY

B.B. is a 68-year-old male with a long history of cigarette smoking (55 pack-years) and an 8-year history of exertional dyspnoea. Five years ago he went to his physician because his breathlessness interfered with activities of daily living. At that time his pulmonary function testing showed airflow obstruction ($FEV_1/FVC = 52\%$) with $FEV_1 = 38\%$ predicted. He was diagnosed with COPD and treated with long-acting bronchodilator medications.

Donald A. Mahler, MD, Professor of Medicine, Dartmouth Medical School, Hanover, New Hampshire, USA

Giorgio L. Scano, MD, Associate Professor in Respiratory Medicine, Department of Internal Medicine, Section of Immunology and Respiratory Medicine, University of Florence, Careggi General Hospital, Florence, Italy

At the present time he describes being 'short of breath' at rest 'most of the time', and experiences breathlessness when walking from one room to another in his residence. When asked to describe his breathlessness, he reports that he has 'trouble getting enough air in.' Upper extremity activities, such as combing his hair, dressing and washing provoke difficulty breathing as well as general fatigue. He is unable to do yard work or even enjoy his hobby of woodworking because his dyspnoea interferes with these activities. B.B. spends most of his time indoors at home watching television: he has little interest in eating, and has lost 5 kg in the past few months.

When questioned, B.B. and his spouse confirm that he becomes anxious and frustrated at various times because he cannot do any activities. B.B. has become reluctant to leave home because he is concerned that 'I will lose control of my breathing.' In fact, he sometimes thinks to himself 'Why bother doing anything?'.

PHYSICAL EXAMINATION

Vital signs
- Respiratory rate: 22 breaths/min
- Heart rate: 110 beats/min
- Blood pressure: 126/76 mmHg
- Oxygen saturation: 87% breathing room air.

General appearance
The patient is seated in a chair, but leans forward supporting his forearms on his thighs just above the knees. His lips are pursed and the sternocleidomastoid muscles are hypertrophied. The chest is 'barrel shaped' and there is inward motion of the lower intercostal spaces during inspiration (Hoover sign). Chest examination reveals diminished intensity of breath sounds with prolonged expiratory time. Heart auscultation reveals diminished intensity of heart sounds. The abdomen is scaphoid and non-tender. The extremities show no clubbing, oedema, or cyanosis. The skin is dry and scaly with ecchymoses on the dorsal aspects of the hands and forearms.

LUNG FUNCTION TESTS AND ARTERIAL BLOOD GASES

Current testing reveals (Table 3.1):
- Obstructive pattern with a FEV_1/FVC ratio <70%.
- Level of severity is 'severe', or Stage IV GOLD, based on FEV_1 = 27% predicted.
- Expiratory flow limitation on flow-volume loop.
- Hyperinflation with increased forced residual capacity (FRC) and total lung capacity (TLC).
- Presence of emphysema based on markedly reduced single-breath diffusing capacity (35% predicted).
- Partial bronchodilator responsiveness as there were increases of 120 ml in FEV_1 and 140 ml in FVC after inhalation of two puffs (180 µg) of salbutamol.

CHEST RADIOGRAPHS

The lateral view shows hyperinflation of the lung fields (flat diaphragm and enlarged retrosternal air space). The posterior–anterior view shows a narrowed cardiac shadow with vertical orientation and diminished vascular markings of the lung parenchyma.

WHY DOES THE PATIENT HAVE BREATHLESSNESS?

A neurophysiological model has been used to explain dyspnoea [10]. In brief, there is a disassociation between the motor command originating from the central nervous system and

Table 3.1 Lung function and arterial blood gases in patient B.B.

	Measured	Percent predicted
Age (years)	68.00	
Height (cm)	186.50	
Weight (kg)	77.70	
FVC (l)	3.53	74
FEV_1 (l)	0.94	27
FEV_1/FVC (%)	27.00	
TLC (l)	10.20	131
FRC (l)	7.50	193
MIP (cm H_2O)	61.00	
Single-breath diffusing capacity (ml/min/mmHg)	6.70	35
Arterial blood gases on room air		
pH	7.41	
$PaCO_2$ (mmHg)	46.00	
PaO_2 (mmHg)	52.00	

FEV_1 = forced expiratory volume in one second; FRC = functional residual capacity; FVC = forced vital capacity; MIP = maximal inspiratory mouth pressure (measured at FRC); $PaCO_2$ = arterial carbon dioxide tension; PaO_2 = arterial oxygen tension; TLC = total lung capacity.

the mechanical response (incoming afferent information from receptors in the airways, lungs, and chest wall structures) of the respiratory system. This 'mismatch' of neural activity and consequent ventilatory output contributes to breathing discomfort or difficulty.

In general, four major mechanisms cause dyspnoea in patients with COPD [10–12]. Specific factors that contributed to B.B.'s breathlessness are highlighted in italics in the following discussion.

Increased ventilatory demand
At rest, this patient has increased ventilation in order to compensate for the *high dead space* due to his airflow obstruction. In addition, neural outflow from the carotid bodies, located at the bifurcation of the common carotid arteries, accounts for up to 15% of resting ventilation [13]. With his *hypoxaemia* (PaO_2 = 52 mmHg), carotid body neural discharge would be marked [14]. Central chemoreceptors, located in the medulla and mid-brain, adjust ventilation to maintain acid–base homeostasis. As the normal pH indicates metabolic compensation, the elevated $PaCO_2$ appeared to be chronic and probably has minimal effect on his breathlessness. Based on the chronicity of his respiratory disease, the patient is likely to be deconditioned. *Deconditioning* is associated with an early and accelerated rise in blood lactate with exertion and imposes an additional respiratory stimulus [10].

Decreased ventilatory capacity
One cause of airflow obstruction in patients with COPD is *increased airway resistance*. With an increase in ventilatory impedance, the level of central respiratory motor output rises in order to achieve the required ventilation. When the level of respiratory effort is out of proportion with the resultant level of ventilation, dyspnoea develops.

Respiratory muscle dysfunction
This patient exhibited *hyperinflation* of the lung fields on his chest radiograph. With overexpanded lungs there is added elastic recoil (i.e. an inspiratory load) as well as shortening

of the vertical muscle fibres of the diaphragm (reduced force-generation capacity) that contribute to dyspnoea.

In addition, many patients with COPD develop *dynamic hyperinflation* with even minimal physical activities [15, 16]. This development can further contribute to the mechanical abnormalities associated with breathing and cause more breathlessness.

Poor nutrition may lead to respiratory muscle weakness and also contribute to breathlessness.

Altered central perception

Dyspnoea has affective dimensions with associated *anxiety*, panic, and *depression* [1, 17]. The patient's emotional response (a direct result of the disability and handicap of COPD) can influence the intensity, quality and duration of breathing discomfort.

DISCUSSION

The following discussion considers various treatments that have been shown to reduce the severity of breathlessness in randomized controlled trials. This approach is organized based on our current understanding of the mechanisms whereby specific therapies relieve dyspnoea (Table 3.2). Certainly, more than one mechanism may account for an improvement in an individual's breathing difficulty. Certain treatments are reviewed in more detail in other chapters of this volume. Our emphasis will be on options that can be used toward the end of a patient's life in order to reduce the severity of breathing discomfort and to provide comfort.

Table 3.2 General treatment strategies to reduce dyspnoea based on physiological mechanisms

Mechanism	Treatment

Reduce ventilatory demand	Oxygen*
	 Exercise training
	 Pharmacological therapy
	   Anxiolytics*
	   Opiates*
	 Alter pulmonary afferent information
	   Chest wall vibration*
	   Fans*

Reduce ventilatory impedance	Reduce hyperinflation
	   Pursed-lips breathing*
	   Volume reduction surgery
	   Non-invasive ventilatory support*
	     (counterbalances elastic recoil)
	 Reduce resistive load
	   Pharmacotherapy (also deflates the lung)*

Improve respiratory muscle function	Nutrition* Positioning* Inspiratory muscle training Non-invasive ventilatory support* (unloads the respiratory muscles)
Alter central perception	Distraction strategies* Attention strategies*

*Appropriate for patients with COPD near the end of life.

REDUCE VENTILATORY DEMAND

Oxygen

Supplemental oxygen therapy clearly reduces the severity of breathlessness in patients with COPD at rest and during activities of daily living [18–22]. The relief of dyspnoea with oxygen use has generally been considered a result of reduced chemoreceptor activity and associated reduced ventilation (V_E) [10]. However, O'Donnell et al. [21] showed that the reduction in dyspnoea *during exercise* was related to decreased blood lactate levels in 11 patients with COPD who had oxygen saturations ≤88% at rest. These investigators reported no differences in the relationship between V_E and dyspnoea whether patients breathed oxygen or room air [21].

Somfay et al. [22] studied 10 patients with COPD who had SaO_2 >93% at rest and >88% during exercise. The improvement in breathlessness during exercise was correlated to the reduced respiratory rate ($r = 0.38$; $P = 0.028$), but was not related to SaO_2 levels or end-expiratory lung volumes (EELV). Oxygen supplementation also led to decreased hyperinflation during exercise [22].

Other possible explanations for reductions in breathlessness with oxygen are an improvement in respiratory muscle function and blunting of any increase in pulmonary artery pressure associated with exertion [10].

Clearly, continuous oxygen should be prescribed for patient B.B. based on his hypoxaemia at rest ($PaO_2 = 52$ mmHg). The FIO_2 should be titrated to achieve an oxygen saturation of 90–92%. There is no evidence that higher FIO_2 levels are beneficial for relief of dyspnoea at rest.

Exercise training

Exercise training is important for the majority of patients with COPD to reverse deconditioning (see Chapter 7). However, the physiological demands of exercise generally exceed the physical ability of most patients with advanced COPD. Many of these patients report that they need to conserve energy in order to perform the necessary activities of daily living. An open discussion with each patient can address whether exercise training as part of a pulmonary rehabilitation programme is appropriate for that individual. Certainly, as the COPD progresses and the end of an individual's life approaches, physical training is no longer appropriate.

The physician and B.B. had a long discussion about exercise training. B.B. reported that he did not have the energy or stamina to do daily exercises because he struggles with each breath during normal daily activities such as combing his hair, bathing and dressing. The physician and B.B. agreed that a physical therapist would be helpful to assist the patient in their passive range of motion.

Fans

The movement of cool air across a patient's face modifies breathing discomfort. It is believed that stimulation of mechanoreceptors on the face or a decrease in the temperature of the facial skin, both of which are mediated by the trigeminal nerve, may alter feedback to the brain and reduce breathlessness [10, 23].

B.B. typically requests that a family member position a fan in the room where he sits and in his bedroom when he sleeps. At times he asks a family member to open the window to allow 'fresh air' into the room.

Anxiolytics

Anxiolytic medications have the potential to relieve dyspnoea by altering the emotional response to dyspnoea. Although various randomized controlled trials have generally failed to show any benefit with benzodiazepines, the subjects in these studies were not selected on the basis of having a diagnosis of anxiety in addition to their breathing difficulty due to COPD [10]. Given the prevalence of severe anxiety in patients who experience substantial breathlessness, it is reasonable to consider a trial of anxiolytic therapy in selected patients.

The physician discussed the possibility that anxiety could worsen dyspnoea with B.B. and his family. All parties agreed that a trial of alprazolam was appropriate.

Opiates

Opiates reduce ventilation and the central processing of neural signals within the central nervous system to reduce the intensity of dyspnoea. In a systematic review, Jennings *et al*. [24] reported that oral or parenteral opioids had a clear effect on relieving the sensation of breathlessness (based on nine studies), but that a nebulized method of delivery was not beneficial (based on three studies). These authors found that the overall effect of oral or parenteral opioids on relief of dyspnoea was 'relatively small' [24]. This may be due to the fact that:

- Small doses of narcotics were used in some studies.
- The prescribed dose of the opiate was not titrated in any of the studies.
- Dosing intervals were probably too long in selected studies.
- A steady state was not reached in trials when only a single dose of a narcotic was used [24].

The physician discussed the use of oral or parenteral opiates with B.B. after all other treatments were tried without adequate relief of his breathlessness at rest. The discussion included the anticipated reduction in breathing discomfort as well as information about the possible side-effects of opiates (e.g. somnolence, constipation, nausea, vomiting and hypercapnia). B.B. agreed with an initial trial of immediate-release oral morphine at a dose of 15 mg. The physician reassured B.B. and his family that the dose: could be repeated every 4 h if needed to achieve relief of breathlessness; could be increased to 30 mg if the 15 mg dose did not achieve the expected benefit; and that a long-acting narcotic could be prescribed to achieve more sustained benefit.

REDUCE VENTILATORY IMPEDANCE

Pursed-lips breathing

Many patients with COPD 'discover' on their own that pursed-lips breathing (PLB) reduces the severity of breathlessness. Alternatively, the patient can be instructed in the technique of PLB by a respiratory or physical therapist.

Two recent studies provide further scientific support for the beneficial effects of PLB on dyspnoea. Bianchi *et al*. [25] showed that the use of PLB, when compared to spontaneous breathing, lengthened expiratory time, reduced EELV of the chest wall, and improved breathlessness at rest in 22 patients with COPD. In a study of eight patients with COPD, Spahija *et al*. [26] found that changes in dyspnoea scores with PLB during exercise were correlated with changes in EELV ($r^2 = 0.82$; $P = 0.002$) and with changes in the mean inspiratory ratio of pleural pressure to the maximal static inspiratory pressure-generating capacity ($r^2 = 0.84$; $P = 0.001$).

B.B.'s physician requested a consultation with a respiratory therapist to review the technique of PLB with the patient, so that he could use it both at rest and during exertion. B.B. reported a sense of control of his breathing using PLB.

Pharmacotherapy

Both short- and long-acting bronchodilators have been shown to reduce the severity of breathlessness based on two distinct stimuli: activities of daily living and during constant work exercise [27]. Combination therapy with a long-acting β-agonist and an inhaled corticosteroid also provide relief of breathlessness [28, 29]. The use of pharmacotherapy in patients with COPD is reviewed in Chapter 7.

Medications that should be prescribed for B.B. to relieve dyspnoea include:

- *Tiotropium*
- *Salmeterol/fluticasone or formoterol/budesonide*
- *Theophylline (if no contraindication)*
- *Salbutamol metered-dose inhaler 'as needed'.*

If B.B. has difficulty performing the appropriate inspiratory manoeuvres in order to deliver the powder or aerosol to the lower respiratory tract, then consideration should be given to use of short-acting bronchodilator solutions administered via nebulization.

Non-invasive ventilation support
The technique is reviewed in Chapter 13 of this volume.

IMPROVE RESPIRATORY MUSCLE FUNCTION

Positioning
Patients with COPD learn from experience that certain positions alter the experience of breathlessness. For example, the leaning forward position with forearms resting on the thighs reduces dyspnoea by enhancing the mechanics of breathing [30].

B.B. was encouraged to lean forward, or to use a walker (at home) or a shopping cart (if he was in a store) to provide support for the shoulder girdle muscles and enhance diaphragmatic function to achieve some relief from breathing discomfort.

Nutrition
Very few investigations of nutritional supplementation have evaluated dyspnoea as an outcome in patients with COPD. The efficacy of nutritional support is reviewed in Chapter 5 of this volume.

Inspiratory muscle training
'Targeted' inspiratory muscle training has clear benefits in the relief from dyspnoea [31, 32]. However, as discussed for exercise training, the physiological demands of inspiratory muscle training are generally excessive for patients with advanced COPD. Thus, inspiratory muscle training is not appropriate for patients with COPD near the end of their life.

ALTER CENTRAL PERCEPTION

Cognitive-behavioural strategies can alter the patient's affective response to the symptom of breathlessness [33]. In general, these therapies appear to enhance the tolerance to and decrease the physiological arousal and psychological distress resulting from dyspnoea. Although there are limited data from randomized controlled trials, these coping strategies are used clinically in the management of breathlessness of affected individuals.

If dyspnoea is relatively brief, acute distraction may be more effective in reducing breathlessness and increasing tolerance [33]. However, attention strategies may be more beneficial if the individual can more actively confront the situation. In general, attentive coping (i.e. symptom monitoring and obtaining information about the symptom) is associated with better adjustment to an illness, whereas avoidance results in higher levels of physical and psychological disability [34].

Distraction strategies
Distraction from an unpleasant sensation, such as difficulty in breathing, can increase the patient's tolerance and reduce the associated distress. With the sudden or acute onset of

Table 3.3 Cognitive-behavioural therapies to reduce dyspnoea (with permission from [17])

> *Distraction strategies*
> 1. Social support
> 2. Relaxation exercises
> 3. Biofeedback
> 4. Music
> 5. Hypnosis
> 6. Guided imagery
> 7. Acupuncture and acupressure
>
> *Attention strategies*
> 1. Symptom monitoring
> 2. Increased knowledge about symptom management

breathlessness, various distraction strategies may be effective in the short term to alleviate or modify dyspnoea (Table 3.3). For example, social support from family members, friends and individuals who have the same disease can provide immense help for the individual in dealing with their breathlessness. The desire for social support may vary from weekly group meetings to periodic use of 'chat rooms' on the Internet. Certainly, the benefits of social support should depend on the preferences of the affected individual.

Relaxation is a useful method to reduce the anxiety and distress that accompany breathing difficulty. Typically, relaxation can be achieved by the patient reducing their respiratory rate and increasing tidal volume – 'taking slow, deep breaths'. Relaxation methods may include a quiet environment, comfortable position, loose clothing, repetition of a word or image in a systematic manner or the systematic tensing and/or relaxing of muscles [33]. Tape recordings can be used to coach patients in relaxation methods. Quiet instrumental music is often used to accompany relaxation techniques.

Hypnosis may modify neural activity in the cerebral cortex and alter the perception of dyspnoea by 'desensitization' [33]. At present, only limited scientific information is available about the possible benefits of acupuncture and acupressure on breathlessness.

Attention strategies
Regular monitoring of the intensity of breathlessness and an individualized action plan are essential features of a symptom management programme [33]. Daily recording of difficulty in breathing in a diary may improve adherence to a treatment regimen because review of this information may help the patient identify patterns of trigger and response to therapy [35].

In addition, increased knowledge of strategies for managing dyspnoea may help the patient and his family members to deal with episodes of breathlessness at home.

The physician suggested to B.B. that a nurse specialist be consulted to help the patient with coping-behavioural strategies. After initially saying, 'No, I am not interested,' B.B. changed his mind. The nurse had several appointments with B.B. and his family; they discussed some of the above distraction and attention strategies. B.B. reported to his physician that he found the use of music, the relaxation tape, and 'chatting' with other COPD sufferers on the Internet to be particularly helpful for relieving his breathlessness.

SUMMARY

Several options can be used toward the end of a patient's life in order to reduce the severity of breathing discomfort and provide comfort:

- Supplemental oxygen therapy
- Positioning of a fan to allow a flow of cool air across the patient's face
- Bronchodilator, anxiolytic and opiate medications
- Pursed-lips breathing
- Non-invasive ventilation
- Cognitive-behavioural strategies (e.g. attention/distraction techniques).

The choice of options should be tailored to the individual and based on the patient's clinical situation and symptom severity. As more than one mechanism may lead to an improvement of the breathing difficulty, physicians, nurses and other caregivers should question each patient about the characteristics of their dyspnoea (onset, frequency, intensity, duration, triggers, provoking activities as well as actions that might provide relief) that affect the individual [36]. Based on the patient's responses, the physician should then individualize the various therapeutic strategies. In general, opiate medications should be considered only when other therapies have been tried but have failed to adequately relieve the patient's breathing difficulty.

Frequent discussions with the patient and their family can establish whether the patient has gained some relief of the breathing discomfort, whether the dose of a medication needs to be adjusted or whether a new treatment should be started.

REFERENCES

1. Connors AF Jr, Dawson NV, Thomas C et al. Outcomes following acute exacerbations of severe chronic obstructive lung disease. The SUPPORT investigators (Study to Understand Prognoses and Preferences for Outcomes and Risks of Treatments). *Am J Respir Crit Care Med* 1996; 154:959–967.
2. Claessens MT, Lynn J, Zhong Z et al. Dying with lung cancer or chronic obstructive pulmonary disease: insights for SUPPORT. Study to Understand Prognosis and Preferences for Outcomes and Risks of Treatments. *J Am Geriatr Soc* 2000; 48:S146–S153.
3. Skilbeck J, Mott L, Page H et al. Palliative care in chronic obstructive airways disease: a needs assessment. *Palliat Med* 1998; 12:245–254.
4. Gore JM, Brophy CJ, Greenstone MA. How well do we care for patients with end stage chronic obstructive pulmonary disease (COPD)? A comparison of palliative care and quality of life in COPD and lung cancer. *Thorax* 2000; 55:1000–1006.
5. Elkington H, White P, Addington-Hall J et al. The healthcare needs of chronic obstructive pulmonary disease patients in the last year of life. *Palliat Med* 2005; 19:485–491.
6. Dudgeon D. Management of dyspnea at the end of life. In: Mahler DA, O'Donnell DE (eds). *Dyspnea: Mechanisms, Measurement, and Management,* 2nd edition. Taylor & Francis, New York, 2005, pp 429–461.
7. Bruera E, Sala R, Spruyt O et al. Nebulized versus subcutaneous morphine for patients with cancer dyspnea: a preliminary study. *J Pain Symptom Manage* 2004; 29:613–618.
8. Bruera E, Macmillan K, Pither J, MacDonald RN. Effects of morphine on the dyspnea of terminal cancer patients. *J Pain Symptom Manage* 1990; 5:341–344.
9. Abernethy AP, Currow DC, Frith P et al. Randomized, double-blind, placebo-controlled crossover trial of sustained release morphine for the management of refractory dyspnea. *Br Med J* 2003; 327:523–528.
10. American Thoracic Society. Dyspnea. Mechanisms, assessment, and management: a consensus statement. *Am J Respir Crit Care Med* 1999; 159:321–340.
11. Mahler DA. Dyspnoea in chronic obstructive pulmonary disease. *Monaldi Arch Chest Dis* 1998; 53:669–671.
12. O'Donnell DA, Webb KA. Mechanisms of dyspnea in COPD. In: Mahler DA, O'Donnell DE (eds). *Dyspnea: Mechanisms, Measurement, and Management,* 2nd edition. Taylor & Francis, New York, 2005, pp 29–58.
13. Lambertsen CJ. *Chemical Control of Respiration at Rest,* 14th edition. Mosby Company, St. Louis, 1980.
14. Briscoe TJ, Purves MJ, Sampson SR. The frequency of nerve impulses in single carotid body chemoreceptor afferent fibres recorded in vivo with intact circulation. *J Physiol London* 1970; 208:121–131.
15. O'Donnell DE, Revill SM, Webb AK. Dynamic hyperinflation and exercise intolerance in chronic obstructive pulmonary disease. *Am J Respir Crit Care Med* 2001; 164:770–777.

16. Gigliotti F, Coli C, Bianchi R et al. Arm exercise and hyperinflation in patients with COPD. Effect of arm training. *Chest* 2005; 128:1225–1232.
17. Carrieri-Kohlman V. Coping and self-management strategies for dyspnea. In: Mahler DA, O'Donnell DE (eds). *Dyspnea: Mechanisms, Measurement, and Management,* 2nd edition. Taylor & Francis, New York, 2005, pp 365–396.
18. Lane R, Crockcroft A, Adams L, Guz A. Arterial oxygen saturation and breathlessness in patients with chronic obstructive airway disease. *Clin Sci* 1987; 76:693–698.
19. Swinburn CR, Mould H, Stone TN et al. Symptomatic benefit of supplemental oxygen in hypoxemic patients with chronic lung disease. *Am Rev Respir Dis* 1991; 143:913–918.
20. Dean NC, Brown JK, Himelman RB et al. Oxygen may improve dyspnea and endurance in patients with chronic obstructive pulmonary disease and only mild hypoxemia. *Am Rev Respir Dis* 1992; 146:941–945.
21. O'Donnell DE, Bain DI, Webb KA. Factors contributing to relief of exertional breathlessness during hyperoxia in chronic airflow limitation. *Am J Respir Crit Care Med* 1997; 155:530–535.
22. Somfay A, Porszasz J, Lee SM, Casaburi R. Dose-response effect of oxygen on hyperinflation and exercise endurance in nonhypoxemic COPD patients. *Eur Respir J* 2001; 18:77–84.
23. Schwartzstein RM, Lahive K, Pope A et al. Cold facial stimulation reduces breathlessness induced in normal subjects. *Am Rev Respir Dis* 1987; 136:58–61.
24. Jennings AL, Davies AN, Higgins JPT et al. A systematic review of the use of opioids in the management of dyspnoea. *Thorax* 2002; 57:939–944.
25. Bianchi R, Gigliotti F, Romagnoli I et al. Chest wall kinematics and breathlessness during pursed-lip breathing in patients with COPD. *Chest* 2004; 125:459–465.
26. Spahija J, de Marchie M, Grassino A. Effects of imposed pursed-lips breathing on respiratory mechanics and dyspnea at rest and during exercise in COPD. *Chest* 2005; 128:640–650.
27. Mahler DA. Dyspnea. In: Celli BR (ed.). *Pharmacotherpay in Chronic Obstructive Pulmonary Disease.* Marcel Dekker, Inc., New York, 2004, pp 145–157.
28. O'Donnell DE, Mahler DA. Effect of bronchodilators and inhaled corticosteroids on dyspnea in COPD. In: Mahler DA, O'Donnell DE (eds). *Dyspnea: Mechanisms, Measurement, and Management,* 2nd edition. Taylor & Francis, New York, 2005, pp 283–300.
29. O'Donnell DE, Sciurba F, Celli B et al. Effect of fluticasone propionate/salmeterol on lung hyperinflation and exercise endurance in COPD. *Chest* 2006; 130:647–656.
30. Sharp JT, Drutz WS, Moisan T et al. Postural relief of dyspnea in severe chronic obstructive pulmonary disease. *Am Rev Respir Dis* 1980; 122:201–211.
31. Lotters F, van Tol B, Kwakkel G, Gosselink R. Effects of controlled inspiratory muscle training in patients with COPD: a meta-analysis. *Eur Respir J* 2002; 20:570–576.
32. Lisboa C, Borzone G. Inspiratory muscle training. In: Mahler DA, O'Donnell DE (eds). *Dyspnea: Mechanisms, Measurement, and Management,* 2nd edition. Taylor & Francis, New York, 2005, pp 321–344.
33. Carrieri-Kohlman V. Coping and self-management strategies for dyspnea. In: Mahler DA, O'Donnell DE (eds). *Dyspnea: Mechanisms, Measurement, and Management,* 2nd edition. Taylor & Francis, New York, 2005, pp 365–396.
34. Keefe FJ, Dunsmore J, Burnett R. Behaviorial and cognitive-behavioral approaches to chronic pain: recent advances and future directions. *J Consult Clin Psychol* 1992; 60:528–536.
35. Burman ME. Health diaries in nursing research and practice. *J Nurs Scholarsh* 1995; 27:147–152.
36. Mahler DA. Diagnosis of dyspnea. In: Mahler DA (ed.). *Dyspnea.* Marcel Dekker, Inc., New York, 1998, pp 221–259.

4

A COPD patient with bronchospasm episodes after the inhalation of tobacco smoke

S. Nardini, G. Invernizzi

BACKGROUND

Chronic obstructive pulmonary disease (COPD) is, according to the recent ERS-ATS guidelines, 'a preventable and treatable disease state characterized by airflow limitation that is not fully reversible' [1].

The disease consists of a progressive decline in lung function (a sort of premature ageing), which is irreversible and causes progressive dyspnoea and disability. Eventually, the respiratory function is so impaired that it cannot supply oxygen and clear carbon dioxide enough to grant survival and the patient dies.

According to the Global Alliance for Respiratory Diseases (GARD) of the World Health Organization, respiratory diseases are the second most important cause of death in the world and COPD accounts for a large proportion of deaths caused by respiratory diseases. In fact, among the 4 million deaths caused by chronic respiratory diseases in 2005, over 3 million deaths were due to COPD. COPD and chronic respiratory diseases are widely under-recognized, under-diagnosed, under-treated and insufficiently prevented: if the existing trend continues, chronic respiratory diseases will increase by 30% in the next 10 years [2].

As already stated, the main cause of COPD is tobacco smoking [3] and its influence appears to be related not only to the age when smoking started (the younger the starting age, the worse the disease), but also to the total number of cigarettes smoked (the higher the number of cigarettes smoked, the faster the decline in FEV_1).

Smoking starts to damage lungs even in the uterus if the mother is a smoker. Smoking during adolescence causes chronic symptoms and reduces lung growth. The lung damage continues and worsens if a young smoker keeps on smoking through adult life, until clinical COPD can be diagnosed.

Other risks for COPD are found in certain working environments [4], and as a consequence of outdoor [5] as well as indoor pollution. For this latter, the situation is different in developing countries (where the pollution is mainly due to biomass combustion for cooking and heating purposes) [6] compared to industrialized ones, where the indoor pollution is mainly generated by environmental tobacco smoke (ETS) [7].

Smoking cessation (SC) can treat COPD. Indeed, so far, only two treatments have been demonstrated to improve (extend) the life expectancy: long-term oxygen therapy and SC. After SC, both symptoms and signs improve. Phlegm and cough as well as the exaggerated

---

Stefano Nardini, MD, Pneumologist, U.O. di Pneumologia, Regione Veneto, Sinistra Piave, Vittorio Veneto, Italy
Giovanni Invernizzi, MD, Allergologist, Tobacco Control Unit, National Tumour Institute and SIMG-Italian College of General Practitioners, Milan, Italy

© Atlas Medical Publishing Ltd 2007

Table 4.1 The '5 As'

1. Ask – ask all patients if they are smokers
2. Advise – advise all smokers to stop smoking, in an individualized way
3. Assess – assess motivation to quit
4. Assist – assist the smoker motivated to quit in his quitting attempt
5. Arrange – arrange follow-up of the patient, managing relapses

decline of FEV_1 (compared to non-smokers) can ameliorate [1]. In the Lung Health Study, the prevalence of respiratory symptoms (chronic cough, chronic sputum, dyspnoea and wheezing) was significantly lower in smokers who successfully ceased smoking [8]. The lowest prevalence of these symptoms was observed among sustained quitters, while continuous smokers had the highest, and intermittent smokers were in the middle. A reduction of the mean decrement of FEV_1 over time was also observed, although there was also a small improvement in FEV_1 during the first year after cessation. Some benefits were also seen in patients who did not succeed in achieving complete and sustained abstinence [9]. These patients had less loss of lung function compared to patients who continued to smoke as before.

A smoker can quit without help, but it is difficult and long-term abstinence is higher when the quitting attempt is aided with medical assistance [10]. Usually, a strong motivation to quit (i.e. a strong desire from the patient to stop his habit) is the best predictor of successful quitting. However, even poorly motivated smokers can be helped and eventually led to quit [11].

The standardized mode of treatment in SC is through the '5 As' treatment (Table 4.1) [12]. Treatment involves the use of drugs. These include the various forms of nicotine replacement therapy (NRT), i.e. patches, gums, inhalers, lozenges as well as bupropion [13]. Overall, such treatments can double the success rate of unassisted attempts.

Some side-effects are common during SC. The most common are depressed mood and weight gain. Patients suffering from chronic respiratory disease are very often depressed, particularly COPD patients. Hence, SC, even if attained, can worsen the health status of these patients, and this can constitute a 'good' reason for the patient to re-commence smoking.

CASE REPORT

Mario R, manager of an international telecommunications company, is an Italian, 57 years of age, with a 'regular' lifestyle. For the last 20 years, his working life has been a largely sedentary one (seated at meetings, in his own office, in taxis or during his frequent flights). He has been a smoker for more than 30 years, having started smoking at age 17, when in high school, and with a current habit of smoking a mean of 15–20 cigarettes per day. When he was 47, he suffered a severe cold, during which he experienced for the first time in his life an unpleasant feeling of breathlessness. After recovering from the cold, he underwent clinical examinations and was diagnosed with COPD, stage 3. In fact, he had a spirometry (after testing with a β_2-agonist, which led to a partial but not complete reversion of the bronchial obstruction) that showed an $FEV_1 < 50\%$ and a ratio between FEV_1 and forced vital capacity under 70%. Notably, the first specialist who visited Mario was not a chest physician but a cardiologist, since the initial diagnosis was one of cardiac disease. Mario underwent SC treatment following the initial diagnosis of COPD. He was treated by his general practitioner with the 5 As treatment, and was administered NRT *via* a patch. He succeeded in quitting smoking almost immediately but, after 2 months, relapsed during a business trip to Denmark, when, while discussing a joint venture over supper in a restaurant where there were many people smoking, his counterpart offered him a cigarette.

In fact, after cessation, he experienced stress, depression and occasional difficulty in concentrating.

He was then referred to a smokers' clinic where, after a treatment with various forms of NRT administered in combination (patch + inhaler + bupropion-SR), he eventually succeeded in quitting smoking.

Currently, he is taking drugs for his disease, with a reasonable level of compliance, and uses anti-muscarinics delivered by a dry powder inhaler once a day, along with long-acting β_2-agonists (LABA) delivered by metered dose inhaler twice a day. He also uses short-acting β_2-agonists (SABA) when required.

Mario is currently taking no drugs for SC and he has been completely abstinent for the last 9 years. He feels no wish to smoke, even when in company with smokers, but, in the last few months, he has experienced breathlessness when in environments polluted with ETS. Initially, he thought that this was only as a result of the annoyance caused by the smell of smoke, but after some time and after experiencing real respiratory distress in such situations, he eventually understood that it was the effect of the smoke (or of something contained in it) that was causing the problem.

He asked his GP about this and was told that the problem probably lay in the particulate matter (PM) carried in the smoke. This PM comprises very small particles, invisible to the naked eye, containing many toxic and hazardous substances, some of which are carcinogenic and almost all of which can irritate the airways. In Mario's case, the airways, already inflamed and restricted, react with a bronchospasm when challenged by PM. This is fortunately treatable with SABA.

In these circumstances, one can understand Mario's great satisfaction when a smoking ban came into force in Italy at the beginning of 2005, prohibiting smoking almost everywhere except in private homes (or places with specially designed ventilation systems) and his even greater joy when he saw that the ban was almost completely complied with [14].

However, the GP has also warned Mario that PM is found not only in tobacco smoke, but also in traffic fumes or from other combustion sources in cities, so that the air breathed in some places can also cause irritation to the airways. Consequently, Mario is currently anxious at the thought of a business trip to Mexico City, where pollution levels are reported to be very high.

DISCUSSION

Can passive smoking cause COPD?
Yes: indeed, ETS composition is qualitatively similar to the smoke actively inhaled by the smoker and can have the same effects. Some studies have shown the effect of inhaled ETS on the lung function of adults. Among these, a review by Jaakkola [15] measured the impact of ETS on COPD and found that out of six studies (three case–control and three longitudinal), *all* showed an increased risk in high ETS exposure categories. In summary, the existing evidence points to an excess risk of 30% for lung cancer and of about 50% for COPD. One study even found that a poorly significant link between ETS and lung cancer was, on the contrary, quite indicative of a link between COPD and ETS. This study showed a relative risk of COPD of 1.80 for men and of 1.57 for women [16].

Is the '5 As' treatment the only evidence-based one for SC?
No: SC treatment can be delivered in a primary care setting as well in a specialized clinic setting. Among the primary care settings, the one most supported by evidence is the GP's office, but SC can also be delivered by nurses, dentists or pharmacists. All these primary care health professionals are entitled to deliver the so-called 5 As (see Table 4.1 and further) [10]. This kind of treatment is not time-consuming (it is also termed short or minimal intervention), but has a low success rate.

Table 4.2 Patient groups eligible for short intervention or treatment in the SC clinic

Level	Patients	Intervention	Staff
First	'Healthy' smokers with tobacco smoking as the only risk factor	Minimal (5 As)	Primary care
Second	Ill or priority (other risk factor) smokers	Intensive	SC clinics

Indeed, SC can be viewed from different perspectives, depending on the level of intervention. There is the *public health perspective*, whose focus is the advantage of the community. Its rationale is that, due to the high smoking prevalence, even if the intervention is not very effective, a great number of people will quit, with a great advantage to the community and a very high cost-effectiveness ratio: this is an example of a short intervention. Then there is the *clinical perspective*, whose focus is the advantage of the individual. From this perspective, the intervention must be very effective. A great quantity of resources (e.g. time, drugs) is concentrated at the same moment on the same person, since in SC, evidence shows that there is a strong dose–response relationship; i.e. the more resources used, the higher the sustained abstinence rate. The SC clinic is an example of this type of intervention: it guarantees a higher success rate but, of course, is more expensive. The cost-effectiveness ratio is still, however, in favour of intervention.

The SC clinic has a dedicated staff to assist a population of patients that is different from that eligible for short intervention (Table 4.2) [17]. It deals with very dependent smokers who are also very motivated to quit, as well as 'difficult' smokers (frequent relapsers, smokers poorly motivated to quit, psychiatric smokers, and so on).

In this setting, the 5 As are expanded to a complete process of diagnosis and treatment. The first step, in the specialized clinic, is aimed at *identifying* a smoker's complete smoking history (age of initiation, number of cigarettes smoked, activity of daily life usually associated with smoking, previous quitting attempts) together with an assessment of nicotine dependence (using the Fagerstrom Tolerance questionnaire) and of the degree of nicotine intake (through dosage of exhaled carbon monoxide). In the second step, the patient receives individualized *advice* to stop smoking, tailored to their habits. The third step (to *assess motivation*) is carried out in the clinic, not with the purpose of treating only motivated patients, but in order to decide how many resources need to be used to elicit motivation and manage that specific patient with an individualized intensive treatment programme. The fourth step (to *assist* the attempt to quite smoking) is the most specific activity of the clinic, and comprizes intensive behavioural assistance, together with updated and managed pharmacological treatment (with different forms of NRT and other drugs, e.g. bupropion). Finally, the fifth step (to *arrange* or organize the follow-up) is carried out very frequently; sometimes on demand or sometimes according to a schedule. The ex-smoker can be contacted by telephone or during a visit or consultation. The items recorded in this follow-up include all problems encountered in maintaining abstinence, including the presence of adverse effects from the cessation of smoking and/or the taking of drugs, as well as the advantages felt by the patient. The physician and nurses teach 'resistance skills' according to the patient's reports and relapses are discussed in depth.

Overall, it is important to keep the patient in touch with the clinic, as tobacco smoking is: *'a chronic disease, which moves through multiple periods of relapse and remission. Like hypertension or COPD, smoking requires ongoing care with counselling advice, support and pharmacotherapy. Relapse is common and simply reflects the chronic nature of the condition, not a failure of the physician or patient'* [10]. Keeping up this contact can be particularly easy if the patient – like

Mario – is already suffering from a chronic condition, since SC is part of the normal management of the disease.

If the patient is not motivated to stop smoking immediately, a 'progressive' approach can be adopted, aimed at reducing gradually the number of cigarettes smoked per day, using NRT as a substitute for nicotine not administered through cigarettes. This approach, which can be referred to as 'reduction-to-stop' consists in the use of pharmacotherapy (usually NRT) to obtain a reduction of at least 50% in the number of cigarettes smoked in the first 6 weeks, further reducing the number in the following weeks, until the patient has ceased smoking completely within 6–9 months [18].

If SC cannot be attained, even after multiple attempts, and after 'reduction-to-stop' has been tried, then a 'harm reduction' approach is advisable, which tries to reduce permanently the number of cigarettes smoked per day using pharmacological therapy (usually NRT). The basic principle is to give the body a certain dose of nicotine without smoking, while permitting a certain number of cigarettes per day [19].

Are the patient's dyspnoea episodes due to passive smoking?
Yes: currently, a cardiac origin has been ruled out. ETS presents health risks for respiratory and cardiovascular diseases [20]. ETS can contribute to air pollution, and has been shown to be responsible for indoor PM levels much higher than official threshold levels for outdoor pollution [21].

Can dyspnoea episodes be predicted after exposure to high levels of pollution?
Yes: air pollution due to PM is a risk factor for respiratory diseases (COPD, asthma and lung cancer) [22–24]. Moreover, each increase of $10\,\mu g/m^3$ in ambient PM levels carries with it a short-term health burden that leads to an increase in morbidity and mortality due to exacerbations or worsening of chronic diseases [25]. For this reason, official annual average PM limits have been set at $40\,\mu g/m^3$ for PM10 in Europe, and at $15\,\mu g/m^3$ for PM2.5 in the US. However, there are reasons to think that these levels are still too high and dangerous to human health [26].

As a matter of fact, PM production by cigarettes has been demonstrated to be much *higher* than the new low-emission cars: an experimental study compared PM production from ecodiesel exhaust and smouldering cigarettes and found the pollution from the latter much heavier [27].

Pollution levels in a given place can easily be estimated using real-time PM levels for most cities that are available on the Internet: this is precisely what Mario did in reference to Mexico City. It is also possible to quantify risk levels for a given pollution level, using the air quality index related to PM2.5 pollution (US-EPA), according to Table 4.3 [28].

How should Mario prepare for his business trip to Mexico City?
He should be advised to avoid staying outdoors for long periods, to avoid outdoor exercising, to avoid the most polluted hours of the day and to try to check the pollution levels on the Internet. A change in drug therapy may also be useful, adding an anti-inflammatory drug and a SABA in the case of respiratory distress.

SUMMARY

Discussing all these issues with the patient is mandatory to help them understand their disease better and manage it optimally. Such an educational effort can include the use of peak expiratory flow (PEF) monitoring to assess pulmonary function.

Table 4.3 Air quality index for particle pollution [28]

Air quality index	Air quality	Health advisory
0–50	Good	None
51–100	Moderate	Unusually sensitive people should consider reducing prolonged or heavy exertion
101–150	Unhealthy for sensitive groups	People with heart or lung disease, older adults, and children should reduce prolonged or heavy exertion
151–200	Unhealthy	People with heart or lung disease, older adults, and children should avoid prolonged or heavy exertion. Everyone else should reduce prolonged or heavy exertion
201–300	Very unhealthy	People with heart or lung disease, older adults, and children should avoid all physical activity outdoors. Everyone else should avoid prolonged or heavy exertion

With these recommendations, Mario's trip, and those of other patients in a similar situation, should cause no undue problems.

REFERENCES

1. American Thoracic Society. European Respiratory Society Standards of diagnosis and management of Patients with COPD Lausanne, 2004. www.ersnet.org.
2. Prevention and Control of Chronic Respiratory Diseases at Country Level – Towards a Global Alliance against Chronic Respiratory Diseases (GARD) based on the WHO Meeting on Prevention and Control of Chronic Respiratory Diseases Geneva, Switzerland, 17–19 June 2004 – WHO/NMH/CHP/CPM/CRA/05.1.
3. US Department of Health and Human Services. The health consequences of smoking: chronic obstructive lung disease. 2004 Revision: pp 463–507. www.cdc.gov/tobacco/sgr/sgr_2004/chapter4.
4. Becklake MR. Occupational exposures: evidence for a causal association with chronic obstructive pulmonary disease. *Am Rev Respir Dis* 1989; 140:S85–S91.
5. Viegi G, Enarson D. Human health effects of air pollution from mobile sources in Europe. *Int J Tuberc Lung Dis* 1998; 2:947–967.
6. Albalak R, Frisancho AR, Keeler GJ. Domestic biomass fuel combustion and chronic bronchitis in two rural Bolivian villages. *Thorax* 1999; 54:1004–1008.
7. Simoni M, Biavati P, Carrozzi L et al. The Po river Delta (North Italy) indoor epidemiological study: home characteristics, indoor pollutants, and subjects' daily activity pattern. *Indoor Air* 1998; 8:70–79.
8. Anthonisen NR, Skeans MA, Wise RA, Manfreda J, Kanner RE, Connett JE; Lung Health Study Research Group. The effects of a smoking cessation intervention on 14.5-year mortality: a randomized clinical trial. *Ann Intern Med* 2005; 142:233–239.
9. Murray RP, Anthonisen NR, Connett JE et al. Effects of multiple attempts to quit smoking and relapses to smoking on pulmonary function. Lung Health Study Research Group. *J Clin Epidemiol* 1998; 51:1317–1326.
10. Fiore MC, Bailey WC, Cohen SJ et al. Treating tobacco use and dependence. Clinical practice guidelines. US Department of Heath and Human services (2000). AHRQ Publication No. 00032.
11. Barbano G, Diamandi A, Nardini S. Long-term abstinence from smoking does not depend on the stage of change. *Eur Respir J* 2005; 26(suppl 49):245s.
12. Raw M, McNeill A, West R. Smoking cessation guidelines for health professionals. A guide to effective smoking cessation interventions for the health care system. *Thorax* 1998; 53(suppl 5):S1–S19.
13. US Department of Health and Human Services. Public health service treating tobacco use and dependence. Clinical practice guideline. AHRQ Publication No. 00-0032, June 2000.

14. Viegi G, Nardini S, Zuccaro PG. Smoking Ban in Italy: lights and shadows after one year. *ERS Bulletin* 2006; 5.
15. Jaakkola MS. Environmental tobacco smoke and health in the elderly. *Eur Respir J* 2002; 19:172–181.
16. Enstrom JE, Kabat GC. Environmental tobacco smoke and tobacco related mortality in a prospective study of Californians 1960–1998. *Br Med J* 2003; 326:1057–1067.
17. Nardini S. The smoking cessation clinic. *Monaldi Arch Chest Dis* 2000; 55:495–501.
18. Nardini S, Carozzi L, Invernizzi G. Smoking Reduction: a new smoking cessation strategy. *Multidiscip Respir Med* 2006; 1.
19. Ramström L, Uranga R, Hendrie A. Social and economic aspects of reduction of tobacco smoking by use of alternative nicotine delivery systems (ANDS). Summary report of a roundtable organized by the UN Focal Point on Tobacco and Health, Geneva, September 1997.
20. The IARC Monograph 83 on involuntary smoking. *IARC Monographs* 2004.
21. Repace JL, Lowrey AH. Indoor air pollution, tobacco smoke, and public health. *Science* 1980; 208:464–472.
22. Invernizzi G, Ruprecht A, Mazza R et al. Real-time measurement of indoor particulate matter originating from environmental tobacco smoke: a pilot study. *Epidemiol Prev* 2002; 26:30–34.
23. Kunzli N. The public health relevance of air pollution abatement. *Eur Respir J* 2002; 20:198–209.
24. Viegi G, Annesi I, Matteelli G. Epidemiology of asthma. *Eur Respir Mon* 2003; 8:1–25.
25. Pope CA III, Burnett RT, Thun MJ et al. Lung cancer, cardiopulmonary mortality, and long-term exposure to fine particulate air pollution *JAMA* 2002; 287:1132–1141.
26. Samet JM, Dominici F, Curriero FC, Coursac I, Zeger SL. Fine particulate air pollution and mortality in 20 U.S. cities, 1987–1994. *N Engl J Med* 2000; 343:1742–1749.
27. Johnson PR, Graham JJ. Fine particulate matter national ambient air quality standards: public health impact on populations in the northeastern United States. *Environ Health Perspect* 2005; 113:1140–1147.
28. Invernizzi G, Ruprecht A, Mazza R et al. Particulate matter from tobacco *versus* diesel car exhaust: an educational perspective. *Tob Control* 2004; 13:305–307.
29. http://airnow.gov/index.cfm?action=particle.airborne#6.

5

Improvement in exercise capacity after correcting calorie uptake in a patient with severe emphysema

A. Del Ponte, S. Marinari

BACKGROUND

The natural history of chronic obstructive pulmonary disease (COPD) patients is often characterized by a progressive deterioration in nutritional status caused by the development of protein calorie malnutrition with loss of muscular mass following as a result [1].

This wasting condition, which commonly leads to a poor prognosis, is not necessarily linked to body weight decrease. In fact, it is possible that a normal or even increased body weight could mask changes in lean body mass [2]. A number of investigators have focused their attention on the importance of better defining the actual amount of lean body mass with more accurate, reproducible and easy-to-perform measurement methods so that initial muscle depletion can be sensitively detected.

To date, numerous validated methods for the estimation of body composition are available, although only a few, such as bioelectrical impedance analysis (BIA), satisfy the requisites of being precise, accurate, reliable, inexpensive and easy-to-use by clinicians. BIA utilizes numerous indices: fat mass (FM; normal value = 22–31%), fat-free mass (FFM; normal value = 69–78%) or more specifically, body cellular mass (BCM; normal value = 40–49%) and phase angle (PA; normal value = 6–8°) and has given us a useful tool for the accurate diagnosis and prognosis of COPD [3].

Three major pathogenetic mechanisms are widely acknowledged to be involved in the lean body mass deterioration of COPD patients:

1. Inadequate energy intake
2. Increase of energy expenditure
3. Alteration of protein synthesis and turnover.

The altered balance between calorie intake and increased energy expenditure seems to be caused particularly by dyspnoea, which produces a consequent reduction of food intake. Respiratory efforts are particularly disabling when eating, because of limited diaphragm movements, resulting in an 'anorexia-like' condition associated with a depressive state [4].

Adriana Del Ponte, MD, Department of Internal Medicine and Aging, Chieti Hospital, Chieti, Italy
Stefano Marinari, MD, Department of Pneumology, San Camillo De Lellis Hospital, Chieti, Italy

© Atlas Medical Publishing Ltd 2007

Moreover, recent studies have highlighted the involvement of the central nervous system in the regulation of appetite influenced by systemic inflammatory mediators. In COPD patients with recurrent acute exacerbations, low levels of circulating leptine are related to body mass index (BMI; normal BMI defined as 18.5–25 kg/m^2) and tumour necrosis factor (TNF). This hormone, released by adipocytes with a feedback mechanism that involves the hypothalamus, is also involved in the regulation of energy balance. C-reactive protein and TNF receptor families are known to affect both energy expenditure and FFM [5, 6]. A few studies reported an increase of 25% in the resting energy expenditure, after body weight was adjusted for BCM [7]. The increased energy expenditure noted in COPD patients, whose mechanisms are not yet fully understood, could make the calorie intake/energy expenditure ratio even worse.

Finally, numerous studies observing the alteration of protein synthesis and turnover have provided a remarkable contribution towards the determination of the origin of muscular mass depletion. The muscle atrophy seen in muscular biopsies taken from these patients could be caused by increased proteolysis and activated enzymes of degradation, with mechanisms that have not yet been clarified [8, 9]. In addition, inflammatory processes seem to play a specific role in the anabolic–hypermetabolic mechanism of muscular cells [10, 11]. Another potential mechanism that may trigger muscle apoptosis is an increased oxidative load determined by free radicals deriving from structurally and biochemically altered peripheral muscles. It is also possible to postulate the role of protracted systemic steroid therapy (self-treatment by patients and not recommended by clinicians), in determining myopathy and muscle fibre atrophy [12].

This nutritional pattern and its consequence of severe malnutrition may, in the long term, result in a substantial reduction in exercise-induced capacity that is generally related to FFM amount and size [13]. In fact, significant relationships have been found between FFM and the distance walked during a 12 min walking test (WT) [14]. Moreover, in COPD patients, both body weight and muscle mass are related to VO_2 peak and the anaerobic threshold [15, 16]. The hypothesized pathogenetic mechanisms seem to involve altered O_2 utilization and oxidative processes that enhance anaerobic metabolism and increase in lactic acid production [17]. It is possible that COPD patients who show reduced lean body mass, such as non-exerted individuals, may present with a serious alteration of the mechanisms involved in the muscular production of energy. This condition is frequently noted in COPD patients who become progressively disabled and unable to satisfy their necessary metabolic requirements.

CASE REPORT

A 66-year-old man (body weight = 62 kg; height = 1.67 m) was admitted to hospital because of severe dyspnoea at a minimal level of effort. In the last few months, his breathing had become more uncomfortable and the patient progressively perceived a marked reduction in exercise tolerance and an increase in muscle weakness. He had a long history of smoking (>20 cigarettes/day) up until 8 years ago.

COPD had been diagnosed 15 years before the admission. At first, breathlessness occurred only with heavy exercise, but in the last few years he had complained of progressive dyspnoea, even with moderate activity. Frequently, breathlessness was associated with a chronic cough, productive of variable amounts of sputum, chest tightness and wheezing over a period of hours to days. This respiratory discomfort had often resulted in poor tolerance to physical exercise.

Furthermore, due to the occurrence of frequent acute episodes of respiratory tract infections in which cough, sputum production and breathlessness were augmented, he had been admitted to hospital on several occasions. During these admissions he had received i.v. antibiotic and i.v. or oral steroid therapy for long periods.

Over the last 6 months, he had noticed an apparent body weight decrease of approximately 5 kg because of the reduced calorie intake resulting from decreased appetite and shortness of breath at meal times.

The patient's medication at the time of admission consisted of inhaled steroids (budesonide), LABA (formoterol) and SABA (salbutamol), used irregularly to relieve symptoms. In the last 3 years the steroid therapy had been the cause of slight fasting hyperglycaemia, yet glycated haemoglobin (HbA1C; normal value <6.1%), which is expressive of metabolic control, had never been over 6.3%.

The patient also had a 4-year history of hypertension, successfully treated with amlodipine. Additional problems included prostatic hypertrophy and frequent constipation. The results of some laboratory tests performed just before admission showed: normal liver and kidney function; complete blood cell count; erythrocyte sedimentation rate (ESR); slight increase of fibrinogen. At that time, urine analysis was negative and HbA1C was not significantly changed (6.2%).

Recent chest radiography showed evidence only of thoracic hyperinflation (e.g. flattening of the diaphragm, tenting of the diaphragm at the rib insertions and increased volume of the retrosternal airspace). An electrocardiogram showed tachycardia (105 bpm), non-specific ST–T wave changes and right axis deviation. At the general physical examination, the patient had a normal body-weight appearance. Shortness of breath was manifested by pursed-lip breathing and the use of accessory muscles for respiration. Blood pressure was normal. The patient was sitting forward; he was diaphoretic and perhaps unable to speak because of severe dyspnoea. Important signs were also paradoxical abdominal and diaphragmatic movements on inspiration, rales and wheezing, but there were no apparent signs of peripheral oedema.

Because of the critical condition of the patient, it was necessary to submit him to an accurate nutritional examination in order to ascertain the presence of signs of malnutrition, i.e. lean body mass loss, if any.

BASIC DIAGNOSTIC ASSESSMENT

All normal diagnostic procedures were performed, including routine haematology and a complete physical examination of the patient. A detailed nutritional history was taken in order to better define the calorie requirements of the patient. After obtaining diaries of the patient's daily calorie intake and calculating his BMI, this was found to be within normal limits at 22 kg/m^2; the measurement of body composition was performed using BIA. The following BIA parameters were obtained: FM = 18.3 kg (32.2%); FFM = 38.7 kg (67.8%); BCM = 17.1 kg (34.7%); PA = 4.0°. The patient was submitted to complete spirometry (pulmonary function tests [PFT]), body plethysmography, DLCO diffusion capacity, and arterial blood gas (ABG) analysis. Resting complete lung function test values showed severe pulmonary obstruction (FEV_1 = 32% of predicted value; FEV_1/FVC = 44%) with severe hyperinflation (TLC = 105% of predicted value; RV = 187% of predicted value) and severe reduction of respiratory muscles strength (MIP = 41 cmH_2O, MEP = 45 cmH_2O). The DLCO value was decreased with slight reduction of DLCO/VA (DLCO = 10.6 ml/min/mmHg; DLCO/VA = 3.62; 71% of predicted value).

ABGs measured at rest breathing room air showed no abnormalities (PaO_2 = 72.4 mmHg; $PaCO_2$ = 43.3 mmHg; O_2 Sat = 95.6%; PA = 7.412°). Sputum was purulent with bacterial respiratory tract infections (Enterobacteria – *Klebsiella*). Exercise tolerance tests were also performed: a 6-minute walking test (6MWT) showed not only a marked decrease in oxygen saturation at the end of the exercise (from 95 to 89%), but also a reduction in the distance walked (210 m). Dyspnoea, evaluated with the Medical Research Council (MRC) scale, was significantly different pre- and post-testing (0 at rest and 3 at 6 min).

Aerobic capacity was also evaluated during a submaximal effort test using an incremental cyclo-ergometer. The test showed a severe reduction of VO_2 peak (15.1 ml/kg/min) and anaerobic threshold (AT = 6.7 ml/kg/min), showing that malnutrition may influence both the aerobic and exercise capacities. An increase of *ventilatory* failure, expressed by the VD/VT ratio (0.29) was also demonstrated.

DIFFERENTIAL DIAGNOSIS

This patient had a fourth acute episode of exacerbation of COPD in the last year, but this was the first time that he had come under our observation. At admission he complained of the progressive and rapid evolution of the pulmonary disease. His opinion was that this severe condition might be secondary both to incorrect therapy, taken irregularly, and to involuntary body weight loss.

Moreover, in the last few years, he had complained of progressive muscle weakness and reduced exercise tolerance, yet physicians had not taken this problem into consideration. Mild diabetes could also have explained the body weight loss and muscle weakness experienced by the patient. It is well-known that peripheral neuropathy, manifested by muscular pain, may be one of the common complications of poorly controlled type 2 diabetes mellitus. Furthermore, the finding of glucose in the urine sample might also have explained both the weight loss and muscle weakness. At the time of our observation, however, the glycated haemoglobin value was not significantly augmented, indicating good glycaemic control and the urine analysis was negative. Therefore, the actual cause of body weight loss seemed to be not related to worsening diabetes mellitus.

Remarkably, the patient had never previously had his body composition evaluated, so the early detection of a lean body mass decrease had not been possible. Therefore, the muscle mass loss observed at the hospital might be one of the primary causes of the frequent episodes of exacerbation of his COPD.

TREATMENT

On the basis of diagnostic tests and the clinical profile, the treatment consisted principally of three different interventions:

1. *Pharmacological intervention* to reduce the airway infection and inflammation, including initially antibiotics and systemic steroids, and successively LABA (formoterol), inhaled steroids (budesonide) and tiotropium bromide, all correctly taken under strict medical control.
2. *Correction of the daily calorie intake* with a proper dietary regimen of 1600 kcal (carbohydrate 55%; protein 15–20%; fat 30–35%). Small and frequent meals were recommended to avoid over ingestion of food, which might cause abdominal pain, fatigue, and limit the degree of diaphragmatic movement.
3. *Adequate physical exercise* (endurance training programme 3 times/week).

The patient was evaluated after 6 months of therapy and a significant improvement of symptoms with a sense of general well-being and better health status was reported. In addition, body weight had increased by 2 kg and exercise capacity had improved, as documented by increases of VO_2 peak (18 ml/mg/min) and anaerobic threshold (9 ml/kg/min).

BIA showed a slight restoration of BCM (18.2 kg) and PA (4.7°). Six-minute walk test (6MWT) showed an increase in the distance walked (324 m) and a smaller decrease in oxygen saturation at the end of the exercise test (from 96 to 92%). The corresponding data are reported in Table 5.1. PFTs showed no significant changes.

SUMMARY

This case report clearly describes the difficulties encountered in the routine management of COPD patients, in whom progressively rapid respiratory decline is often observed,

Table 5.1 Effects of the 6-month programme of adequate correction of daily calorie intake and physical exercise (endurance training) on some principal anthropometric, body composition and physical performance parameters observed in a 66-year-old COPD male patient

	BMI	BCM (kg)	PA (°)	VO_2 max (ml/mg/min)	AT (ml/kg/min)	6MWT (m)	SaO_2 pre-6MWT (%)	SaO_2 post-6MWT (%)
Baseline	22	17.1	4.0	15.1	6.7	210	95	89
After treatment	23	18.2	4.7	18.0	9.0	324	96	92

AT = anaerobic threshold; BCM = body cellular mass (normal value = 40–49%); BMI = body mass index (normal = 18.5–25 kg/m^2); PA = phase angle (normal value = 6–8°); SaO_2 = % arterial oxygen saturation measured by pulse oximetry; VO_2 max = the maximum amount of oxygen that can be removed from circulating blood; 6MWT = 6-minute walk test.

especially if involuntary and even slight body weight loss occurs. Therefore, the assessment of BMI (kg/m^2), which is the easiest measure of nutritional screening and in particular the evaluation of body composition are necessary to follow the natural course of the disease and, possibly, prevent future complications. This measurement is obtained using a validated, simple and inexpensive method, namely BIA. The estimate of lean body mass, expressed by FFM, BCM and PA, provides more information than the BMI on the prognosis of the obstructive pulmonary disease. In fact, FFM was found to be an independent predictor of survival in a large group of clinically stable COPD patients admitted to a rehabilitation program [18] and is directly related to mortality [19].

Assessment of body composition may also help to better understand peripheral and respiratory muscle weakness, reduced exercise capacity and decreased sense of well-being perceived by the patient, as in this case.

In addition to these symptoms, the lean body mass depletion observed in this patient could have caused the recurrent inflammatory processes (COPD exacerbations) that had occurred in the last few years and that had resulted in several hospitalizations.

In the course of our observations, and later on, the patient experienced a significant restoration not only of respiratory and peripheral muscle function but also of exercise capacity. Moreover, he perceived an overall improvement in health status after appropriate pharmacological therapy, nutritional intervention (which in this case consisted of adaptations of the patient's adequate daily calorie intake), and a rehabilitation programme. In fact, the patient participated in an exercise programme of endurance training that resulted in a greater restoration of lean body mass (increased BCM and PA) than fat storage.

For these reasons, in COPD, the prevention of lean body mass loss should be addressed as soon as possible, even in the presence of normal BMI, to avoid the deleterious consequences of a chronic and disabling disease. In the view of the authors, early evaluation of body composition should be considered routine practice in the examination of COPD patients.

REFERENCES

1. De Benedetto F, Del Ponte A, Marinari S et al. In COPD patients body weight excess can mask lean tissue depletion: a simple method of estimation. *Mon Arch Chest Dis* 2000; 55:273–278.
2. De Benedetto F, Bitti G, D'Intino D et al. Body weight alone is not an index of nutritional imbalance in the natural course of COPD. *Monaldi Arch Chest Dis* 1993; 5:541–542.

3. Rodriguez-Roisin R, MacNee W. Pathophysiology of chronic obstructive pulmonary disease. *Eur Respir Monogr* 1998; 3:107–126.
4. Gray-Donald K, Carrey MA, Larsh HW. The nutritional status of patients with chronic obstructive pulmonary disease. *Clin Invest Med* 1998; 21:135–141.
5. Li YP, Schwartz RJ, Waddell ID *et al*. Skeletal muscle myocytes undergo protein loss and reactive oxygen-mediated NF-kappaB activation in response to tumor necrosis factor alpha. *FASEB J* 1998; 12:871–880.
6. Pouw EM, Schols AM, Deutz NE *et al*. Plasma and muscle amino acid levels in relation to resting energy expenditure and inflammation in stable chronic obstructive pulmonary disease. *Am Respir Crit Care Med* 1998; 158:797–801.
7. Goldstein S, Askanazi J, Weissman C *et al*. Energy expenditure in patients with chronic obstructive pulmonary disease. *Chest* 1987; 2:91.
8. Mitch WE, Goldberg AL. Mechanism of muscle wasting. The role of ubiquitin-proteasome pathway. *N Engl J Med* 1996; 335:1897–1905.
9. Jagoe RT, Goldberg AL. What do we really know about ubiqitin-proteasome pathway in muscle atrophy? *Curr Opin Clin Nutr Metab Care* 2001; 4:183–190.
10. Guttridge DC, Mayo MW, Madrid LW *et al*. NF-kappaB-induced loss of MyoD messenger RNA: possible role in muscle decay and cachexia. *Science* 2000; 289:2363–2366.
11. Langen RC, Schols AM, Kelders MC *et al*. Inflammatory citokines inhibit myogenic differentiation through activation of nuclear factor-kappaB. *FASEB J* 2001; 15:1169–1180.
12. Van Balkom RH, Van Der Heijden HF, Van Herwaarden CL, Dekhuijzen PN. Corticosteroid induced myopathy of the respiratory muscles. *Neth J Med* 1994; 45:114–122.
13. Toth MJ, Goran MI, Ades PA *et al*. Examination of data normalization procedures for expressing peak VO_2 data. *J Appl Physiol* 1993; 75:2288–2292.
14. Schols AM, Mostert R, Soeters PB *et al*. Body composition and exercise performance in patients with chronic obstructive pulmonary disease. *Thorax* 1991; 46:695–699.
15. Palange P, Forte S, Felli A *et al*. Nutritional state and exercise tolerance in patients with COPD. *Chest* 1995; 107:1206–1212.
16. Baarends E, Schols AMWJ, Mostert R *et al*. Peak exercise response in relation to tissue depletion in patients with chronic obstructive pulmonary disease. *Eur Respir J* 1997; 10:2807–2813.
17. Maltais F, Simard A, Simard C *et al*. Oxidative capacity of the skeletal muscle and lactic acid kinetics during exercise in normal subjects and in patients with COPD. *Am J Respir Crit Care Med* 1996; 153:288–293.
18. Schols AM, Broekhuizen R, Weling-Scheepers CA *et al*. Body composition and mortality in chronic obstructive pulmonary disease. *Am J Clin Nutr* 2005; 82:53–59.
19. Vestbo J, Prescott E, Almdal T *et al*. Body mass, fat-free body mass, and prognosis in patients with chronic obstructive pulmonary disease from a random population sample. *Am J Respir Crit Care Med* 2006; 173:79–83.

6

A 36-year-old patient with stage I – GOLD misdiagnosed as asthma

I. Cerveri, R. Nimiano, J. Vestbo

BACKGROUND

Despite clear and updated guidelines for asthma [1] and chronic obstructive pulmonary disease (COPD) [2, 3], the differential diagnosis can sometimes be difficult. In order to properly identify and reduce risk factors and initiate appropriate management, it is particularly important to distinguish COPD from asthma at an early stage of the disease [4–8]. In a recent review entitled *'Is it asthma or COPD? The answer determines proper therapy for chronic airflow obstruction'* the authors outline an approach to differential diagnosis that should result in better evaluation, therapy, and quality of life in these patients [9]. Asthma and COPD have important similarities and differences [10]. Both are chronic inflammatory diseases that involve the small airways and cause airflow limitation, both result from gene–environment interactions, and both are usually characterized by mucus and some degree of bronchoconstriction. However, the two diseases also have striking differences. Different anatomical sites are involved: COPD affects both the airways and the parenchyma, whereas asthma affects only the airways. Both diseases involve the small airways responsible for much of the physiological impairment. The most important difference is probably the nature of inflammation: it is primarily eosinophilic and CD4-driven in asthma and neutrophilic and CD8-driven in COPD. It is mainly this difference that affects the response to pharmacological agents and particularly to steroids [11]. Moreover, particularly in the elderly, diagnosis can be especially problematic as the two diseases sometimes coexist. Indeed, individuals with asthma who smoke or are exposed to other noxious agents that can cause COPD may be more prone to develop COPD in addition to pre-existing asthma [2, 12].

CASE REPORT

MC is a 36-year-old woman with a diagnosis of asthma since childhood. In April 2005, the family doctor referred her to our hospital because of chronic cough and episodic wheeze. She was born in Naples and has been living in Milan since age 6; she comes from a family of low socio-economic status (SES) and had completed her full time education at age 14. Thereafter, she was employed as a cleaner, first in a private home and then in a school. Since

---

Isa Cerveri, MD, Consultant Pulmonologist, Department of Respiratory Diseases, IRCCS Policlinico San Matteo, University of Pavia, Pavia, Italy

Rosanna Nimiano, MD, Consultant Pneumologist, Department of Respiratory Diseases, Fondazione IRCSS Policlinico S. Matteo, Universita de Pavia, Pavia, Italy

Jørgen Vestbo, MD, PhD, Professor of Respiratory Medicine, University of Manchester, North West Lung Centre, Wythenshawe Hospital, Manchester, UK

© Atlas Medical Publishing Ltd 2007

age 18 she smoked approximately one pack of cigarettes per day up until about 5 years ago; since then she has continually tried to cut down smoking to half a pack per day – on many days she now smokes less than 10 cigarettes per day – and she is currently trying to stop smoking. She is very worried about weight gain as a result of smoking cessation and reports that she has already gained 3 kg simply due to smoking reduction. She has no family history of asthma; both her mother and father were heavy smokers. Her mother died of cancer at age 65 and her father of emphysema and chronic respiratory failure at age 63. Her elder sister, a non-smoking housewife, and her own husband, a light smoker, have never suffered from respiratory symptoms.

Her early past medical history was negative. When she moved from Naples to Milan she developed 'winter bronchitis' and frequent post-infective episodes of insidious cough and wheeze, which resulted in significant periods of absence from school. The patient reported that she was hospitalized for dyspnoea and wheeze and was diagnosed as having asthma at age 8. Subsequently, she was hospitalized for 'pneumonia' at age 11. During and after puberty, symptoms – particularly wheezing – improved, even though she still complained on most mornings of cough after drinking coffee and smoking the first cigarette of the day. During winter, she also suffered from frequent episodes of nasal obstruction with nasal discharge and sinus pain. She ignored these symptoms for many years but tried to reduce smoking. Last winter she suffered from an exacerbation of chronic cough and phlegm with severe wheeze, fever and dyspnoea. On that occasion, she received antibiotics, inhaled steroids and long acting β_2-agonists; after 3 weeks she complained that the inhaled steroids were ineffective and stopped therapy, taking only β_2-agonists when needed. She did not visit her family doctor until April 2005 when they both agreed on the need for a specialist visit. At the hospital evaluation, she reported persistent cough and phlegm in the morning, occasionally accompanied by wheezing related to the cigarettes smoked the previous evening. Moreover, she reported that she was not limited in her activities of daily living but partially limited in her professional activities. She did not practise any sport or engage in any moderate or heavy physical exercise.

On physical examination, the patient was moderately obese, with normal blood pressure. Breath and heart sounds were normal and she had no elevated JVP or oedema.

After the clinical examination she underwent lung function testing, methacholine challenge test, skin-prick tests, routine laboratory tests with total and specific immunoglobulin (Ig)E and blood and induced sputum counts of eosinophils. The α_1-antitrypsin level was also measured.

The patient's pulmonary function tests, including lung volume measurements, diffusion test and methacholine test, are summarized in Table 6.1. Baseline FEV_1 was in the normal range (2.44 l, 81% of predicted) while there was an increased residual volume due to mild hyperinflation (2.04 l, 125%); DLCO was in the normal range. After salbutamol, FEV_1 (70 ml, 3%) and FVC (150 ml, 4%) did not change significantly, while residual volume (RV) decreased slightly (210 ml, −10%). The post-bronchodilator FEV_1/FVC was 65%. These tests revealed mild airflow obstruction with no significant response to an inhaled β_2-agonist bronchodilator. The methacholine challenge test, carried out the following day, showed the presence of mild BHR (PD_{20} FEV_1 = 800 µg).

She had a negative skin-prick test for a standard aeroallergen panel, undetectable specific IgE for a panel of the most common inhalant allergens, and total IgE in the normal range. Complete blood counts and induced sputum cell counts did not demonstrate any increase in eosinophils. The α_1-antitrypsin level was within the normal range.

At this point the differential diagnoses were intrinsic mild persistent asthma, COPD stage I, and bronchiectases. High-resolution computed tomography (HRCT) scan excluded the presence of emphysema or bronchiectases. Thus, she was treated for 3 weeks with low doses of inhaled corticosteroids and β_2-agonists as needed to assess the reversibility of obstruction after long-term anti-inflammatory therapy.

Table 6.1 Pulmonary function tests at the initial assessment

	Pre-bronchodilator		Post-bronchodilator	
	Absolute value	Percentage of predicted	Absolute value	Change percent of baseline
FVC, l	3.70	106	3.85	4
FEV_1, l	2.44	81	2.51	3
FEV_1/FVC, %	66	–	65	–
RV, l	2.04	125	1.83	−10
TLC, l	5.74	113	5.68	−1
DLCO, mmol/(kPa/s)	8.80	98	–	–
PD_{20} FEV_1, µg	800	–	–	–

At the re-evaluation, no significant improvement in the respiratory symptoms was reported and no change in lung volumes or pre- and post-bronchodilator flow-volume curve was observed. The evaluation of all clinical and functional data, along with the negative response of more chronic therapy with β_2-agonists and inhaled steroids led to the diagnosis of COPD. According to the spirometric values, the disease was classified as mild. The patient was extensively informed about her disease, its natural history, and the important role of risk factors. She was invited to participate in a smoking cessation programme, advised to prevent exposure to dust by wearing a face mask while working, and instructed about how to treat occasional wheeze and prevent exacerbations.

DISCUSSION

This young woman with a history and findings of respiratory symptoms led us to consider a diagnosis of either persistent asthma or mild COPD. Several of the features of both history and findings led to a final diagnosis of mild COPD but obviously – as in most aspects of medicine – the choice of tests and their interpretation can be questioned.

In the differentiation, the combined pattern of previous and current risk factors, symptoms, and findings from lung function tests and other laboratory tests is used, and these points are discussed separately below.

RISK FACTORS

'Risk factor' is a term clinicians have taken over from epidemiology. Traditionally, a risk factor is an aspect of personal behaviour or lifestyle, an environmental exposure, or an inborn or inherited characteristic which, on the basis of epidemiological evidence, is known to be associated with a health-related condition considered important to prevent. However, in daily terminology a risk factor is often referred to as an attribute or an exposure that increases the likelihood of disease – in our patient asthma or COPD. Asthma and COPD can to some extent be distinguished in terms of the major risk factors associated with each condition. Nevertheless, some important putative risk factors are common to both diseases; e.g. smoking, air pollution, some occupational exposures, and adenovirus infections. Young age, a family history of asthma, and presence of atopy may help in pointing to a diagnosis of asthma, whereas increasing age, cigarette smoking, and exposure to occupational hazards may point to a diagnosis of COPD. Women are more likely than men to be diagnosed with asthma, given a history of breathlessness and cough [13]; the traditionally low incidence of smoking in females could explain the bias against diagnosing COPD in this group. However, there are epidemiological studies suggesting that women are more susceptible to smoking than men regarding risk of COPD [14] and we are indeed seeing a change in gender distribution in COPD in the current period.

For genetic factors, there is a strong association between α_1-antitrypsin deficiency and the development of emphysema and thus COPD. This genetic disorder serves as the model for emphysema, but it is important to underline that patients with α_1-antitrypsin deficiency may have only slightly reduced lung function and can present with mucus hypersecretion and wheeze, mimicking bronchial asthma [8]. As in COPD, allergic asthma may also be inherited, although the lack of precise asthma phenotypes has so far resulted in significant obstacles to genetic studies.

Our patient came from a background of low SES. Low SES is generally regarded as a strong risk factor for COPD [15], although not necessarily for asthma although a low SES often will increase risk of both under-diagnosis and under-treatment of asthma. It is not quite clear which component of a low SES leads to the increased risk for COPD but recurrent lower respiratory tract infections and poor nutrition have been suggested as playing an important role.

SYMPTOMS

Despite differences in the underlying pathophysiology of COPD and asthma, several distinctive symptoms are shared between the two diseases – making differential diagnosis more difficult for the clinician.

The hallmark symptom of COPD is shortness of breath on exertion. Both the progressive airflow limitation and the static as well as dynamic hyperinflation lead to breathlessness when exercising, and eventually at rest. In addition, many COPD patients suffer from chronic cough, often with sputum production, both attributed to chronic bronchitis. Repeated and increasingly frequent exacerbations in COPD are associated with increased inflammation and deterioration of lung function and health status.

Asthma patients often present with wheeze, shortness of breath, chest tightness, and cough. Asthma patients more often than COPD patients will have nocturnal symptoms. The underlying inflammation is associated with exacerbations.

As both conditions have several major symptoms in common, symptoms alone are not sufficient to make a differential diagnosis. Variability of symptoms, including frequent night awakenings, or a history of wheezing is more indicative of asthma and chronic sputum production is more suggestive of COPD; however, even experienced clinicians will often refer to pattern recognition, clinical judgement and similar terms when describing how they deduce a diagnosis from symptoms description. Coexistent conditions, such as respiratory infections or mild bronchiectases, can further complicate diagnosis.

Lung function tests

In COPD, a post-bronchodilator $FEV_1/FVC < 70\%$ confirms the presence of COPD [2, 3]. Until recently, the presence or absence of reversibility of the airway obstruction was thought to be the major distinction between asthma and COPD with reversible airflow obstruction being the hallmark of asthma and lack of reversibility being the hallmark of COPD. Over the past few years, this concept has changed appreciably [10]. It can now be stated that the bronchodilator responses in asthma and COPD differ both quantitatively and in their spirometric patterns. Patients with asthma more frequently improve their FEV_1 by >200 ml and show an increase in FEV_1 alone or both in FVC and FEV_1, whereas patients with COPD, particularly when severe, show most commonly an increase only in FVC [16, 17]. Bronchodilator responsiveness in COPD patients is a continuous variable, and classifying patients as responders or non-responders can be misleading [18]. The test of acute bronchodilator response has limited diagnostic value in separating asthma and COPD, limited value for assessing choice of treatment, and no prognostic value [19].

BHR has long been recognized as a hallmark of chronic asthma. Less is known about the prevalence and mechanisms of hyperreactivity in COPD. Certainly, BHR is different in the two diseases: it is a more inherent feature in asthma than in COPD, although not occurring in all asthmatic subjects. At the same airway calibre, asthmatic patients generally have a higher BHR and they are more reactive to the indirect stimuli (AMP, eucapnic hyperventilation, hypertonic saline etc.) than COPD patients. However, BHR is probably not merely a reflection of chronically reduced airway calibre in COPD where it, at least in some patients, may also represent a pathophysiological abnormality that contributes to the phenotype [20, 21]. In epidemiology, BHR is a significant determinant of prognosis in COPD but the clinical implication of these findings is not fully clear [22].

Laboratory tests
High total and specific serum levels of IgE as well as an increased serum and sputum number of eosinophils may contribute in the differential diagnosis between asthma and COPD. However, any treatment with corticosteroids will blunt the eosinophils in asthma, and COPD patients may have eosinophilia during exacerbations either as a reaction to an infectious micro-organism or as yet another abnormal inflammatory reaction. The new non-invasive markers, such as exhaled nitric oxide, may also assist but they do not yet appear ready for routine clinical practice [23]. Similarly, a recent paper has stated that current routine analysis procedures to assess endobronchial biopsy specimens are not sufficiently discriminatory, although specific histopathological features of asthma and COPD probably exist [24].

SUMMARY

Our young woman with shortness of breath, productive cough, wheeze and airflow limitation will continue to provide a challenge. Her prognosis is highly dependent on her making a change in lifestyle, as smoking cessation at this stage is crucial. She will require continued follow-up to ensure that her lung function does not deteriorate further and that her symptoms are well controlled. Given her previous lack of success in stopping smoking it must realistically be anticipated that she may progress in her COPD; in this case she will need advice on vaccination, exercise/rehabilitation and proper medication.

In parallel with this case report, a large number of other young women and men will present to their family doctors with similar stories and symptoms, challenging them for a correct diagnosis.

REFERENCES

1. Global Initiative for Asthma. Global strategy for asthma management and prevention: NHLBI/WHO workshop report. Updated 2004. National Heart, Lung, and Blood Institute, Bethesda, MD, 2004.
2. Global Initiative for Chronic Obstructive Lung Disease. Global Strategy for the Diagnosis, Management and Prevention of Chronic Obstructive Pulmonary Disease. NHLBI/WHO workshop report. National Heart, Lung and Blood Institute, Bethesda, April 2001, Update of the Management Sections, GOLD website (www.goldcopd.com). Updated 2004.
3. American Thoracic Society (New York, USA) and European Respiratory Society (Lausanne, Switzerland). Standards for Diagnosis and Management of patients with COPD. American Thoracic Society (ATS) and European Respiratory Society (ERS). 2004. http://www.thoracic.org/copd/pdf/copddoc.pdf.
4. Guerra S. Overlap of asthma and chronic obstructive pulmonary disease. *Curr Opin Pulm Med* 2005; 11:7–13.
5. Cerveri I, Accordini S, Corsico A et al. Chronic cough and phlegm in young adults. *Eur Respir J* 2003; 22:413–417.
6. De Marco R, Accordini S, Cerveri I et al. An international survey of chronic obstructive pulmonary disease in young adults according to GOLD stages. *Thorax* 2004; 59:120–125.

7. Vestbo J. COPD in the ECRHS. *Thorax* 2004; 59:89–90.
8. Petty TL. COPD: Clinical phenotypes. *Pulm Pharmacol Ther* 2002; 15:341–351.
9. Martinez FJ, Standiford C, Gay SE. Is it asthma or COPD? The answer determines proper therapy for chronic airflow obstruction. *Postgrad Med* 2005; 117:19–26.
10. Buist AS. Similarities and differences between asthma and chronic obstructive pulmonary disease: treatment and early outcomes. *Eur Respir J* 2003; 21:30s–35s.
11. Decramer M, Selroos O. Asthma and COPD: differences and similarities. With special reference to the usefulness of budesonide/formoterol in a single inhaler (Symbicort®) in both diseases. *Int J Clin Pract* 2005; 59:385–398.
12. Lange P, Parner J, Vestbo J, Jensen G, Schnohr P. A 15-year follow-up of ventilatory function in adults with asthma. *N Engl J Med* 1998; 339:1194–1200.
13. Chapman K, Tashkin D, Pye D. Gender bias in the diagnosis of COPD. *Chest* 2001; 119:1691–1695.
14. Prescott E, Bjerg AM, Andersen PK, Lange P, Vestbo J. Gender differences in smoking effects on lung function and risk of hospitalization for COPD: results from a Danish longitudinal population study. *Eur Respir J* 1997; 10:822–827.
15. Prescott E, Vestbo J. Socioeconomic status and chronic obstructive pulmonary disease. *Thorax* 1999; 54:737–741.
16. Donohue JF. Therapeutic responses in asthma and COPD. Bronchodilators. *Chest* 2004; 126:125s–137s.
17. Cerveri I, Pellegrino R, Dore R et al. Mechanisms for isolated volume response to a bronchodilator in patients with COPD. *J Appl Physiol* 2000; 88:1989–1995.
18. Calverley PMA, Burge PS, Spencer S et al. Bronchodilator reversibility testing in chronic obstructive pulmonary disease. *Thorax* 2003; 58:659–664.
19. Chhabra SK. Acute bronchodilator response has limited value in differentiating bronchial asthma from COPD. *J Asthma* 2005; 42:367–372.
20. Grootendorst DC, Rabe KF. Mechanisms of bronchial hyperreactivity in asthma and chronic obstructive pulmonary disease. *Proc Am Thorac Soc* 2004; 1:77–87.
21. Hansen EF, Vestbo J. Bronchodilator reversibility in COPD: the roguish but harmless little brother of airway hyperresponsiveness? *Eur Respir J* 2005; 26:6–7.
22. Vestbo J, Hansen EF. Airway hyper-responsiveness and COPD mortality. *Thorax* 2001; 56:s11–s14.
23. Kharitonov SA. Exhaled markers of inflammatory lung diseases: ready for routine monitoring? *Swiss Med Wkly* 2004; 134:175–192.
24. Bourdin A, Serre I, Flamme H et al. Can endobronchial biopsy analysis be recommended to discriminate between asthma and COPD in routine practice? *Thorax* 2004; 59:488–493.

7

A 68-year-old patient with COPD

T. Troosters, R. Casaburi

BACKGROUND

Dyspnoea, especially during exercise, is one of the cardinal complaints of patients consulting a medical doctor. Accurate diagnosis is often difficult and clinicians may need to distinguish between acute and chronic cardiac or respiratory disorders or metabolic or psychosomatic disorders. In addition, treatment of the symptoms of dyspnoea is not always straightforward. In a patient with chronic obstructive pulmonary disease (COPD) – as the one described in the present case report – bronchodilators may represent just a first step in the comprehensive management of dyspnoea. The reason why bronchodilators may fail in alleviating the symptoms of dyspnoea is that factors outside the lung may contribute to symptom perception or to the ventilatory requirements during exercise. Deconditioning and the consequent skeletal muscle abnormalities are common contributors to enhanced ventilatory needs. Therefore, in patients with limited ventilatory function, this contributes to symptoms of dyspnoea during mild exercise. Other factors include hypoxaemia, obesity, dynamic hyperinflation, respiratory muscle weakness and the perception of dyspnoea. Once identified, these factors can be tackled by a comprehensive and multidisciplinary pulmonary rehabilitation programme [1, 2]. In addition to a systematic improvement of dyspnoea, pulmonary rehabilitation has benefits in terms of enhanced exercise tolerance, muscle function, improved health-related quality of life and psychological morbidity (anxiety and depression). Reduced exacerbation rates and reduced utilization of healthcare recourses are other important benefits of pulmonary rehabilitation. Such programmes are individually tailored to the patient's needs and stem from accurate diagnostic testing. The present case report discusses the relevant diagnostic steps and describes the pulmonary rehabilitation programme that could be set up for this patient.

CASE REPORT

CLINICAL PRESENTATION

A 68-year-old patient, a smoker of 70 pack-years until 2 years ago, with known COPD, visits the out-patient clinic. The lung function obtained 15 min after bronchodilation is displayed in Table 7.1 along with the office spirometry from the time of COPD diagnosis (in the year 2000). His main complaint is *shortness of breath* with light household work and while climbing one flight of stairs. He is concerned about this problem and the breathlessness preoccupies him.

Thierry Troosters, PT, PhD, Associate Professor, Rehabilitation Sciences, Faculty of Kinesiology and Rehabilitation Sciences, Respiratory Division, Katholieke Universiteit Leuven, Leuven, Belgium

Richard Casaburi, MD, PhD, Rehabilitation Clinical Trials Center, Los Angeles Biomedical Research Institute at Harbor-UCLA Medical Center, Torrance, California, USA

© Atlas Medical Publishing Ltd 2007

Table 7.1 Anthropometric data, lung function and arterial blood gases (breathing room air)

	Diagnosis	Discharge	Present		Percentage of predicted
			pre	post	
Weight, kg	90	92	93		
Height, cm	170	170	170		
BMI, kg/m²	31.1	31.8	32.0		
Spirometry					
FEV_1, l	1.41	1.32	1.33	1.35	47
FVC, l	3.70	3.49	3.13	3.58	97
IC, l	–	1.61	1.53	1.74	68
Static lung volumes (whole body plethysmography)					
TLC, l	–	–	–	6.65	110
FRC, l	–	–	–	4.91	140
Lung diffusion capacity					
TL, CO, mmol · kPa⁻¹ min⁻¹	–	–	–	4.85	58
Arterial blood gases while breathing room air					
PaO_2, mmHg	–	70	72		
SaO_2, %	–	94	95		
$PaCO_2$, mmHg	–	43	44		
HCO_3^-, mmol/l	–	24	25		
pH	–	7.42	7.41		

The data at diagnosis pertain to an office spirometry conducted by the GP in the year 2000. The data at discharge pertain to the data obtained on the discharge day of the last hospital admission of this patient (one month ago). The current (2005) data are obtained at this out-patient consultation before and after inhalation of a bronchodilator (400 µg salbutamol with a spacer). Predicted normal values are those proposed by the European Respiratory Society [92].

Careful questioning revealed that the complaints of dyspnoea increased after a hospital admission for an acute exacerbation of COPD 1 month ago. The patient was discharged after being treated for an infectious exacerbation. Continuing dyspnoea at home while attempting to carry out activities of daily living and helping his wife with household activities was treated by his general practitioner (GP) with methylprednisolone (40 mg/day for 4 days). Subsequently, the dose was reduced gradually to 36 and 32 mg/day after 4 and 8 days, respectively. Since the dyspnoea complaints did not improve, his GP sent the patient for consultation to the chest physician in hospital. A consultation was scheduled within 10 days, but in the meantime, the GP maintained the dose of methylprednisolone at 32 mg/day.

Inhaled medications at the present time are tiotropium daily, and a twice-daily combination of a long-acting β_2-agonist (salmeterol, 50 µg) and fluticasone (250 µg).

On auscultation there was mild wheezing but no abnormalities. A chest X-ray showed no evidence of pulmonary infiltrates.

DIFFERENTIAL DIAGNOSIS

In the context of the present case, the following differential diagnosis of the patient's complaint was considered:

Table 7.2 Respiratory and peripheral muscle strength

	Absolute value	Percentage of predicted
PI_{max}, cmH_2O	52	46
PE_{max}, cmH_2O	118	60
Quadriceps force, Nm	96	49
Hand grip force, N	36	87

Inspiratory (PI_{max}) and expiratory (PE_{max}) mouth pressures, lower limb strength (quadriceps force in Nm) and hand grip force (in N). Predicted normal values are those proposed by Rochester and Arora [93] for respiratory pressures, by Mathiowetz et al. [94] for hand grip strength, and by Decramer et al. [42].

- New exacerbation.
- Worsening of lung function.
- Other reason for the dyspnoea including:
  - psychosomatic problems;
  - sleep apnoea;
  - deconditioning;
  - respiratory muscle problem;
  - cardiac congestion.

The latter was excluded from the differential diagnosis list based on the presence of a relatively normal echocardiogram performed as part of the assessments during his recent hospital admission and the absence of clinical features of heart failure both in the clinical examination (no oedema, no abnormal jugular vein distention) and on auscultation (no crackles). Sleep apnoea was excluded by a polysomnograph that was performed at the end of the patient's last hospital admission.

ASSESSMENT AND LABORATORY TESTING OF THE PATIENT

A summary of the tests performed at the consultation are given in Tables 7.1 and 7.2. In this patient, static and dynamic lung volumes were assessed, revealing hyperinflation and severe COPD (GOLD III). There was no significant reversibility of FEV_1 with acute administration of albuterol. Interestingly, FVC and inspiratory capacity increased with bronchodilators. Decline in lung function appeared to be as anticipated [3] when the current data were compared with office spirometry from March 2000 (FEV_1 and FVC declined by approximately 15–20 ml/year). Lung diffusion capacity was moderately impaired.

Lung function testing was complemented by the assessment of leg and respiratory muscle strength. This was assessed using maximum volitional manoeuvres. These tests are not currently commonly used in clinical practice, but normal values can be predicted based on age and gender (for respiratory pressures) [4] or based on age, gender, and anthropometric variables (for quadriceps force). Patients need to be cooperative and the traces from the tests should be checked for appropriate force development (i.e. rapid achievement of peak torque or pressure). Further information on how measurements of respiratory and peripheral muscle function can be made in clinical practice is available elsewhere [5, 6].

These tests revealed moderately reduced inspiratory pressures, a sign of inspiratory muscle dysfunction, and significant quadriceps weakness. Since dyspnoea complaints were related mainly to exertion, a cardiopulmonary exercise test was scheduled. The results of this test are displayed in Table 7.3. A 6-min walking test was also performed to evaluate functional exercise tolerance.

Table 7.3 Summary of relevant data obtained in the maximal incremental exercise test and the 6-min walking test

	Unloaded	Peak	Percentage of predicted
Incremental maximal cycle ergometry			
Work, W		70	54
VO_2, ml/min	480	1230	68
VCO_2, ml/min	398	1373	
Lactate, mEq/l	1.0	5.7	
V_E, l/min	18.2	54.3	101
HR, beats/min	95	138	90
SpO_2, %	98	96	
Borg dyspnoea	1.5	5	
Borg fatigue	1	7	
6-min walking test (best of 2 encouraged tests)	Rest	6-min	
Walking distance, m		380	62
SaO_2, %	98	94	
HR, beats/min	89	139	
Borg dyspnoea (points 0–10)	0.5	7	
Borg fatigue (points 0–10)	0.5	4	

When relevant data are expressed as percentage of the predicted normal value (for peak work rate and peak oxygen consumption) the values proposed by Jones et al. [95], for peak ventilation 40 × FEV_1, the patient's measured MVV was 59 l/min. Peak heart rate was predicted based on age as 220 − age. Oxygen saturation is measured with a finger pulse oximeter probe. Dyspnoea and fatigue are measured on a 10-point modified Borg symptom scale.

KEY POINTS IN THE SPECIFIC ANALYSIS OF THE PATIENT'S COMPLAINT

Our analysis focused on the activity pattern of the patient. The quantity and quality of the activities the patient pursues is important in determining whether the patient may be suffering from deconditioning. Guidelines for maintenance of optimal health were reviewed recently [7]. It is clear that reduced physical activity is a driver of deconditioning, even in healthy subjects [8]. Evaluation of the physical activity level should therefore be a key element in a clinician's consultation. True assessment of the physical activity level may be difficult. Indeed, patients may severely overestimate their true physical activity level [9]. Unfortunately, simple activity monitors, such as pedometers, are relatively unreliable in patients who adopt a slow walking speed [10]. Multiaxial accelerometers are more precise measurement tools [11]. As assessment of activities is currently not available in most clinical practices, we would advise engaging relatives in this part of the analysis, to give as accurate a view as possible.

From the analysis of the present patient, we determined that walking activities were restricted to walking inside the house (one flight of stairs) with twice-weekly short walks outdoors. The walking pace was judged by the partner as slow, with frequent rests because of shortness of breath. Virtually all social contacts took place in the patient's house. His hobby is soccer, which he watches on television and follows carefully in the newspapers. Formal activity monitoring using a Dynaport activity monitor revealed the following (per day) [12]:

- Walking time: 21 min
- Standing time: 48 min

- Sitting time: 397 min
- Lying time: 254 min

This activity distribution is commonly seen in patients with COPD [12], especially in patients discharged from hospital after being treated for an acute exacerbation of COPD [13, 14].

LABORATORY ASSESSMENT

A venous blood sample was taken and analysed for C-reactive protein as a marker for systemic inflammation. The value was 3.02 mg/l. This is compatible with some degree of systemic inflammation, but compared to the values obtained during the exacerbation (108 mg/l in the emergency room; 4.03 mg/l at discharge in this patient during his last hospital admission), it is low. Haemoglobin content was within normal limits at 14.6 g/dl. Although not present in this patient, anaemia frequently occurs in patients with COPD and is often an unrecognized problem [15]. Since haemoglobin concentration is directly linked to oxygen delivery, it is obvious that anaemia could contribute to exercise intolerance and dyspnoea [16]. It is important to realize that anaemia is especially prevalent in patients recently admitted to hospital, but can also occur in all stages of COPD [17]. Furthermore, anaemic COPD patients have significantly greater utilization of healthcare resources [18].

Testosterone levels were low in this patient (total testosterone: 103 ng/dl; free testosterone: 3 ng/dl). This is considerably lower than that in normal subjects of a comparable age [19]. Such low testosterone levels are associated with skeletal muscle weakness.

INTERPRETATION OF THE CARDIOPULMONARY EXERCISE TESTING IN THIS PATIENT

A maximal incremental cardiopulmonary exercise test is vital in patients with activity-induced dyspnoea [20]. Exercise tolerance is only poorly related to lung function impairment [21] and an incremental exercise test allows investigation of the factors that contribute to exercise intolerance and – in the case of this patient – exercise-related dyspnoea.

The exercise test was carried out on a cycle ergometer. After 3 min of unloaded cycling, the work rate was increased by 10 W each minute. This yielded an exercise test of 10 min duration. In these tests, the peak work rate should be reached in 7–12 min [22].

Table 7.3 shows that exercise tolerance is clearly impaired in this patient. Peak exercise performance (peak work rate and VO_2 of 54% and 68% of that predicted, respectively) and functional exercise tolerance (6-min walking distance = 62% of the predicted value) were both reduced.

At the end of the test, the patient had significant cardiac reserve (14 beats/min reserve), but no ventilatory reserve. The observed peak ventilation was 54.3 l/min compared with a predicted peak V_E (calculated as $40 \times FEV_1$) of 50 l/min and measured maximum voluntary ventilation of 59 l/min. Dyspnoea is further enhanced by significant dynamic hyperinflation (Figure 7.1). No significant reduction in oxygen saturation was observed during incremental exercise. In this patient, no arterial blood gas values were obtained during exercise. It is of note that exercise-induced hypoxia may have been more pronounced had the exercise test been conducted on a treadmill [23]. The patient had subjectively more complaints of leg muscle fatigue than of dyspnoea, but interrupted the test because of both dyspnoea and leg fatigue.

Although the inability to further increase ventilation is clearly the most obvious limiting factor during exercise and the factor that contributes most significantly to the sensation of dyspnoea, clinicians should be aware that the patient has an increased ventilatory need during exercise. Factors that contribute to the increased ventilatory needs in COPD include:

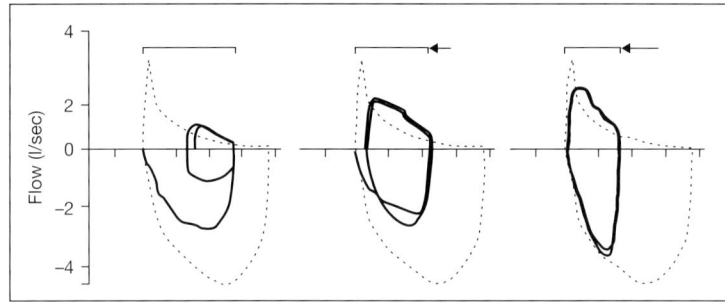

Figure 7.1 Flow volume loops during exercise. Flow volume loops obtained at rest (left panel), at moderate exercise (50 W, middle) and at maximal exercise (right). Resting maximal flow volume loop is displayed as a dashed line in every graph. Tidal breathing is displayed as a solid line. The inspiratory capacity is indicated above each panel. The reduction in inspiratory capacity compared to baseline (dynamic hyperinflation) is indicated by the arrow.

- High dead space ventilation through adoption of a rapid shallow breathing pattern or increased physiological dead space.
- Deconditioning with early lactic acidosis.
- Hypoxia increasing ventilatory drive through stimulation of the carotid bodies or indirectly by promoting early lactate release from the working muscles.
- Exercise-induced pulmonary hypertension.

The present patient clearly has an early onset of lactate accumulation. The lactate level at the peak work rate of 70 W is elevated compared to age-matched control subjects at comparable work rates. Early lactate increase contributes to enhanced ventilation. In healthy subjects, a 1 mEq/l lactate reduction results in a 7.2 l/min reduction in ventilation. In patients with COPD, it has been estimated that a 1 mEq/l reduction in lactate translates to a 2.5 l/min reduction in minute ventilation [24]. An early rise in blood lactate is a typical feature of skeletal muscle deconditioning and may contribute to the frequently-reported symptoms of leg fatigue during cycling in COPD [25, 26].

A consequence of the increased ventilatory demand is dynamic hyperinflation during exercise, as detected in laboratory exercise testing by a reduction in inspiratory capacity. Dynamic hyperinflation is not surprising in the current patient as it is typically seen in patients with reduced resting inspiratory capacity [27] and patients with resting flow limitation [28]. Dynamic hyperinflation exacerbates the symptoms of dyspnoea in patients with COPD [29]. Dynamic hyperinflation in the present patient is illustrated in Figure 7.1.

During the 6-min walking test, symptoms of dyspnoea were more prominent than during the cycle ergometer test. This is in line with recent studies that have compared cycling and walking exercises. During walking there is significantly less lactate production for a given VO_2. This results in less skeletal muscle fatigue during walking [30, 31]. Consequently, walking is associated with higher dyspnoea compared to cycling [31]. It is important to notice the larger arterial oxygen desaturation during the 6-min walk test compared to the incremental cycling test, which is commonly observed in COPD [32]. This is not surprising, as during a 6-min walking test, patients often perform exercise for several minutes at near maximal oxygen consumption [33]. When the patient is encouraged to exert maximal effort, the test may be a clinically useful one to assess the maximum sustainable exercise capacity [34]. In addition, recent studies suggest that patients with a walking distance <400 m are likely to be very inactive in daily life [12].

DISCUSSION

WHY ASSESS PERIPHERAL AND RESPIRATORY MUSCLE STRENGTH IN THIS PATIENT WHO PRESENTS WITH DYSPNOEA?

Skeletal muscle weakness is a common feature in patients with stable COPD [6, 19, 35]. In the out-patient clinic of the University Hospital in Leuven, the average quadriceps force of COPD patients screened is approximately 75% of the predicted normal value. Quadriceps weakness is generally proportional to the reduction of mid-thigh cross-sectional area (CSA) [36], which can be assessed with computerized tomography. Skeletal muscle weakness has been associated with important clinical features such as exercise intolerance [21, 25] and increased utilization of healthcare resources [37]. In addition, patients with a low CSA had significantly worse survival compared to patients with similar lung function, but preserved (i.e. >70 cm^2) CSA. This is especially true in patients with an FEV$_1$ below 50% of the predicted value, as in the present patient.

This patient has a medical history that would specifically invite careful assessment of peripheral muscle function. The patient presents with an inactive lifestyle. In addition, his recent exacerbations and hospital admission may have induced further reduction in quadriceps force [38]. During and after hospital admission, the patient was treated with relatively high doses of methylprednisolone. Although one short course of steroid administration in stable patients does not usually lead to the development of quadriceps dysfunction [39], oral corticosteroids, used continuously or in bursts, may induce myopathy [40–42]. The present patient received at least two burst therapies of methylprednisolone of which the first was for treatment of an acute exacerbation. The patient's GP prescribed oral corticoids to counter the dyspnoea. This treatment was maintained until the consultation.

Low testosterone levels as seen in the present patient are also frequently associated with skeletal muscle weakness [19]. Since patients with peripheral muscle weakness respond favourably to exercise training interventions [43], it is important to investigate this feature in patients with COPD.

Respiratory muscle force is not always impaired in patients with COPD. In fact, at comparable lung volumes, the maximal static inspiratory pressure (PI$_{max}$) is often preserved in COPD compared to control subjects [44]. Nevertheless, reduced PI$_{max}$ has been associated with increased breathlessness. Symptoms of dyspnoea can be improved by inspiratory muscle training (IMT) [45, 46]. The transfer of increased inspiratory muscle function towards improved exercise tolerance is much more controversial. Many studies have not shown an improved exercise tolerance after IMT [47, 48]. In patients with more pronounced respiratory muscle weakness, IMT may lead to additional effects on functional exercise capacity when added to a more general exercise training programme. It should be noted, however, that evidence from appropriately powered studies is lacking.

SUMMARY OF THE PATIENT'S CASE AND POTENTIAL TREATMENT OPTIONS

This patient with GOLD III stage COPD has a history of recent acute exacerbations. Dyspnoea is clearly related to impaired lung function and hyperinflation. No important gas exchange abnormalities were observed at rest and during exercise. The enhanced complaints of dyspnoea are, however, not entirely explained by a worsening of airflow obstruction. On the contrary, the lung function of the patient seems to have recovered when compared with past assessments. Other sources of dyspnoea were therefore considered. There was no evidence for worsening cardiac status, nor was there evidence for pulmonary hypertension. Further assessment, including exercise testing and peripheral muscle testing, indicated severe deconditioning and skeletal muscle weakness. The respiratory muscles were also significantly affected. The combination of reduced ventilatory capacity (reduced maximum voluntary ventilation and flow limitation) and increased ventilatory requirements when performing exercise are typical components of exercise-induced dyspnoea in patients with COPD.

TREATMENT PLAN

Optimizing medications

When corticosteroids are used, the potential benefits (improvement in lung function and prevention of consecutive exacerbations [49]) must be balanced with the potential side-effects. In this case no improvement of the lung function was seen with oral corticosteroid treatment. The further use of oral steroids must be carefully considered and avoided if at all possible. Increasing complaints of dyspnoea were treated by increased doses of methylprednisolone in this case. Corticoid-induced myopathy is frequently observed in patients with COPD and asthma [40, 42]. In fact, the diaphragm seems particularly vulnerable to corticosteroid-induced damage when patients receive bursts of steroids [41, 50–52]. When a patient presents with increasing dyspnoea while being treated with corticosteroids, clinicians should always consider respiratory muscle weakness as a potential cause of the dyspnoea. Tapering corticosteroid treatment in combination with specific training of the respiratory and peripheral muscles may lead to a reversal of symptoms.

The patient was maximally treated with bronchodilators including long-acting anticholinergic and β_2-agonist inhalers, and inhaled corticosteroids. He was asked to bring his medication to subsequent visits so that adherence to the medication regimen could be verified. Many patients make mistakes in handling inhaling devices, including metered-dose inhalers and the Handihaler device which delivers tiotropium [53]. Optimal medication has a clear effect on rehabilitation outcome [54]. When optimally treated, less dynamic hyperinflation is observed [55]. Since dynamic hyperinflation is a key factor contributing to exercise limitation in this patient, the benefits of optimizing inhalation strategies and medication adherence may be expected.

Another key factor in the management of this patient's medication is optimizing self-management skills concerning rescue medication and dealing with increased symptoms by providing action plans. These measures have been shown to significantly reduce the number of re-admissions in patients with severe COPD [56].

Exercise training

The patient was offered participation in a pulmonary rehabilitation programme. In this program, the emphasis was on the reconditioning of the patient, with the improvement of skeletal muscle function one of the most important goals. Exercise training was carried out three times weekly and training programmes typically consisted of whole body exercises (cycling or walking) complemented with resistance training [2]. In the rehabilitation centres of the authors, training is carried out at a relatively high intensity (i.e. initially at approximately 70% of the peak work rate or at 50 W in the present patient). An endurance test carried out at this work rate during the first training session revealed that the patient could only carry out exercise for 4.5 min at this intensity, yielding a Borg score of 5 for dyspnoea and 6 for fatigue. Exercise training was therefore carried out as an interval training programme on a bicycle, which was well supported by the patient, with symptom scores systematically around 5/10 at the end of the session. Weekly adjustments of the work rate were made [57–60].

In addition to cycling, walking exercises were introduced. This is done since walking is of immediate benefit in the patient's daily life. Since part of the training effects of pulmonary rehabilitation are achieved by increasing movement efficiency [61], walking is an important part of a clinical rehabilitation programme. One relatively small study has confirmed that the addition of specific activity training resulted in a reduction in the symptoms of dyspnoea in daily life [62]. Walking exercises, however, result in significantly less stress to the working lower limb muscles. As mentioned above, this is manifested by significantly lower skeletal muscle fatigue observed after walking [30, 31], and less lactate production [23, 33]. Although they have not been compared head-to-head, cycling exercises may result in more training effects in the skeletal muscle due to skeletal muscle overload. More details on how to establish a training programme, duration and intensity can be found elsewhere [2, 63].

Why does whole body exercise training reduce dyspnoea?
Several factors may reduce dyspnoea sensation on exertion after exercise training. Firstly, due to improved muscle bioenergetics [64] and enhanced activity of oxidative enzymes [65], less lactate is produced at identical oxygen consumption levels. This may translate into reduced ventilatory requirements. Alveolar ventilation at a given total ventilation may be increased by adopting a slower breathing pattern with a larger tidal volume [66]. As a consequence of the reduced ventilatory needs with slower expiration, less dynamic hyperinflation may occur [67]. This may in turn translate into an additional benefit in lowered dyspnoea, even at identical ventilation levels [68].

Targeting the skeletal muscle
Another key aspect of exercise training in the present patient is resistance training. The patient suffers from clear skeletal muscle weakness and resistance training is a powerful means to reverse this [59, 69, 70]. The addition of resistance training to a conventional endurance training programme may enhance the improvement in skeletal muscle force [71, 72]. Resistance training is generally carried out at a percentage of the maximal load that can be lifted or displaced once (1 repetition maximum, or 1 RM). Most published studies have used training at 70% of the 1 RM [59, 69, 72]. The direct link between improved muscle function and dyspnoea is not completely understood, but studies looking at resistance training found a consistent improvement in dyspnoea during daily life [73]. The most likely mechanism is the improvement in muscle function. Unfortunately, in patients with COPD, no comparisons of endurance vs. resistance training have been done at the molecular level. In frail but otherwise healthy subjects, aerobic capacity of the muscle [74] or whole body [75] was increased after resistance training. A recent systematic review, however, remained inconclusive in regard to the wider applicability of these results due to the many different training protocols applied and the large differences in outcome measures [76].

Anabolic stimulants may amplify the results of resistance training in selected patients. Testosterone levels are reduced in the present patient, and he may therefore be a candidate for testosterone supplements [70]. Intramuscular testosterone therapy aimed at restoring physiological testosterone levels may enhance the strength gain achieved by resistance training. In one study, anabolic steroids were of particular benefit in patients who received corticosteroid treatment [77]. Testosterone leads to significant weight gain; this gain is strictly fat-free mass. In line with testosterone's known lipolytic effects, a recent study showed significant reduction in abdominal fat in patients receiving testosterone supplements [70]. In another study, no change in fat mass was observed [77]. If the patient does not readily respond to the resistance training stimulus, testosterone supplements may be considered as an adjunct to training. It should be stressed, however, that both the long-term safety and efficacy of testosterone supplementation have not been studied in COPD.

INSPIRATORY MUSCLE TRAINING

IMT is a much debated part of pulmonary rehabilitation programmes [45]. The effect of IMT on functional improvement is not clear in the general patient with COPD. However, as mentioned above, in the present case the addition of carefully administered IMT may be worthwhile. Firstly, the present patient has clear respiratory muscle weakness (PI_{max} only

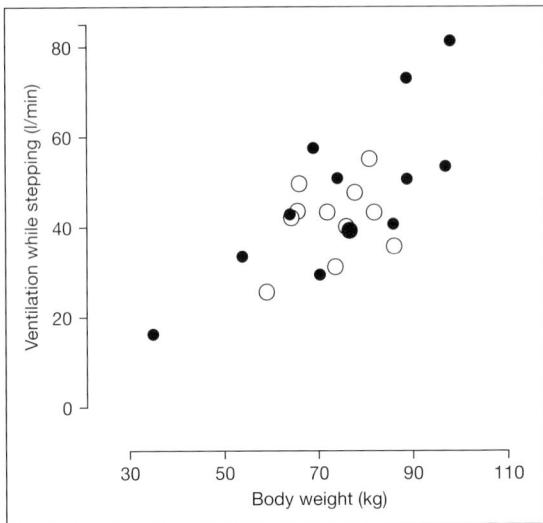

Figure 7.2 Relation between body weight and ventilatory needs during stepping at a fixed pace (18 steps per minute). In patients with COPD (closed symbols: FEV_1 45 ± 19% predicted, VO_2 peak 15 ml/min/kg) and healthy control subjects (open circles: FEV_1 110 ± 8% predicted, VO_2 peak 29 ± 5 ml/min/kg) (unpublished observation).

52 cmH$_2$O, or just 46% of the predicted level). In addition, the main complaint of the patient is shortness of breath. IMT also consistently improves symptoms of dyspnoea during daily life [45]. Although the evidence is not categorical, it has been suggested that in patients with inspiratory muscle weakness, IMT may elicit increased functional exercise tolerance [45]. It is clear that studies with more power are needed to further fine-tune the indications – if any – for resistive IMT. An interesting recent study showed that persistent IMT may reduce hospital admissions in patients with COPD and inspiratory muscle weakness [78]. The training intensity of the IMT is critical and should be carefully controlled [46]. The minimal training intensity is 30–40% of the peak inspiratory pressure. At one of the authors' centres (University Hospital, Leuven), patients with overt inspiratory muscle weakness carry out daily IMT at 40% of PI_{max} for 30 min/day. This training is added to a conventional pulmonary rehabilitation programme. The breathing exercises, using a threshold loading device, are regularly supervised but patients essentially carry out the training at home.

OTHER DISCIPLINES THAT MAY CONTRIBUTE SIGNIFICANTLY TO THE REHABILITATION OF THIS PATIENT

Nutritional intervention

An important feature in the rehabilitation process of the current patient is nutritional advice. The patient is overweight (body mass index [BMI] = 32 kg/m^2). Since there is a clear relationship between the ventilation requirement for weight-bearing activities of daily life and body weight, it is important to attempt to decrease body weight in patients with dyspnoea. The relation between ventilation and body weight is illustrated in Figure 7.2. This figure represents the minute ventilation needed to carry out stair climbing at a fixed pace. From Figure 7.2, it is clear that a loss in body weight will result in the reduction of ventilatory needs during weight-bearing activities of daily living (ADL). A similar relation between body weight and ventilatory needs during walking has been shown [33]. Similarly, another study has shown that an increase in fat mass, without change in fat-free mass (muscle), as a result of the administration of a progestational appetite stimulant, led to the deterioration of walking distance in COPD [79].

In the overweight patient, nutritional advice should be aimed at weight (particularily fat) loss, but it is crucial to maintain – or even further enhance – fat-free mass. Surprisingly little attention has been given to obese COPD patients. This is largely due to the fact that non-volitional weight loss resulting in low BMI and/or a low fat-free mass index is an important negative prognostic factor in COPD [80–84]. Although obesity is less important in the prognosis of patients with COPD, it is a factor that contributes to symptoms during ambulation and weight-bearing activities. Interestingly, abdominal obesity is prevalent in patients with COPD [85] and it does not exclude the presence of quadriceps muscle weakness.

Breathing exercises and walking aids

Although the patient is 'preoccupied by the problem of dyspnoea' it is not readily clear that he will benefit from breathing exercises. In patients with hyperinflation, exercises such as diaphragmatic breathing may have an adverse effect on the work of breathing [86]. Pursed-lips breathing (PLB) may be of benefit in this patient. PLB is variably effective in reducing dyspnoea during exercise [87, 88] and is particularly effective if the end expiratory lung volume can be reduced by applying the technique [87, 89].

Walking aids have also been used to increase ambulation of COPD patients and to reduce symptoms during walking [90, 91]. The present patient also walked further (+36 m) in a 6-min walking test when using a wheeled walking aid (rollator) and symptoms of dyspnoea and fatigue both reduced by one point on the Borg scale. With appropriate training, the patient learned to transfer part of his body weight to the rollator. In addition, rollators increase slightly the peak ventilatory capacity of a patient with COPD [91]. The patient gained outdoor walking ability when using the rollator. The basket on the rollator was also a useful place to put groceries so that he could keep his arms braced for walking, rather than for carrying bags on his return from shopping.

SUMMARY

In the present patient, the increasing complaints of dyspnoea were most likely to be as a result of deconditioning rather than deterioration of pulmonary function. This became obvious when exercise tests were conducted. Significant peripheral and respiratory muscle weakness, as well as abdominal obesity, also contributed to the symptoms.

Treatment consists of exercise training, including endurance, interval and resistance exercises. In addition, nutritional counselling is necessary in an attempt to reduce fat mass, without loss in fat-free mass.

A wheeled walking aid enhanced the mobility of the patient, which allowed him to walk further outdoors, with fewer symptoms.

From this case it is clear that – apart from enhancing medication inhaling strategies – none of the proposed interventions directly alter lung function in the present patient. Rather, they are aimed at reducing ventilatory requirements, increasing ventilatory efficiency and enhancing respiratory muscle pump function.

REFERENCES

1. Nici L, Donner C, Wouters E *et al*. American Thoracic Society/European Respiratory Society statement on pulmonary rehabilitation. *Am J Respir Crit Care Med* 2006; 173:1390–1413.
2. Troosters T, Casaburi R, Gosselink R *et al*. Pulmonary rehabilitation in chronic obstructive pulmonary disease. *Am J Respir Crit Care Med* 2005; 172:19–38.
3. Anthonisen NR, Connett JE, Murray RP. Smoking and lung function of Lung Health Study participants after 11 years. *Am J Respir Crit Care Med* 2002; 166:675–679.

4. Troosters T, Gosselink R, Decramer M. Respiratory muscle assessment. *Eur Respir Mon* 2005; 31:71.
5. ATS/ERS statement on respiratory muscle testing. *Am J Respir Crit Care Med* 2002; 166:518–624.
6. Skeletal muscle dysfunction in chronic obstructive pulmonary disease. A statement of the American Thoracic Society and European Respiratory Society. *Am J Respir Crit Care Med* 1999; 159(pt 2):S1–S40.
7. Blair SN, Lamonte MJ, Nichaman MZ. The evolution of physical activity recommendations: how much is enough? *Am J Clin Nutr* 2004; 79:913S–920S.
8. Jackson AS, Kampert JB, Barlow CE et al. Longitudinal changes in cardiorespiratory fitness: measurement error or true change? *Med Sci Sports Exerc* 2004; 36:1175–1180.
9. Pitta F, Troosters T, Spruit M et al. Activity monitoring for assessment of physical activities of daily life in patients with COPD. *Arch Phys Med Rehabil* 2005; 86:1979–1985.
10. Cyarto EV, Myers AM, Tudor-Locke C. Pedometer accuracy in nursing home and community-dwelling older adults. *Med Sci Sports Exerc* 2004; 36:205–209.
11. Pitta F, Troosters T, Probst V et al. Quantifying physical activity in daily life with questionnaires and motion sensors in COPD. *Eur Respir J* 2006; 27:1040–1055.
12. Pitta F, Troosters T, Spruit MA et al. Characteristics of physical activities in daily life in chronic obstructive pulmonary disease. *Am J Respir Crit Care Med* 2005; 171:972–977.
13. Pitta F, Troosters T, Probst V et al. Physical activity and hospitalization for an exacerbation of chronic obstructive pulmonary disease. *Chest* (in press).
14. Donaldson GC, Wilkinson TM, Hurst JR et al. Exacerbations and time spent outdoors in chronic obstructive pulmonary disease. *Am J Respir Crit Care Med* 2005; 171:446–452.
15. John M, Hoernig S, Doehner W et al. Anemia and inflammation in COPD. *Chest* 2005; 127:825–829.
16. Kalra PR, Bolger AP, Francis DP et al. Effect of anemia on exercise tolerance in chronic heart failure in men. *Am J Cardiol* 2003; 91:888–891.
17. John M, Lange A, Hoernig S et al. Prevalence of anemia in chronic obstructive pulmonary disease: comparison to other chronic diseases. *Int J Cardiol* 2005; 111:365–370.
18. Ershler WB, Chen K, Reyes EB et al. Economic burden of patients with anemia in selected diseases. *Value Health* 2005; 8:629–638.
19. van Vliet M, Spruit MA, Verleden G et al. Hypogonadism, quadriceps weakness, and exercise intolerance in chronic obstructive pulmonary disease. *Am J Respir Crit Care Med* 2005; 172:1105–1111.
20. ATS/ACCP statement on cardiopulmonary exercise testing. *Am J Respir Crit Care Med* 2003; 167:211–277.
21. Gosselink R, Troosters T, Decramer M. Peripheral muscle weakness contributes to exercise limitation in COPD. *Am J Respir Crit Care Med* 1996; 153:976–980.
22. Wasserman K, Hansen JE, Sue DJ et al. *Principles of Exercise Testing and Interpretation*, 2nd edition. Williams & Wilkins, Philadelphia, 1994, p 479.
23. Christensen CC, Ryg MS, Edvardsen A et al. Effect of exercise mode on oxygen uptake and blood gases in COPD patients. *Respir Med* 2004; 98:656–660.
24. Casaburi R, Patessio A, Ioli F et al. Reductions in exercise lactic acidosis and ventilation as a result of exercise training in patients with obstructive lung disease. *Am Rev Respir Dis* 1991; 143:9–18.
25. Hamilton AL, Killian KJ, Summers E et al. Muscle strength, symptom intensity, and exercise capacity in patients with cardiorespiratory disorders. *Am J Respir Crit Care Med* 1995; 152(pt 1):2021–2031.
26. Saey D, Michaud A, Couillard A et al. Contractile fatigue, muscle morphometry, and blood lactate in chronic obstructive pulmonary disease. *Am J Respir Crit Care Med* 2005; 171:1109–1115.
27. O'Donnell DE, Revill SM, Webb KA. Dynamic hyperinflation and exercise intolerance in chronic obstructive pulmonary disease. *Am J Respir Crit Care Med* 2001; 164:770–777.
28. Diaz O, Villafranca C, Ghezzo H et al. Role of inspiratory capacity on exercise tolerance in COPD patients with and without tidal expiratory flow limitation at rest. *Eur Respir J* 2000; 16:269–275.
29. Palange P, Valli G, Onorati P et al. Effect of heliox on lung dynamic hyperinflation, dyspnea, and exercise endurance capacity in COPD patients. *J Appl Physiol* 2004; 97:1637–1642.
30. Man WD, Soliman MG, Gearing J et al. Symptoms and quadriceps fatiguability following walking and cycling in COPD. *Am J Respir Crit Care Med* 2003; 168:562–567.
31. Pepin V, Saey D, Whittom F et al. Walking versus cycling: sensitivity to bronchodilation in chronic obstructive pulmonary disease. *Am J Respir Crit Care Med* 2005; 172:1517–1522.
32. Poulain M, Durand F, Palomba B et al. 6-minute walk testing is more sensitive than maximal incremental cycle testing for detecting oxygen desaturation in patients with COPD. *Chest* 2003; 123:1401–1407.
33. Troosters T, Vilaro J, Rabinovich RA et al. Physiological responses to six minute walking test in COPD patients. *Eur Respir J* 2002; 20:564–569.

34. Casas A, Vilaro J, Rabinovich R et al. Encouraged 6-min walking test indicates maximum sustainable exercise in COPD patients. *Chest* 2005; 128:55–61.
35. Man WD, Hopkinson NS, Harraf F et al. Abdominal muscle and quadriceps strength in chronic obstructive pulmonary disease. *Thorax* 2005; 60:718–722.
36. Bernard S, LeBlanc P, Whittom F et al. Peripheral muscle weakness in patients with chronic obstructive pulmonary disease. *Am J Respir Crit Care Med* 1998; 158:629–634.
37. Decramer M, Gosselink R, Troosters T et al. Muscle weakness is related to utilization of health care resources in COPD patients. *Eur Respir J* 1997; 10:417–423.
38. Spruit M, Gosselink R, Troosters T et al. Muscle force during an acute exacerbation in hospitalised COPD patients and its relationship with CXCL8 and IGF-1. *Thorax* 2003; 58:752–756.
39. Hopkinson NS, Man WD, Dayer MJ et al. Acute effect of oral steroids on muscle function in chronic obstructive pulmonary disease. *Eur Respir J* 2004; 24:137–142.
40. Decramer M, Lacquet LM, Fagard R et al. Corticosteroids contribute to muscle weakness in chronic airflow obstruction. *Am J Respir Crit Care Med* 1994; 150:11–16.
41. Gayan-Ramirez G, Bisschop A, Decramer M. Repetitive burst methylprednisolone treatment affects rat diaphragm more than continuous dose treatment. *Am J Respir Crit Care Med* 1995; 151:A812.
42. Decramer M, de Bock V, Dom R. Functional and histologic picture of steroid-induced myopathy in chronic obstructive pulmonary disease. *Am J Respir Crit Care Med* 1996; 153(pt 1):1958–1964.
43. Troosters T, Gosselink R, Decramer M. Exercise training in COPD; how to distinguish responders from nonresponders. *J Cardiopulm Rehabil* 2001; 21:10–17.
44. Similowski T, Yan S, Gauthier AP et al. Contractile properties of the human diaphragm during chronic hyperinflation. *N Engl J Med* 1991; 325:917–923.
45. Lotters F, Van Tol B, Kwakkel G et al. Effects of controlled inspiratory muscle training in patients with COPD: a meta-analysis. *Eur Respir J* 2002; 20:570–576.
46. Geddes EL, Reid WD, Crowe J et al. Inspiratory muscle training in adults with chronic obstructive pulmonary disease: a systematic review. *Respir Med* 2005; 99:1440–1458.
47. Ramirez-Sarmiento A, Orozco-Levi M, Guell R et al. Inspiratory muscle training in patients with chronic obstructive pulmonary disease: structural adaptation and physiologic outcomes. *Am J Respir Crit Care Med* 2002; 166:1491–1497.
48. Larson JL, Covey MK, Wirtz SE et al. Cycle ergometer and inspiratory muscle training in chronic obstructive pulmonary disease. *Am J Respir Crit Care Med* 1999; 160:500–507.
49. Niewoehner DE, Erbland ML, Deupree RH et al. Effect of systemic glucocorticoids on exacerbations of chronic obstructive pulmonary disease. Department of Veterans Affairs Cooperative Study Group. *N Engl J Med* 1999; 340:1941–1947.
50. Dekhuijzen PN, Gayan-Ramirez G, de Bock V et al. Triamcinolone and prednisolone affect contractile properties and histopathology of rat diaphragm differently. *J Clin Invest* 1993; 92:1534–1542.
51. Dekhuijzen PN, Gayan-Ramirez G, Bisschop A et al. Rat diaphragm contractility and histopathology are affected differently by low dose treatment with methylprednisolone and deflazacort. *Eur Respir J* 1995; 8:824–830.
52. Dekhuijzen PN, Gayan-Ramirez G, Bisschop A et al. Corticosteroid treatment and nutritional deprivation cause a different pattern of atrophy in rat diaphragm. *J Appl Physiol* 1995; 78:629–637.
53. Dahl R, Backer V, Ollgaard B et al. Assessment of patient performance of the HandiHaler compared with the metered dose inhaler four weeks after instruction. *Respir Med* 2003; 97:1126–1133.
54. Casaburi R, Kukafka D, Cooper CB et al. Improvement in exercise tolerance with the combination of tiotropium and pulmonary rehabilitation in patients with COPD. *Chest* 2005; 127:809–817.
55. O'Donnell DE, Fluge T, Gerken F et al. Effects of tiotropium on lung hyperinflation, dyspnoea and exercise tolerance in COPD. *Eur Respir J* 2004; 23:832–840.
56. Bourbeau J, Julien M, Maltais F et al. Reduction of hospital utilization in patients with chronic obstructive pulmonary disease: a disease-specific self-management intervention. *Arch Intern Med* 2003; 163:585–591.
57. Troosters T, Gosselink R, Decramer M. Short- and long-term effects of outpatient rehabilitation in patients with chronic obstructive pulmonary disease: a randomized trial. *Am J Med* 2000; 109:207–212.
58. Emtner M, Porszasz J, Burns M et al. Benefits of supplemental oxygen in exercise training in non-hypoxemic COPD patients. *Am J Respir Crit Care Med* 2003; 168:1034–1042.
59. Spruit MA, Gosselink R, Troosters T et al. Resistance versus endurance training in patients with COPD and skeletal muscle weakness. *Eur Respir J* 2002; 19:1072–1078.
60. Maltais F, LeBlanc P, Jobin J. Intensity of training and physiological adaptation in patients with chronic obstructive pulmonary disease. *Am J Respir Crit Care Med* 1997; 155:555–561.

61. Normandin EA, McCusker C, Connors M et al. An evaluation of two approaches to exercise conditioning in pulmonary rehabilitation. *Chest* 2002; 121:1085–1091.
62. Norweg AM, Whiteson J, Malgady R et al. The effectiveness of different combinations of pulmonary rehabilitation program components: a randomized controlled trial. *Chest* 2005; 128:663–672.
63. ATS-ERS statement on pulmonary rehabilitation. *Am J Respir Crit Care Med* 2005; revised.
64. Sala E, Roca J, Marrades RM et al. Effects of endurance training on skeletal muscle bioenergetics in chronic obstructive pulmonary disease. *Am J Respir Crit Care Med* 1999; 159:1726–1734.
65. Maltais F, LeBlanc P, Simard C et al. Skeletal muscle adaptation to endurance training in patients with chronic obstructive pulmonary disease. *Am J Respir Crit Care Med* 1996; 154(pt 1):442–447.
66. Casaburi R, Porszasz J, Burns MR et al. Physiologic benefits of exercise training in rehabilitation of patients with severe chronic obstructive pulmonary disease. *Am J Respir Crit Care Med* 1997; 155:1541–1551.
67. Porszasz J, Emtner M, Goto S et al. Exercise training decreases ventilatory requirements and exercise-induced hyperinflation at submaximal intensities in patients with COPD. *Chest* 2005; 128:2025–2034.
68. O'Donnell DE, Bain DJ, Webb KA. Factors contributing to relief of exertional breathlessness during hyperoxia in chronic airflow limitation. *Am J Respir Crit Care Med* 1997; 155:530–535.
69. Simpson K, Killian K, McCartney N et al. Randomised controlled trial of weightlifting exercise in patients with chronic airflow limitation. *Thorax* 1992; 47:70–75.
70. Casaburi R, Bhasin S, Cosentino L et al. Anabolic effects of testosterone replacement and strength training in men with COPD. *Am J Respir Crit Care Med* 2004; 170:870–878.
71. Ortega F, Toral J, Cejudo P et al. Comparison of effects of strength and endurance training in patients with chronic obstructive pulmonary disease. *Am J Respir Crit Care Med* 2002; 166:669–674.
72. Bernard S, Whittom F, LeBlanc P et al. Aerobic and strength training in patients with chronic obstructive pulmonary disease. *Am J Respir Crit Care Med* 1999; 159:896–901.
73. Puhan MA, Schunemann HJ, Frey M et al. How should COPD patients exercise during respiratory rehabilitation? Comparison of exercise modalities and intensities to treat skeletal muscle dysfunction. *Thorax* 2005; 60:367–375.
74. Jubrias SA, Esselman PC, Price LB et al. Large energetic adaptations of elderly muscle to resistance and endurance training. *J Appl Physiol* 2001; 90:1663–1670.
75. Vincent KR, Braith RW, Feldman RA et al. Improved cardiorespiratory endurance following 6 months of resistance exercise in elderly men and women. *Arch Intern Med* 2002; 162:673–678.
76. Harris BA. The influence of endurance and resistance exercise on muscle capillarization in the elderly: a review. *Acta Physiol Scand* 2005; 185:89–97.
77. Creutzberg EC, Wouters EF, Mostert R et al. A role for anabolic steroids in the rehabilitation of patients with COPD? A double-blind, placebo-controlled, randomized trial. *Chest* 2003; 124:1733–1742.
78. Beckerman M, Magadle R, Weiner M et al. The effects of 1 year of specific inspiratory muscle training in patients with COPD. *Chest* 2005; 128:3177–3182.
79. Weisberg J, Wanger J, Olson J et al. Megestrol acetate stimulates weight gain and ventilation in underweight COPD patients. *Chest* 2002; 121:1070–1078.
80. Schols AM, Soeters PB, Dingemans AM et al. Prevalence and characteristics of nutritional depletion in patients with stable COPD eligible for pulmonary rehabilitation. *Am Rev Respir Dis* 1993; 147:1151–1156.
81. Engelen MP, Schols AM, Baken WC et al. Nutritional depletion in relation to respiratory and peripheral skeletal muscle function in out-patients with COPD. *Eur Respir J* 1994; 7:1793–1797.
82. Schols AM, Slangen J, Volovics L et al. Weight loss is a reversible factor in the prognosis of chronic obstructive pulmonary disease. *Am J Respir Crit Care Med* 1998; 157(pt 1):1791–1797.
83. Prescott E, Almdal T, Mikkelsen KL et al. Prognostic value of weight change in chronic obstructive pulmonary disease: results from the Copenhagen City Heart Study. *Eur Respir J* 2002; 20:539–544.
84. Schols AM, Broekhuizen R, Weling-Scheepers CA et al. Body composition and mortality in chronic obstructive pulmonary disease. *Am J Clin Nutr* 2005; 82:53–59.
85. Marquis K, Maltais F, Duguay V et al. The metabolic syndrome in patients with chronic obstructive pulmonary disease. *J Cardiopulm Rehabil* 2005; 25:226–232.
86. Gosselink RA, Wagenaar RC, Rijswijk H et al. Diaphragmatic breathing reduces efficiency of breathing in patients with chronic obstructive pulmonary disease. *Am J Respir Crit Care Med* 1995; 151:1136–1142.
87. Spahija J, de Marchie M, Grassino A. Effects of imposed pursed-lips breathing on respiratory mechanics and dyspnea at rest and during exercise in COPD. *Chest* 2005; 128:640–650.

88. Garrod R, Dallimore K, Cook J *et al.* An evaluation of the acute impact of pursed lips breathing on walking distance in nonspontaneous pursed lips breathing chronic obstructive pulmonary disease patients. *Chron Respir Dis* 2005; 2:67–72.
89. Bianchi R, Gigliotti F, Romagnoli I *et al.* Chest wall kinematics and breathlessness during pursed-lip breathing in patients with COPD. *Chest* 2004; 125:459–465.
90. Solway S, Brooks D, Lau L *et al.* The short-term effect of a rollator on functional exercise capacity among individuals with severe COPD. *Chest* 2002; 122:56–65.
91. Probst V, Troosters T, Coosemans I *et al.* Mechanisms of improvement in exercise capacity using a rollator in COPD. *Chest* 2004; 126:1102–1107.
92. Quanjer PH, Tammeling GJ, Cotes JE *et al.* Lung volumes and forced ventilatory flows. Report Working Party Standardization of Lung Function Tests, European Community for Steel and Coal. Official Statement of the European Respiratory Society. *Eur Respir J Suppl* 1993; 16:5–40.
93. Rochester DF, Arora NS. Respiratory muscle failure. *Med Clin North Am* 1983; 67:573–597.
94. Mathiowetz V, Kashman N, Volland G *et al.* Grip and pinch strength: normative data for adults. *Arch Phys Med Rehabil* 1985; 66:69–74.
95. Jones NL, Makrides L, Hitchcock C *et al.* Normal standards for an incremental progressive cycle ergometer test. *Am Rev Respir Dis* 1985; 131:700–708.

8

Clinical approach to a COPD patient with muscle hypotrophy

F. De Benedetto, S. Marinari, E. F. M. Wouters

BACKGROUND

Chronic obstructive pulmonary disease (COPD) is a leading cause of mortality worldwide, with an increasing morbidity over the last year of life. There is an accumulating body of scientific evidence that documents the importance of body weight decrease and malnutrition as factors influencing the survival of these patients [1]. Therefore, recent guidelines on COPD management [2] include a chapter on 'nutrition' as one of the principal components of the disease and an important recent study shows the need for investigation of this component to better evaluate the prognosis of these patients [3].

The first observation of this phenomenon goes back to about 20 years, when some authors showed that in hospitalized and exacerbated COPD patients, many (40–60%) were underweight [4, 5]. Some years later, studies on large cohorts of COPD patients confirmed the presence of malnutrition in a stable phase of the disease, especially when severe [6, 7]. In a previous work, the authors have underlined the importance of estimating body composition, which can provide more information on the evaluation of lean body mass [8].

In fact, the diagnostic application of methods for evaluating body composition have allowed the identification, in these patients, of a decrease in fat-free mass (FFM) related to muscular mass loss, in the presence of normal body weight [8, 9].

A clear relationship between muscular mass loss and airway obstruction has not been demonstrated, although body weight loss and being underweight may be associated with emphysema and diffusing capacity reduction [10, 11], confirming the classic image of the so-called 'pink puffer', with peripheral skeletal muscle hypotrophy.

The main possible causes of malnutrition are:

- Inadequate energy and nutrient intake;
- Increased energy expenditure;
- Alteration of protein turnover.

Symptoms of COPD, in particular dyspnoea, could influence calorie intake through the limitation of diaphragm movement; therefore appetite sensation could be influenced by the low leptine levels observed in COPD patients [12], which correlate with an inflammatory pattern alteration.

Fernando De Benedetto, MD, Director, Department of Pneumology, San Camillo De Lellis Hospital, Chieti, Italy
Stefano Marinari, MD, Department of Pneumology, San Camillo De Lellis Hospital, Chieti, Italy
Emiel F. M. Wouters, MD, PhD, Professor of Medicine, University Hospital Maastricht, Department of Respiratory Medicine, Maastricht, The Netherlands

© Atlas Medical Publishing Ltd 2007

Moreover, some experimental studies [13] have shown an increase of activity-related energy expenditure that could explain body weight loss in the presence of adequate calorie intake.

Several recent studies, performed to investigate the role of chronic systemic inflammation, have demonstrated the influence of high levels of tumour necrosis factor alpha (TNFα) on protein turnover increase [14].

Agustí et al. [15] demonstrated that increased apoptosis occurs in the skeletal muscle of underweight COPD patients and that this may limit their exercise tolerance. Ageing, inactivity due to the limited exercise tolerance, arterial hypoxaemia, smoking history and steroid-induced myopathy have all been advocated as possible causes of apoptosis, but none of them appears to be the actual or potential trigger. Other mechanisms could be postulated, such as oxidative stress, systemic inflammation and mitochondrial abnormalities. With regard to this theory, structural and biochemical alterations of peripheral muscles, such as decreased mitochondrial number, size and function, faster glycogen utilization with lactic acid production and slower metabolism of free fatty acid were demonstrated [16]. In addition, it is possible to hypothesize damage due to the metabolic alteration caused by a chronically reduced oxygen supply to the exercising muscles as a result of reduced arterial oxygen content and inadequate cardiovascular adaptation.

Pharmacological influences may also have an influence on muscular hypotrophy. In particular, chronic systemic steroid therapy, taken continuously or in cycles during disease exacerbations, could result in acute myopathy with rhabdomyolysis and/or chronic muscular damage with muscular cell type IIB atrophy [17] and probably muscular energy reduction with an imbalance between glycolitic and oxidative metabolism [18].

The more evident consequences of body weight loss and muscle wasting are:

- Increased dyspnoea;
- Reduced exercise capacity;
- Worsening of quality of life (QoL).

It has already been established that, in COPD patients, a significant correlation exists between nutritional status and exercise tolerance. This correlation was demonstrated both through the walking test and respiratory effort test. In line with this, several studies have demonstrated that the biochemical and structural alterations of muscles can negatively influence muscular effort and maximal and submaximal exercise capacity [19, 20].

Finally, it is well-known that a worsening nutritional status can influence immunological function by compromising cell-mediated immunity. Moreover, a relevant cause of immunodepression in COPD patients is the alteration of antibacterial pulmonary phagocytosis with reduced activation of lymphocytes and macrophages. The increase in the number and intensity of exacerbations seems to be associated with the involvement of inflammatory mediators – for instance, C-reactive protein and body mass index (BMI) may predict outcome in end-stage respiratory failure [21].

CASE REPORT

A 69-year-old man was admitted to the Rehabilitation Unit because of severe dyspnoea and peripheral muscular weakness. He had no cough or variation in sputum in the last month. The increase in dyspnoea had been gradual, but in the last months, it had reduced the patient to a sedentary lifestyle, with a consequent marked worsening of his QoL.

The patient was a textile dealer and had a history of heavy smoking until 10 years ago (30 pack-years). The first diagnosis of COPD was 20 years earlier when he was submitted for respiratory functional evaluation because of exertional dyspnoea. In recent years, he had noticed a progression of dyspnoea induced by only mild effort.

His body weight had gradually decreased (by about 4 kg in the last 2 years) and in the last few months he had shown a progressive reduction of peripheral muscle strength. In the last 2 years, he had been hospitalized five times because of COPD exacerbations. During the last hospitalization, about 2 months ago, he received treatment with oxygen because of severe respiratory failure but this therapy was interrupted at discharge.

The patient had a long history of arterial hypertension and parossistic episodes of atrial fibrillation with two consequent hospitalizations. Previous cardiac therapy, including amiodarone, had resulted in a thyroid disease with hormone dysfunction. For this reason, amiodarone had been discontinued 6 months ago and replaced with verapamil. Recurrent atrial fibrillation episodes have also resulted in the discontinuation of treatment with formoterol.

BASIC DIAGNOSTIC ASSESSMENT

At the general physical examination, the patient showed a significant reduction of muscular mass, especially in the periphery. Body weight was 57 kg and height was 1.72 m (BMI = 19 kg/m^2).

Thoracic examination showed a severe reduction of vesicular murmur and diffuse hypertympanic sounds on percussion. No signs of exacerbation were observed. Cardiac examination showed a normal rhythm with a pulse of 86 bpm, and blood pressure was 140/80 mmHg.

Laboratory tests performed at hospital admission showed normal values for liver and kidney function, ESR, urine analysis and serum electrolytes with a slight reduction in serum proteins. Blood cell count showed a slight increase in the red cell count and haematocrit. Thyroid hormone evaluation and thyroid stimulating hormone level were normal.

An electrocardiogram showed a sinus rhythm with left ventricular hypertrophy and right bundle-branch block.

Chest radiography showed a thoracic hyperinflation with increased retrosternal airspace. A specimen of arterial blood showed: PaO_2 = 66.2 mmHg, $PaCO_2$ = 41.7 mmHg, pH = 7.410 and O_2 saturation = 93%.

The patient was also submitted for lung function testing. Resting complete lung function testing values showed severe pulmonary obstruction (FEV_1 = 25% of predicted value; FEV_1/FVC = 33%) with severe hyperinflation (TLC = 98% of predicted value; RV = 157% of predicted value) and severe reduction of respiratory muscle strength (MIP = 38 cmH$_2$O, MEP = 39 cmH$_2$O). DLCO value was decreased with slight reduction of DLCO/VA (DLCO = 12.1 ml/min/mmHg; DLCO/VA = 3.25, 67% of the predicted value). The main functional characteristics are reported in Table 8.1.

Because of the low BMI, measurements of body composition were also carried out to provide a means of estimating protein calorie malnutrition, if present. Bioelectrical impedance analysis demonstrated a marked lean body mass loss, expressed by a decreased body cellular mass (BCM) and phase angle (PA)[22] (Table 8.2).

Thus, to overcome problems associated with hypermetabolism, which could be responsible for the body weight loss, an estimation of energy requirements was performed by means of the assessment of resting energy expenditure (REE) by indirect calorimetry. This showed increased values (REE = 1600 kg/day).

Exercise capacity tests were performed by means of the 6-minute walk test (6MWT), which showed a marked reduction of the distance walked: after 140 m in 3 min, the test was interrupted because of marked dyspnoea and oxygen desaturation (O_2 at 95% at baseline compared with 86% at the end of the test). The MRC scale showed elevated resting values (degree 1) that worsened at the end of the test to degree 4.

In addition, evaluation of QoL by means of the St George's Respiratory Questionnaire was performed. The global score of 84.6 was evidence of a poor lifestyle.

Table 8.1 Main functional characteristics of patient

PaO$_2$ (mmHg)	PaCO$_2$ (mmHg)	FEV$_1$ (% predicted)	TLC (% predicted)	VR (% predicted)	MIP (cmH$_2$O)	MEP (cmH$_2$O)	DLCO (ml/min/mmHg)
66.2	41.7	25	98	157	38	39	12.1

Table 8.2 Results of anthropometric measurement and bioimpedance analysis

BMI	FM (%)	FFM (%)	BCM (%)	PA (°)
19	35.5	64.5	32.8	4.2

BCM = body cellular mass (normal value = 40–49%); BMI = body mass index (normal = 18.5–25 kg/m^2); FFM = fat-free mass (normal value = 69–78%); FM = fat mass (normal value = 22–31%); PA = phase angle (normal value = 6–8°).

DIFFERENTIAL DIAGNOSIS

The clinical history of this patient is typical: progressive body weight decrease and expression of protein calorie malnutrition characterized by muscular hypotrophy. This condition is often the result of the expected disequilibrium between metabolic requirements and energy expenditure. Moreover, it is generally present in several wasting diseases, such as heart, liver and kidney failure, hormonal diseases, severe infectious disease (e.g. HIV), cancer or prolonged periods of complete physical inactivity, especially if calorie intake is diminished, as in ageing. These conditions had all been excluded on the basis of the global clinical evaluation of the patient, except for the history of amiodarone-induced thyroid hyperfunction that may have contributed to body weight loss due to a hypermetabolic state.

TREATMENT

The patient's therapy included:

1. Confirmation of the previous pharmacological treatment of the respiratory disease.
2. Nutritional management with a dietary regimen of at least an additional 800 kcal, calculated on the basis of energy requirements (2200 kcal in total; carbohydrate 50–55%; protein 15–20%; fat 25–30%).
3. Eventual administration of anabolic steroids (nandrolone decanoate) for 8 weeks.
4. A 1-month intensive rehabilitation programme followed by 3 days/week of physical training.

Thyroid function monitoring was also recommended.

After 4 months, although significant variations of the respiratory function and arterial blood gases (ABGs) were not evidenced, the patient nevertheless perceived a notable improvement in his dyspnoea at rest and a global sense of well-being. The nutritional evaluation showed an increase of body weight (61 kg; BMI = 20.6 kg/m^2) accompanied by a restoration of FFM, PA and BCM.

The full 6MWT was completed, with a net increase in the distance walked (240 m), but no improvement in the exercise-induced oxygen saturation (81% at 6 min).

DISCUSSION

This case report clearly illustrates the challenges in the daily management of COPD patients that need to be met in order to improve health and functional status. Involuntary weight loss always has to be considered an alarming signal in the clinical course of COPD. The criteria commonly used to define such weight loss are a weight loss greater than 10% of the normal 'habitual' weight in the past 6 months or greater than 5% within the last month. It should be noted, however, that any period of involuntary weight loss that cannot be attributed to daily fluctuations should be taken into consideration.

The assessment of BMI is the simplest mode of nutritional screening. Based on the BMI, patients are divided into underweight (BMI $< 21\,kg/m^2$; age > 50 years), normal weight (BMI of 21–$25\,kg/m^2$) and overweight (BMI of 25–$30\,kg/m^2$). Our patient is therefore clearly at risk! Indeed, survival studies in selected groups of patients with COPD and in population-based studies have consistently shown higher COPD-related mortality rates in underweight and normal weight patients than in overweight and even obese patients [1, 23, 24]. This relation is different from the U-shaped survival curve that is commonly reported for BMI in larger population-based studies. This discrepancy can be attributed to the specific adverse effects of an excess of metabolically and functionally active FFM on mortality in these patients that is not reflected in the BMI. Previous studies have already reported that a small mid-thigh cross-sectional area, as measured by computed tomography scanning, is associated with increased mortality risk [25]. Others reported that FFM provides information to assist prognosis beyond that provided by BMI: FFM was found to be an independent predictor of survival in a large group of clinically stable COPD patients admitted to a rehabilitation program [26]. Other studies have also demonstrated that depletion of FFM is a common problem in COPD – about 25% of clinically stable COPD patients demonstrate a marked loss of muscle mass [27]. The assessment of BMI and particularly FFM should therefore be integrated into the work-up of *every* COPD patient. Assessment of body composition can be very helpful in understanding peripheral and respiratory muscle weakness [28, 29], exercise capacity [30, 31] and reduced health status [32]. Others have reported an associated loss of FFM and bone mineral density in COPD patients [33].

Weight loss and, particularly, loss of fat mass, occurs if energy expenditure exceeds a patient's dietary intake. More specifically, muscle wasting itself is a consequence of an imbalance between protein synthesis and protein breakdown. Impairments in total energy balance and protein metabolism may occur simultaneously, but these processes can also be dissociated. In the case reported in this chapter, an increase in REE was found. It is important for clinical practice to be aware that total energy expenditure can be divided into three components:

1. REE.
2. Diet-induced thermogenesis.
3. Physical activity-induced thermogenesis.

Many reports have focused on REE measurements in COPD. Besides the established role of systemic inflammation, the work of breathing is evaluated as a possible factor contributing to the increase in REE [34–37]. Recent studies have focused attention on the activity-related energy expenditure in patients with COPD. It has been demonstrated that, particularly in these patients, the activity-related energy expenditure is increased [13]. Several factors may account for these changes. Part of the increased oxygen consumption during exercise may be related to inefficient ventilation in the presence of increased ventilatory demand, especially under conditions of dynamic hyperinflation [38]. Furthermore, inefficient muscle metabolism may contribute to an increase in activity-related energy expenditure. Besides disturbances in energy balance, several studies have provided evidence for the involvement of inflammatory processes in the pathogenesis of tissue depletion [39–43].

Considering energy imbalance in the pathogenesis of weight loss in COPD patients, restoration of this energy equilibrium has to be considered as a first step in the management of these patients.

The first clinical trials investigating the effectiveness of nutritional intervention consisted of nutritional supplementation by means of oral liquid supplements or enteral nutrition. All short-term studies [44, 45] of 2–3 weeks' duration showed a significant increase in body weight and respiratory muscle function. This short-term effectiveness is probably partly related to repletion of muscle water, electrolytes and cellular energy states besides reconstitution of muscle protein nitrogen. Only one study addressed the immune response to short-term nutritional intervention in nine patients with advanced COPD [46]. Refeeding and weight gain were associated with a significant increase in absolute lymphocyte count and with an increase in reactivity to skin test antigens after 21 days of refeeding.

Significant improvements not only in respiratory and peripheral skeletal muscle function, but also in exercise capacity and health-related QoL, were observed in one in-patient [47] and one out-patient [48] study after 3 months of oral supplementation (by approximately 1000 kcal daily). In other out-patient studies, however, despite a similar nutritional supplementation regimen, the average weight gain was less than 1.5 kg in 8 weeks [49, 50]. Besides non-compliance and biological characteristics, the poor treatment response may be attributed at least partly to the inadequate initial assessment of energy requirements and to the observation that the patients were taking supplements instead of their regular meals. Despite the positive outcome of nutritional supplementation in a controlled setting, the progressive character of weight loss in COPD demands appropriate feeding strategies to allow sustained out-patient nutritional intervention.

From a functional point of view, we have advocated combining nutritional support with an anabolic stimulus. The effects of a daily nutritional supplement as an integrated part of a pulmonary rehabilitation programme indeed resulted in significant weight gain (0.4 kg/week), despite a daily supplementation level which was much less than in most previous out-patient studies [51]. The combination of nutritional support and exercise not only increased body weight, but also resulted in a significant improvement of FFM and respiratory muscle strength [51]. The clinical relevance of the response to treatment was shown in a *post hoc* survival analysis of this study, which demonstrated that weight gain and an increase in respiratory muscle strength were associated with significantly increased survival rates [1].

From a practical point of view, nutritional supplementation should be considered in specific subgroups of COPD patients, namely weight-losing patients, particularly those who are underweight or have a normal body weight, and patients with a depletion in FFM. Nutritional intervention should initially consist of adaptations of the patient's normal dietary habits.

Nutritional support should be given as energy-dense supplements well divided during the day to avoid loss of appetite and adverse metabolic and ventilatory efforts resulting from a high caloric load. It was long believed that, due to their ventilatory limitation, patients with respiratory disease should consume a fat-rich diet to decrease their carbon dioxide load, but scientific evidence of this is scarce and unconvincing. More recent reports show that patients experience less dyspnoea after a liquid carbohydrate-rich supplement compared to an equicaloric fat-rich supplement [52]. This may not be surprising since gastric emptying time is significantly higher after an equicaloric fat-rich than a carbohydrate-rich supplement [53]. Furthermore, it has been found that the reduced dietary intake of COPD patients during the acute phase of an exacerbation is characterized by a restricted fat intake. Based on data in other chronic wasting conditions, daily protein intake should be at least 1.5 mg/kg body weight to allow optimal protein synthesis. Where feasible, patients should participate in an exercise programme in order to stimulate an anabolic response rather than fat storage. In view of the adverse effects of inactivity and the pulmonary limitations on exercise capacity, most exercise programmes consist predominantly of endurance training. However, since nutritional depletion affects muscle strength at least as much as endurance, a combination of endurance and strength training may be particularly effective in depleted COPD patients. For the severely depleted patients unable to perform exercise training, even simple strength manoeuvres combined with activities of daily living training and energy conservation techniques may be effective. Exercise not only improves the effectiveness of nutritional therapy, but also stimulates appetite. If weight gain and functional improvement occur, therapy is continued or moved to a maintenance regimen. If the desired response is not seen, it may be necessary to identify compliance issues. If compliance is not the problem, more calories may be needed *via* supplements or by enteral routes. Nevertheless, one should recognize that, even then, some patients may not show the intended improvements due to underlying mechanisms of weight loss that are unable to be reversed merely by caloric supplementation.

The difficulties encountered in nutritional support have led investigators to study alternative methods, in particular adjuvant treatment with recombinant human growth hormone (rhGH). Administration of this hormone induces lipolysis, protein anabolism and muscle growth, either directly or through insulin-like growth factor-1. Two uncontrolled studies reported the effects of rhGH in nutritionally-depleted patients with COPD [54, 55]. Administration of rhGH for 8 days (0.03 mg/kg/day subcutaneously for 4 days, then 0.06 mg/kg/day for another 4 days) failed to increase respiratory and peripheral skeletal muscle strength in COPD patients. In contrast, an increase in inspiratory muscle strength was reported after 3 weeks of treatment with rhGH (0.05 mg/kg/day subcutaneously). Using a similar treatment regimen but in a placebo-controlled fashion, the effects of administration of rhGH on body composition, resting metabolic rate and functional capacity in underweight COPD patients in a stable clinical condition were studied [56]. Although FFM increased significantly during the 3-week treatment period, no improvement was seen in muscle function and exercise capacity and it even decreased in the treatment group. Furthermore, a significant increase in the resting metabolic rate was observed. The effects of anabolic steroids have been investigated as adjuvant therapy in COPD. Nutritional repletion in combination with supportive treatment with the anabolic steroid nandrolone decanoate (males 50 mg i.m. every 2 weeks; females 25 mg i.m. every 2 weeks) was studied for 8 weeks in patients undergoing an in-patient pulmonary rehabilitation programme [51]. Despite weight gains similar to the group receiving nutritional support only, measurements of body composition indicated a favourable distribution of the body weight gain toward a larger increase in FFM and a larger improvement in respiratory muscle strength in the group additionally treated with a short course of anabolic steroids.

SUMMARY

In summary, despite the variable results of clinical trials of nutritional supplementation in COPD, the adverse effects of weight loss on exercise tolerance, health status and mortality are such that, at the very least, efforts to prevent weight loss are warranted in the routine management of patients with COPD. Assessment of muscle mass or FFM should be part of the evaluation of all patients suffering from COPD, and stimulation of the skeletal muscles has to be an important part in the optimal management of these patients.

REFERENCES

1. Schols AM, Slangen J, Volovics L, Wouters EF. Weight loss is a reversible factor in the prognosis of chronic obstructive pulmonary disease. *Am J Respir Crit Care Med* 1998; 157:1791–1797.
2. Celli BR, MacNee W. Standards for the diagnosis and treatment of patients with COPD: a summary of the ATS/ERS position paper. *Eur Respir J* 2004; 23:932–946.
3. Celli BR, Cote CG, Marin JM *et al*. The body-mass index, airflow obstruction, dyspnea, and exercise capacity index in chronic obstructive pulmonary disease. *N Engl J Med* 2004; 350:1005–1012.

4. Hunter AM, Carey MA, Larsh HW. The nutritional status of patients with chronic obstructive pulmonary disease. *Am Rev Respir Dis* 1981; 124:376–381.
5. Driver AG, McAlevy MT, Smith JL. Nutritional assessment of patients with chronic obstructive pulmonary disease and acute respiratory failure. *Chest* 1982; 82:568–571.
6. De Benedetto F, Bitti G, D'Intino D, Marinari S, Del Ponte A. Body weight alone is not an index of nutritional imbalance in the natural course of chronic obstructive lung disease. *Monaldi Arch Chest Dis* 1993; 48:541–542.
7. Schols AM, Soeters PB, Dingemans AM, Mostert R, Frantzen PJ, Wouters EF. Prevalence and characteristics of nutritional depletion in patients with stable COPD eligible for pulmonary rehabilitation. *Am Rev Respir Dis* 1993; 147:1151–1156.
8. De Benedetto F, Cervone L, Cisternino R et al. Nutritional status in severe COPD: traditional and new methods in the field assessment. *World Congress on Home Care* 1989.
9. De Benedetto F, Del Ponte A, Marinari S. In COPD patients body weight excess can mask lean tissue depletion: a simple method of estimation. *Monaldi Arch Chest* 2000; 55:273–278.
10. Engelen MP, Schols AM, Lamers RJ, Wouters EF. Different patterns of chronic tissue wasting among patients with chronic obstructive pulmonary disease. *Clin Nutr* 1999; 18:275–280.
11. Engelen MP, Schols AM, Baken WC, Wesseling GJ, Wouters EF. Nutritional depletion in relation to respiratory and peripheral skeletal muscle function in out-patients with COPD. *Eur Respir J* 1994; 7:1793–1797.
12. Takabatake N, Nakamura H, Abe S et al. Circulating leptin in patients with chronic obstructive pulmonary disease. *Am J Respir Crit Care Med* 1999; 159:1215–1219.
13. Baarends EM, Schols AM, Pannemans DL, Westerterp KR, Wouters EF. Total free living energy expenditure in patients with severe chronic obstructive pulmonary disease. *Am J Respir Crit Care Med* 1997; 155:549–554.
14. Debigare R, Cote CH, Maltais F. Peripheral muscle wasting in chronic obstructive pulmonary disease. Clinical relevance and mechanisms. *Am J Respir Crit Care Med* 2001; 164:1712–1717.
15. Agustí AG, Sauleda J, Miralles C et al. Skeletal muscle apoptosis and weight loss in chronic obstructive pulmonary disease. *Am J Respir Crit Care Med* 2002; 166:485–489.
16. Holloszy JO, Coyle EF. Adaptations of skeletal muscle to endurance exercise and their metabolic consequences. *J Appl Physiol* 1984; 56:831–838.
17. van Balkom RH, van der Heijden HF, van Herwaarden CL, Dekhuijzen PN. Corticosteroid-induced myopathy of the respiratory muscles. *Neth J Med* 1994; 45:114–122.
18. Koerts-de Lang E, Schols AM, Rooyackers OE, Gayan-Ramirez G, Decramer M, Wouters EF. Different effects of corticosteroid-induced muscle wasting compared with undernutrition on rat diaphragm energy metabolism. *Eur J Appl Physiol* 2000; 82:493–498.
19. Schols AM, Mostert R, Soeters PB, Wouters EF. Body composition and exercise performance in patients with chronic obstructive pulmonary disease. *Thorax* 1991; 46:695–699.
20. Palange P, Forte S, Onorati P et al. Effect of reduced body weight on muscle aerobic capacity in patients with COPD. *Chest* 1998; 114:12–18.
21. Cano NJ, Pichard C, Roth H et al. C-reactive protein and body mass index predict outcome in end-stage respiratory failure. *Chest* 2004; 126:540–546.
22. Savino F, Cresi F, Grasso G, Oggero R, Silvestro L. The Biagram vector: a graphical relation between reactance and phase angle measured by bioelectrical analysis in infants. *Ann Nutr Metab* 2004; 48:84–89.
23. Landbo C, Prescott E, Lange P, Vestbo J, Almdal TP. Prognostic value of nutritional status in chronic obstructive pulmonary disease. *Am J Respir Crit Care Med* 1999; 160:1856–1861.
24. Gray Donald K, Gibbons L, Shapiro SH, Macklem PT, Martin JG. Nutritional status and mortality in chronic obstructive pulmonary disease. *Am J Respir Crit Care Med* 1996; 153:961–966.
25. Marquis K, Debigare R, Lacasse Y et al. Midthigh muscle cross-sectional area is a better predictor of mortality than body mass index in patients with chronic obstructive pulmonary disease. *Am J Respir Crit Care Med* 2002; 166:809–813.
26. Schols AM, Broekhuizen R, Weling-Scheepers CA, Wouters EF. Body composition and mortality in chronic obstructive pulmonary disease. *Am J Clin Nutr* 2005; 82:53–59.
27. Vermeeren M, Creutzberg E, Schols A et al. Prevalence of nutritional depletion in a large out-patient population of patients with COPD. *Respir Med* 2006; 100:1349–1355.
28. Engelen MP, Schols AM, Does JD, Wouters EF. Skeletal muscle weakness is associated with wasting of extremity fat-free mass but not with airflow obstruction in patients with chronic obstructive pulmonary disease. *Am J Clin Nutr* 2000; 71:733–738.

29. Gosker HR, Lencer NH, Franssen FM, van der Vusse GJ, Wouters EF, Schols AM. Striking similarities in systemic factors contributing to decreased exercise capacity in patients with severe chronic heart failure or COPD. *Chest* 2003; 123:1416–1424.
30. Baarends EM, Schols AM, Mostert R, Wouters EF. Peak exercise response in relation to tissue depletion in patients with chronic obstructive pulmonary disease. *Eur Respir J* 1997; 10:2807–2813.
31. Palange P, Forte S, Felli A, Galassetti P, Serra P, Carlone S. Nutritional state and exercise tolerance in patients with COPD. *Chest* 1995; 107:1206–1212.
32. Mostert R, Goris A, Weling-Scheepers C, Wouters EF, Schols AM. Tissue depletion and health related quality of life in patients with chronic obstructive pulmonary disease. *Respir Med* 2000; 94:859–867.
33. Bolton CE, Ionescu AA, Shiels KM *et al*. Associated loss of fat-free mass and bone mineral density in chronic obstructive pulmonary disease. *Am J Respir Crit Care Med* 2004; 170:1286–1293.
34. Jounieaux V, Mayeux I. Oxygen cost of breathing in patients with emphysema or chronic bronchitis in acute respiratory failure [see comments]. *Am J Respir Crit Care Med* 1995; 152:2181–2184.
35. Hamilton AL, Killian KJ, Summers E, Jones NL. Muscle strength, symptom intensity, and exercise capacity in patients with cardiorespiratory disorders. *Am J Respir Crit Care Med* 1995; 152:2021–2031.
36. Baarends EM, Schols AM, Nusmeier CM, van der Grinten CP, Wouters EF. Breathing efficiency during inspiratory threshold loading in patients with chronic obstructive pulmonary disease. *Clin Physiol* 1998; 18:235–244.
37. Sridhar MK, Carter R, Lean ME, Banham SW. Resting energy expenditure and nutritional state of patients with increased oxygen cost of breathing due to emphysema, scoliosis and thoracoplasty. *Thorax* 1994; 49:781–785.
38. Baarends EM, Schols AM, Akkermans MA, Wouters EF. Decreased mechanical efficiency in clinically stable patients with COPD. *Thorax* 1997; 52:981–986.
39. Di Francia M, Barbier D, Mege JL, Orehek J. Tumor necrosis factor-alpha levels and weight loss in chronic obstructive pulmonary disease. *Am J Respir Crit Care Med* 1994; 150:1453–1455.
40. Godoy de I, Donahoe M, Calhoun WJ, Mancino J, Rogers RM. Elevated TNF-alpha production by peripheral blood monocytes of weight-losing COPD patients. *Am J Respir Crit Care Med* 1996; 153:633–637.
41. Nguyen LT, Bedu M, Caillaud D *et al*. Increased resting energy expenditure is related to plasma TNF-alpha concentration in stable COPD patients. *Clin Nutr* 1999; 18:269–274.
42. Schols AM, Buurman WA, Staal van den Brekel AJ, Dentener MA, Wouters EF. Evidence for a relation between metabolic derangements and increased levels of inflammatory mediators in a subgroup of patients with chronic obstructive pulmonary disease. *Thorax* 1996; 51:819–824.
43. Eid AA, Ionescu AA, Nixon LS *et al*. Inflammatory response and body composition in chronic obstructive pulmonary disease. *Am J Respir Crit Care Med* 2001; 164:1414–1418.
44. Whittaker JS, Ryan CF, Buckley PA, Road JD. The effects of refeeding on peripheral and respiratory muscle function in malnourished chronic obstructive pulmonary disease patients. *Am Rev Respir Dis* 1990; 142:283–288.
45. Wilson DO, Rogers RM, Sanders MH, Pennock BE, Reilly JJ. Nutritional intervention in malnourished patients with emphysema. *Am Rev Respir Dis* 1986; 134:672–677.
46. Fuenzalida CE, Petty TL, Jones ML *et al*. The immune response to short-term nutritional intervention in advanced chronic obstructive pulmonary disease. *Am Rev Respir Dis* 1990; 142:49–56.
47. Rogers RM, Donahoe M, Costantino J. Physiologic effects of oral supplemental feeding in malnourished patients with chronic obstructive pulmonary disease. A randomized control study. *Am Rev Respir Dis* 1992; 146:1511–1517.
48. Efthimiou J, Fleming J, Gomes C, Spiro SG. The effect of supplementary oral nutrition in poorly nourished patients with chronic obstructive pulmonary disease. *Am Rev Respir Dis* 1988; 137:1075–1082.
49. Knowles JB, Fairbarn MS, Wiggs BJ, Chan-Yan C, Pardy RL. Dietary supplementation and respiratory muscle performance in patients with COPD. *Chest* 1988; 93:977–983.
50. Otte KE, Ahlburg P, D'Amore F, Stellfeld M. Nutritional repletion in malnourished patients with emphysema. *JPEN J Parenter Enteral Nutr* 1989; 13:152–156.
51. Schols AM, Soeters PB, Mostert R, Pluymers RJ, Wouters EF. Physiologic effects of nutritional support and anabolic steroids in patients with chronic obstructive pulmonary disease. A placebo-controlled randomized trial. *Am J Respir Crit Care Med* 1995; 152:1268–1274.
52. Vermeeren MAP, Wouters EFM, Geraerts-Keeris AJW, Schols AMWJ. Nutritional support in patients with chronic obstructive pulmonary disease during hospitalization for an acute exacerbation; a randomized controlled feasibility trial. *Clin Nutr* 2004; 23:1184–1192.

53. Akrabawi SS, Mobarhan S, Stoltz RR, Ferguson PW. Gastric emptying, pulmonary function, gas exchange, and respiratory quotient after feeding a moderate versus high fat enteral formula meal in chronic obstructive pulmonary disease patients. *Nutrition* 1996; 12:260–265.
54. Pape GS, Friedman M, Underwood LE, Clemmons DR. The effect of growth hormone on weight gain and pulmonary function in patients with chronic obstructive lung disease. *Chest* 1991; 99:1495–1500.
55. Suchner U, Rothkopf MM, Stanislaus G, Elwyn DH, Kvetan V, Askanazi J. Growth hormone and pulmonary disease. Metabolic effects in patients receiving parenteral nutrition. *Arch Intern Med* 1990; 150:1225–1230.
56. Burdet L, de Muralt B, Schutz Y, Pichard C, Fitting JW. Administration of growth hormone to underweight patients with chronic obstructive pulmonary disease. A prospective, randomized, controlled study. *Am J Respir Crit Care Med* 1997; 156:1800–1806.

9

Improvement of function and health status in a severely disabled patient with COPD

P. W. Jones, M. Rosa Güell Rous

BACKGROUND

The position paper of the American Thoracic Society and the European Respiratory Society (ATS/ERS) defines chronic obstructive pulmonary disease (COPD) as a preventable, treatable disease state characterized by an airflow limitation that is not fully reversible. The airflow limitation is usually progressive and is associated with an abnormal inflammatory response of the lungs to noxious particles and gases, mainly cigarette smoke [1].

The clinical expression of these pathophysiological changes is mucus hypersecretion, airflow limitation, lung overinflation, gas exchange abnormalities, pulmonary hypertension and systemic effects such as cachexia, loss of lean body mass, and disturbances of mood state. The systemic consequences that lead to muscle wasting and fatigue are now recognized to be very important. Superimposed on these chronic changes are the acute changes associated with an exacerbation, which appear to be more frequent in patients with severe airway obstruction [2].

Cough with chronic sputum expectoration are the characteristic features of the chronic bronchitis element of COPD, but the most important symptoms are breathlessness and fatigue. Whilst breathlessness is a very well-known characteristic of COPD, fatigue may be frequently as important [3, 4]. The consequent loss of autonomy and severe level of disability have a major impact on the patient's Health-Related Quality of Life (HRQoL) and lead to a growing dependence on health services.

COPD has a progressive and insidious course, and it is frequently not diagnosed until the disease is quite advanced. The diagnosis is suspected from the clinical history – a smoker or ex-smoker with a history of at least 10 pack-years (20 cigarettes a day for 10 years) who nearly always has a chronic cough with or without expectoration, and dyspnoea. There may be a history of episodes of bronchial infection. The dyspnoea is usually of progressive onset and, even in patients who present for the first time with an acute exacerbation, there will always be a history (for at least 2 years) of breathlessness on hills, stairs, or when hurrying on the level. The diagnosis is confirmed using spirometry, but whilst the FEV_1 plays a central role in the diagnosis of COPD, and is used in staging of the disease, it is only weakly related to impaired health and physical disability. Most classifications of COPD depend on the severity of airway obstruction [1, 5–8], but the recognition that other effects in COPD are

---

Paul W. Jones, PhD, FRCP, Department of Respiratory Medicine, St George's Hospital Medical School, London, UK
M. Rosa Güell Rous, MD, Department of Pneumology, Hospital de la Santa Creu i Sant Pau, Barcelona, Spain

© Atlas Medical Publishing Ltd 2007

equally important has led to the development of a multidimensional grading system (the BODE index) that assesses both the respiratory and systemic expression of COPD in order to improve classification, and to predict outcome [8]. This index is a more accurate predictor of risk of death than the FEV_1.

COPD is a progressive disease, even in patients who stop smoking. In people with COPD who continue to smoke, the FEV_1 declines typically by 60 ml/year. In ex-smokers it is lower than this, but does not return to the level of decline of people who have never smoked. This picture is derived from studies in populations of patients, but in individuals (even smokers with COPD) the rate of decline is too low, relative to the repeatability of the measurement, to detect changes in individual patients, unless these are carried out over several years. In patients treated with short-acting bronchodilators, health status has been reported to deteriorate by a clinically significant amount every 14 months [9]. This level of deterioration in health status score is detectable by patients and physicians [10]. It appears that, unlike FEV_1, progression of symptomatic deterioration may be detectable in individual patients over a period of 1–2 years.

The reasons for the progressive deterioration in health are not fully understood, but FEV_1 decline is a factor, as is the frequency of exacerbations. These may have complex effects. It is known that health status takes many weeks to recover following a single exacerbation, even in patients who have not been admitted to hospital [11]. Some patients appear to recover lung function incompletely following an exacerbation [12], and there is some evidence that frequent exacerbations may be associated with faster loss of FEV_1. However the major impact of exacerbations may be through effects on muscle function. Quadriceps weakness is known to occur following an exacerbation, probably through a cytokine-mediated action, but disuse atrophy of muscles may occur due to the prolonged period of reduced activity that is now known to occur following an exacerbation [12]. Exacerbations are reported more frequently in patients with more severe airways obstruction [2], although it is not yet known whether this apparent increase is due to more exacerbations *per se* or to the fact that increased severity of airways obstruction makes the patient more likely to seek medical attention.

A picture of COPD is emerging in which there is a progressive cycle of decline, particularly involving exacerbations and exercise capacity (Figure 9.1). This suggests that careful attention should be paid to rehabilitation, exacerbation prevention, and treatment of acute exacerbations to speed recovery during the acute phase and then during the recovery phase.

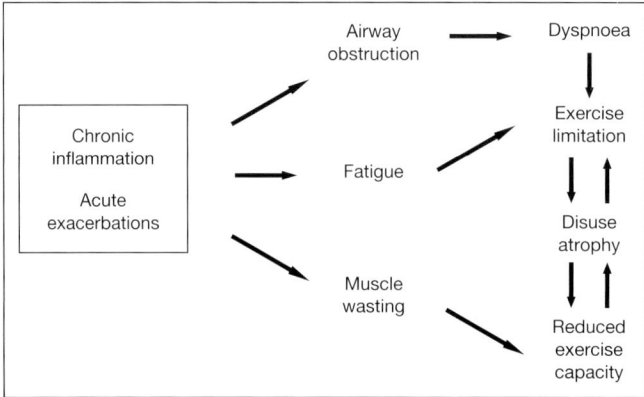

Figure 9.1 Pathways in COPD that lead to progressive decline in exercise capacity.

CASE REPORT

A 62-year-old male with progressive dyspnoea was sent to the referral hospital to participate in a pulmonary rehabilitation (PR) programme, 1 month after a severe exacerbation due to respiratory infection. On presentation with that exacerbation he had respiratory failure (PaO_2: 56 mmHg and $PaCO_2$: 45 mmHg) and required hospitalization. He was discharged home on continuous treatment with a long-acting β_2-agonist, tiotropium and inhaled corticosteroids (ICSs).

At his assessment for rehabilitation, he was found to be an ex-smoker of 50 packs of cigarettes per year, but had stopped smoking 1 year ago. He had a 10-year history of daily morning cough and sputum production. Over the last 2 years, he had developed slowly worsening dyspnoea and at the time of examination he was unable to walk quickly or climb more than one flight of stairs. He also reported one or two exacerbations of symptoms each winter, with increased sputum production of a deep yellow colour, together with wheezing and dyspnoea.

Physical examination revealed a patient with shortness of breath, increase in the respiratory muscle work, pursed-lips breathing and neck vein distention. Pulmonary auscultation revealed decreased breath sounds and expiratory wheezes. His pulse was regular. He had hepatomegaly of 3 cm and leg oedema was also observed. His Medical Research Council (MRC) Scale dyspnoea grade was 3.

Chest radiology showed overinflation of lungs with flattening of diaphragmatic domes, enlarged hilar pulmonary arteries, and no cardiomegaly. The computed tomography (CT) scan revealed centrolobular emphysema signs with overinflation and small areas of abnormally low attenuation near the vessels in the centre of the secondary lung lobules. It also revealed enlarged, pulmonary arteries, and bronchial dilatations and cystic spaces on the lower lobules of both lungs, suggesting bronchiectasis.

Laboratory tests showed glycaemia of 150 mmol/l, haematocrit 55% and haemoglobin 17 dl/g. All other parameters were within the normal range.

The electrocardiogram showed an atrial rhythm, a right axis deviation and a P wave of 2.5 mm. The echocardiogram demonstrated a left ventricle and left atrial of normal size and function, and the ejection fraction was 65%. The right ventricle was dilated and pulmonary arterial pressure was slightly increased with a value of 50 mmHg.

Pulmonary function tests showed a severe airflow limitation with a forced vital capacity (FVC) of 2.89 l (71% of predicted normal), FEV_1 of 0.63 l (22% of predicted normal) and FEV_1/FVC of 22%. The FEV_1 increased by 14% with bronchodilator. His lung volumes showed air trapping with a residual volume (RV) of 3.85 l (180% of predicted normal), TLC of 6.74 l (118% of predicted normal), RV/TLC of 57% and a slight decrease in the transfer factor for carbon monoxide (66% of predicted normal) with a DL/VA of 80% of the reference value. Arterial blood gases showed a mild hypoxaemia with normocapnia: $PaO_2 = 67$ mmHg; $PaCO_2 = 44$ mmHg; pH = 7.38 and a slight increase in the alveolar–arterial difference: $P(A-a)O_2 = 30.5$ mmHg.

He walked 240 m during the 6-min walk test. Dyspnoea during exercise was assessed using the Borg scale and increased from 2 at rest to 8 at the end of exercise.

Assessment of health status using the St George's Respiratory Questionnaire (SGRQ) showed a significant impairment of health status; 16.5 units in the symptom domain, 53.6 units in the activity domain, 34.2 units in impacts and a total score of 37.2 units.

The patient participated in a multidisciplinary rehabilitation programme in a group with five other patients. They received education sessions, chest physiotherapy and muscular training. Education sessions consisted of two 45–60-min sessions conducted by the programme physiotherapist. In the first session, a video related to basic knowledge of the pulmonary system and pulmonary disease was shown, followed by a group discussion with the patients. The second session was related to training in inhalator management. Chest physiotherapy consisted of eight sessions of breathing retraining, relaxation techniques and postural drainage. The patients then performed the exercise programme three times a week. The programme included respiratory muscle training and upper and lower extremity training. Respiratory muscle training consisted of two 15-min sessions – one at the hospital in the morning and the second at home in the evening – with a Threshold® device. The inspiratory pressure was set at 40% of the PI_{max}. Arm training consisted of a 30-min weight-lifting session; starting with 1 kg (0.5 kg in each hand) the patient progressively increased 2 kg each week until peak tolerance. Lower extremity training consisted of a 30-min session of pedalling on a cycle ergometer, at 60% of the W_{max} reached in the progressive effort test.

ASSESSMENT AFTER TREATMENT

The patient was re-assessed 3 months after the rehabilitation programme. He reported a great improvement in symptoms. Dyspnoea assessed by the MRC scale decreased from grade 3 to 2. His walking distance during the 6-min walk test increased from 240 to 325 m, and scores on the Borg dyspnoea scale at the end of exercise decreased from 8 to 4. The SGRQ scores improved by a clinically significant amount: symptoms score decreased from 16.5 to 7.7 units; activity from 53.6 to 53.5 units; impact from 34.2 to 26.7 units; and the total score from 37.2 to 31.7 units.

DISCUSSION

The management of stable COPD patients can be split into three main components:

- Symptomatic therapy;
- Pulmonary rehabilitation;
- Exacerbation: treatment and prevention.

SYMPTOMATIC THERAPY

First-line symptomatic therapy is a short-acting bronchodilator (or combination of short-acting $β_2$-agonist and ipratropium), but many patients find that their dyspnoea is inadequately controlled by this treatment alone. Long-acting bronchodilators are the next step, and the choice lies between a long-acting $β_2$-agonist (LABA) and tiotropium (the only long-acting antimuscarinic agent). Recent evidence suggests that there may be an additive effect on lung function of combining a LABA with tiotropium [13].

Clinical trials have shown that dyspnoea and health status may improve with long-acting bronchodilators when measured with questionnaires such as the transition dyspnoea index (TDI) [14] and SGRQ [15]. However, such clinical trial results do not help the practising clinician identify whether their particular patient has improved with treatment. The correlation between health status gain and improvement in FEV_1 is too weak to permit spirometry to be used to identify symptomatic benefit. Questionnaires such as the TDI and SGRQ are too complex to use in routine practice. In addition, they may not be suitable for use in individual patients since they were developed and validated in populations of patients, and may not have the properties needed to assess HRQoL benefits in the daily lives of individual patients.

The clue to assessment of benefit from symptomatic therapy lies in the objective of the treatment itself. If a patient notices benefit and thinks that it is worthwhile, then it should be judged clinically significant *for that patient*. This is easy to do in the clinic by asking the patient if they have noticed a change with the treatment and what that change was. Often, patients can only remember one example of benefit, but are able to make a judgement very readily as to whether it was big enough to be worthwhile. Equally, they can report that it made no difference. Research has shown that patients' retrospective estimate of treatment efficacy correlates well with changes in SGRQ score [16].

PULMONARY REHABILITATION

PR has proved extremely valuable in COPD patients. Systematic reviews of a number of randomized trials have demonstrated small to moderate improvements in functional exercise capacity and HRQoL in patients with COPD undergoing PR [17–20]. There is also evidence from a few studies, controlled [21, 22] and uncontrolled [23–26], that PR impacts positively on health expenditure, mainly by reducing the number of hospitalizations.

The main component of PR is muscular training. Exercise training focused on lower extremities has been clearly shown to improve effort capacity and HRQoL in COPD patients [17–20, 27], even when the intensity of training is low [28]. Exercise training not only improves symptoms but also changes muscular structure [29]. Relatively few studies have assessed improvement in muscular arm strength after training. However, upper limb activity has notable metabolic and ventilatory consequences [30]. Some studies have shown that PR programmes that include specific arm exercise improve muscular function in upper extremities and respiratory muscle function with lower metabolic cost [17–20, 31]. A few studies have analysed the benefits of upper extremity training alone [31] and shown a significant improvement in strength and endurance of these muscles [17–20, 31].

There is some controversy related to respiratory muscle training. Findings from two meta-analyses [32, 33] and two recent randomized studies [34, 35] suggest that respiratory muscle training can improve respiratory muscle strength when it ensures generation of adequate mouth pressure. Some randomized studies also show that this kind of training can intensify the beneficial effects of general muscle training, in terms of HRQoL and exercise capacity, when it is combined with general exercise reconditioning [33, 36]. The improvement in respiratory muscle function with specific training is related to inspiratory muscle weakness [33].

Other components of PR, such as education and self-management, chest physiotherapy or psychosocial support, are much more controversial. Educational programmes that include only knowledge about disease do not improve health status [37, 38], but when a programme includes self-management it seems to be more effective, mainly by reducing the risk for re-admission after hospitalization, as Bourbeau et al. [26] showed. Evidence regarding the impact of breathing retraining and chest physiotherapy on HRQoL or exercise capacity is weaker [18]. The true value of these techniques has not yet been established. Clinical trials involving diaphragmatic breathing, pursed-lips breathing and exercise are very scarce and such treatments do not seem effective, although one study showed that a period of breathing retraining and chest physiotherapy combined with low-level exercise may have beneficial effects on exercise capacity and HRQoL independent of more structured exercise training [22]. The benefits of psychological interventions included in PR programmes are controversial. Several studies have evaluated psychosocial interventions in COPD patients [17], but few have analysed the impact of PR on psychosocial issues when no specific psychosocial interventions are performed. Those that have examined psychological issues have focused on the effects of PR on depression and anxiety [39–44]. Some of these studies have suggested that PR programmes reduce anxiety and depression [39–44] while others did not find such differences [40]. A recent randomized trial has shown that PR may decrease psychosocial morbidity in COPD patients, other than depression and anxiety, even when no specific psychosocial intervention is performed [45].

Table 9.1 Indications for hospitalization of patients with a COPD exacerbation (with permission from [1])

- The presence of high-risk comorbid conditions, including pneumonia, cardiac arrhythmia, congestive heart failure, diabetes mellitus, renal or liver failure
- Inadequate response of symptoms to out-patient management
- Marked increase in dyspnoea
- Inability to eat or sleep due to symptoms
- Worsening hypoxaemia
- Worsening hypercapnia
- Changes in mental status
- Inability of the patient to care for her/himself (lack of home support)
- Uncertain diagnosis
- Inadequate home care

Few studies have examined the benefits of PR over the long term. Ries *et al.* [46] found that the improvements persisted for 1 year. Other studies have employed some kind of maintenance techniques, but the benefits lasted no longer than 1 or 2 years [17, 47–49], probably because the maintenance programmes were not sufficiently intense. One randomized controlled trial of PR in 60 severe COPD patients showed that patients can obtain benefits, in terms of exercise capacity and HRQoL, that persist for a period of 2 years after the programme. One factor in maintaining improvement may have been the psychological and social support received by patients participating in a self-help association for chronic respiratory patients organized with the assistance of the rehabilitation team [22].

TREATMENT OF EXACERBATIONS

There is no agreement concerning the classification of COPD exacerbation. The ATS/ERS standards have proposed an operational classification of severity according to the clinical relevance of the episode: Level I, treated at home; Level II, requires hospitalization; Level III, leads to respiratory failure [1]. The standards also include guidelines for patient hospitalization (Table 9.1). The treatment of COPD exacerbation should include pharmacological treatment, oxygen therapy when indicated, and assisted ventilation if necessary. Pharmacological treatment of patients with a COPD exacerbation is based upon the use of nebulized salbutamol and ipratropium. The use of oral glucocorticosteroids for patients treated in a hospital setting is supported by findings from randomized trials [1, 50–52]. Oxygen therapy should be used when there is respiratory failure. The aim of in-patient oxygen therapy is to maintain $PaO_2 \geq 60$ mmHg to preserve cellular oxygenation. It is important to monitor the $PaCO_2$ to prevent the risk of CO_2 retention and respiratory acidosis. Finally, assisted ventilation should be considered when there is respiratory acidosis and hypercapnia despite optimal pharmacological and oxygen therapy. Mechanical ventilation may be invasive or non-invasive. Non-invasive ventilation is preferable because it is as efficient as invasive ventilation but has fewer complications, as several authors have demonstrated [53–55].

PREVENTION OF EXACERBATIONS

The patient described in the case study was moving into a stage of his disease during which he was experiencing regular acute exacerbations that were sufficiently severe to require hospital admission. It was important to prevent or reduce the number of these exacerbations. Immunization against influenza is recommended for all people over the age of 65 years, and this applies especially to patients with COPD. Guidelines are also now recommending pneumococcal immunization for COPD patients. In terms of specific COPD therapy, there is evidence that tiotropium may reduce exacerbations [56], but the evidence for LABA is less consistent. Until recently, the strongest evidence that prophylactic therapy may reduce exacerbations came from the 3-year ISOLDE trial of fluticasone [57]. More recently there is convincing evidence for a reduction in exacerbations with a combination of LABA and inhaled corticosteroid (ICS) therapy [58–60]. The use of ICS in COPD is very different from the use of long-acting bronchodilators. Those agents are given for symptomatic benefit, which can be assessed symptomatically as already discussed. By contrast, ICS should be given prophylactically, so they are prescribed long-term, on the basis of the probability of benefit. These drugs reduce the rate at which health status gets worse over time [9], and much of this appears to be due to a reduction in exacerbation rate [61]. Clearly, the patients who are most likely to benefit are those with frequent exacerbations. The reduction in exacerbations appears to be marginally greater when ICS are combined with LABA, but the ICS effect appears to be the dominant component in reducing exacerbations.

The role of PR after an exacerbation in COPD patients is not well established, although a recent study by Man *et al.* [62] showed that an early PR program in the recovery period after hospital admission is more efficient in terms of exercise capacity and HRQoL than usual care.

SUMMARY

For most patients, COPD is a progressive disease in which there is evidence for complex pathophysiological interactions between systems and possibly the development of a downward spiral that involves lung function, exacerbations, exercise capacity and skeletal muscle strength. As a result, each patient requires a comprehensive management package tailored specifically for them, in which all components of treatment – symptomatic therapy, prophylaxis against exacerbations, treatment of exacerbations and pulmonary rehabilitation – are combined. The encouraging message is that there is now a strong evidence base for therapies that can have beneficial effects on all these important areas of the disease. Whilst it cannot be cured, there is much that can now be done to improve symptoms and slow down the effects of the disease.

REFERENCES

1. Celli B, MacNee W. Standards for the diagnosis and treatment of patients with COPD: a summary of the ATS/ERS position paper. ATS/ERS TASK FORCE. *Eur Respir J* 2004; 23:932–946.
2. Jones PW, Willits LR, Burge PS, Calverley PMA. Disease severity and the effect of fluticasone proprionate on chronic obstructive pulmonary disease exacerbations. *Eur Respir J* 2003; 21:1–6.
3. Guyatt GH, Townsend M, Berman LB, Pugsley SO. Quality of life in patients with chronic airflow limitation. *Br J Dis Chest* 1987; 81:45–54.
4. Killian KJ, Summers E, Jones NL, Campbell E. Dyspnea and leg effort during incremental cycle ergometry. *Am Rev Respir Dis* 1992; 145:1339–1345.
5. Standards for the diagnosis and care of patients with chronic obstructive pulmonary disease. ATS statement. *Am J Respir Crit Care Med* 1995; 152(suppl):S77–S120.
6. Siafakas NM, Vermeire P, Pride NB *et al.*; on behalf of the Task Force. Optimal assessment and management of chronic obstructive pulmonary disease (COPD). Consensus statement ERS. *Eur Respir J* 1995; 8:1398–1420.
7. Pauwels RA, Buist AS, Calverley PMA, Jenkins CR, Hurd S; on behalf of the GOLD Scientific Committee. GOLD: Global initiative for chronic Obstructive Lung Disease. National Institutes of Health. National Heart, Lung, and Blood Institute. *Am J Respir Crit Care Med* 2001; 163:1256–1276.
8. Celli BR, Cote CG, Marin JM *et al.* The body-mass index, airflow obstruction, dyspnea, and exercise capacity index in chronic obstructive pulmonary disease. *N Engl J Med* 2004; 350:1005–1012.
9. Spencer S, Calverley PMA, Burge PS, Jones PW. Health status deterioration in patients with chronic obstructive pulmonary disease. *Am J Respir Crit Care Med* 2001; 163:122–128.
10. Jones PW. Interpreting thresholds for a clinically significant changes in health status in asthma and COPD. *Eur Respir J* 2002; 19:398–404.
11. Seemungal TA, Donaldson GC, Bhowmik A, Jeffries DJ, Wedzicha JA. Time course and recovery of exacerbations in patients with chronic obstructive pulmonary disease. *Am J Respir Crit Care Med* 2000; 161:1608–1613.

12. Donaldson GC, Wilkinson TMA, Hurst JR, Perera WR, Wedzicha JA. Exacerbations and time spent outdoors in chronic obstructive pulmonary disease. *Am J Respir Crit Care Med* 2005; 171:446–452.
13. van Noord JA, Aumann JL, Janssens E et al. Comparison of tiotropium once daily, formoterol twice daily and both combined once daily in patients with COPD. *Eur Respir J* 2005; 26:214–222.
14. Mahler DA, Weinberg DH, Wells CK, Feinstein AR. Measurements of dyspnea. Contents, interobserver correlates of two new clinical indices. *Chest* 1984; 85:751–758.
15. Jones PW, Quirk FH, Baveystock CM, Littlejohns P. A self-complete measure for chronic airflow limitation – the St George's Respiratory Questionnaire. *Am Rev Respir Dis* 1992; 145:1321–1327.
16. Jones PW, Bosh TK. Changes in quality of life in COPD patients treated with salmeterol. *Am J Respir Crit Care Med* 1997; 155:1283–1289.
17. ACCP/AACVPR Pulmonary Rehabilitation Guidelines Panel. Pulmonary rehabilitation. Joint ACCP/AACVPR Evidence-Based Guidelines. *Chest* 1997; 112:1363–1396.
18. British Thoracic Society. Standards of Care Subcommittee on Pulmonary Rehabilitation. Pulmonary Rehabilitation. *Thorax* 2001; 56:827–834.
19. Lacasse Y, Brosseau L, Milne S et al. Pulmonary rehabilitation for chronic obstructive pulmonary disease. *Cochrane Database Syst Rev* 2002; CD003793.
20. Nice L, Donner CI, Wouters E et al. American Thoracic Society/European Respiratory Society statement on pulmonary rehabilitation. *Am J Respir Crit Care Med* 2006; 173:1390–1413.
21. Griffiths TL, Burr ML, Campbell JA et al. Results at 1 year of outpatient multidisciplinary pulmonary rehabilitation: a randomised controlled trial. *Lancet* 2000; 355:362–368.
22. Guell R, Casan P, Belda J et al. Long term effects of outpatient rehabilitation of COPD: a randomised trial. *Chest* 2000; 117:976–983.
23. Young P, Dewse M, Fergusson W et al. Improvements in outcomes for chronic obstructive pulmonary disease (COPD) attributable to a hospital-based respiratory rehabilitation program. *Aust N Z J Med* 1999; 29:59–65.
24. Stewart DG, Drake DF, Robertson C et al. Benefits of an inpatient pulmonary rehabilitation program: a prospective analysis. *Arch Phys Med Rehabil* 2001; 82:347–352.
25. Hui KP, Hewitt AB. A simple pulmonary rehabilitation program improves health outcomes and reduces hospital utilization in patients with COPD. *Chest* 2003; 124:94–97.
26. Bourbeau J, Julien M, Maltais F et al. Reduction of hospital utilization in patients with chronic obstructive pulmonary disease: a disease-specific self-management intervention. *Arch Intern Med* 2003; 163:585–591.
27. Troosters T, Casaburi R, Gosselink R et al. Pulmonary rehabilitation in chronic obstructive pulmonary disease. State of the art. *Am J Respir Crit Care Med* 2005; 172:19–38.
28. Maltais F, Leblanc P, Jobin J et al. Intensity of training and physiologic adaptation in patients with chronic obstructive pulmonary disease. *Am J Respir Crit Care Med* 1997; 155:555–561.
29. Maltais F, Leblanc P, Simard C et al. Skeletal muscle adaptation to endurance training in patients with chronic obstructive pulmonary disease. *Am J Respir Crit Care Med* 1996; 154:442–447.
30. Martinez FJ, Couser JI, Celli BR. Respiratory response to arm elevation in patients with chronic airflow obstruction. *Am Rev Respir Dis* 1991; 143:476–480.
31. Martinez FJ, Vogel PD, Dupont DN, Stanopoulos I, Gray A, Beamis JF. Supported arm exercise vs unsupported arm exercise in the rehabilitation of patients with severe chronic airflow obstruction. *Chest* 1993; 103:1397–1402.
32. Smith K, Cook D, Guyatt GH, Madharan J, Oxman AD. Respiratory muscle training in chronic airflow limitation: a meta-analysis. *Am Rev Respir Dis* 1992; 145:533–539.
33. Lötters F, van Tol B, Kwakkel G, Gosselink R. Effects of controlled inspiratory muscle training in patients with COPD: a meta-analysis. *Eur Respir J* 2002; 20:570–576.
34. Weiner P, Magadle R, Beckerman M, Weiner M, Berar-Yanay N. Comparison of specific expiratory, inspiratory and combined muscle training programs in COPD. *Chest* 2003; 124:1357–1364.
35. Ramirez-Sarmiento A, Orozco-Levi M, Güell R et al. Inspiratory muscle training in patients with chronic obstructive pulmonary disease. *Am J Respir Crit Care Med* 2002; 166:1491–1497.
36. Weiner P, Azgad Y, Ganam R. Inspiratory muscle training combined with general exercise reconditioning in patients with COPD. *Chest* 1992; 102:1351–1356.
37. Sassi Dambron DE, Eakin EG, Ries AL, Kaplan RM. Treatment of dyspnea in COPD: a controlled clinical trial of dyspnea management strategies. *Chest* 1995; 107:724–729.
38. Gallefoss F, Bakke PS, Rsgaard PK. Quality of life assessment after patient education in a randomized controlled study on asthma and chronic obstructive pulmonary disease. *Am J Respir Crit Care Med* 1999; 159:812–817.

39. Dekhuijzen PRN, Beek MML, Folgering HTM et al. Psychological changes during pulmonary rehabilitation and target-flow inspiratory muscle training in COPD patients with a ventilatory limitation during exercise. *Int J Rehabil Res* 1990; 13:109–117.
40. Ries AL, Kaplan RM, Limberg TM et al. Effects of pulmonary rehabilitation on physiologic and psychosocial outcomes in patients with chronic obstructive pulmonary disease. *Ann Intern Med* 1995; 122:823–832.
41. Eiser N, West C, Evans S et al. Effects of psychotherapy in moderately severe COPD: a pilot study. *Eur Respir J* 1997; 10:1581–1584.
42. Withers NJ, Rudkin ST, White RJ. Anxiety and depression in severe chronic obstructive pulmonary disease: the effect of pulmonary rehabilitation. *J Cardiopulm Rehabil* 1999; 19:362–365.
43. Godoy DV, Godoy RF. A randomized controlled trial of the effect of psychotherapy on anxiety and depression in chronic obstructive pulmonary disease. *Arch Phys Med Rehabil* 2003; 84:1154–1157.
44. Garuti G, Cilione C, Dell'Orso D et al. Impact of comprehensive pulmonary rehabilitation on anxiety and depression in hospitalized COPD patients. *Monaldi Arch Chest Dis* 2003; 59:56–61.
45. Güell R, Resqueti V, Sangneis M et al. Impact of pulmonary rehabilitation on psychosocial morbidity in patients with severe COPD. *Chest* 2006; 129:899–904.
46. Ries AL, Kaplan TM, Myers R et al. Maintenance after pulmonary rehabilitation in chronic lung disease: a randomized trial. *Am J Respir Crit Care Med* 2003; 167:880–888.
47. Singh SJ, Smith DL, Hyland ME et al. A short outpatient pulmonary rehabilitation program: immediate and longer-term effects on exercise performance and quality of life. *Respir Med* 1998; 92:1146–1154.
48. Troosters T, Grosselink R, Decramer M. Short and long-term effects of outpatient rehabilitation in patients with chronic obstructive pulmonary disease: a randomized trial. *Am J Med* 2000; 109:207–212.
49. Strijbos JH, Postma DS, van Altena R et al. A comparison between an outpatient hospital-based pulmonary rehabilitation program and a home-care pulmonary rehabilitation program in patients with COPD. A follow-up of 18 months. *Chest* 1996; 109:366–372.
50. Thompson WH, Nielson CP, Carvalho P et al. Controlled trial of oral prednisone in outpatients with acute COPD exacerbation. *Am J Respir Crit Care Med* 1996; 154:407–412.
51. Niewhoeher DD, Erbland ML, Deupree RH et al. Effect of systemic glucocorticoids on exacerbations of chronic obstructive pulmonary disease. Department of Veterans Affairs Cooperaive Study Group. *N Engl J Med* 1999; 340:1941–1947.
52. Davies L, Angus RM, Calverley PM. Oral corticosteroids in patients admitted to hospital with exacerbations of chronic obstructive pulmonary disease: a prospective randomized controlled trial. *Lancet* 1999; 345:456–460.
53. Diaz O, Ilesia R, Ferrer M. Effects of non invasive ventilation on pulmonary gas exchange and hemodynamics during acute hypercapnic exacerbations of chronic obstructive pulmonary disease. *Am J Respir Crit Care Med* 1997; 156:1840–1845.
54. Anton A, Guell R, Gomez J et al. Predicting the result of non-invasive ventilation in severe acute exacerbations of patients with chronic airflow limitation. *Chest* 2000; 117:828–833.
55. Plant PK, Owen JL, Elliot MW. Non-invasive ventilation in acute exacerbations of chronic obstructive pulmonary disease: long-term survival and predictors of in-hospital outcome. *Thorax* 2001; 56:708–712.
56. Niewoehner DE, Rice K, Cote C et al. Prevention of exacerbations of chronic obstructive pulmonary disease with tiotropium, a once-daily inhaled anticholinergic bronchodilator: a randomized trial. *Ann Intern Med* 2005; 143:317–326.
57. Burge PS, Calverley PM, Jones PW, Spencer S, Anderson JA, Maslen TK. Randomised, double blind, placebo controlled study of fluticasone propionate in patients with moderate to severe chronic obstructive pulmonary disease: the ISOLDE trial. *Br Med J* 2000; 320:1297–1303.
58. Calverley PMA, Boonsawat W, Cseke Z, Zhong N, Peterson S, Olsson H. Maintenance therapy with budesonide and formoterol in chronic obstructive pulmonary disease. *Eur Respir J* 2003; 22:912–919.
59. Calverley PMA, Pauwels R, Vestbo J, Jones PW, Pride N, Gulsvick A. Combined salmeterol and fluticasone in the treatment of chronic obstructive pulmonary disease. *Lancet* 2003; 361:449.
60. Szafranski W, Cukier A, Ramirez A et al. Efficacy and safety of budesonide/formoterol in the management of chronic obstructive pulmonary disease. *Eur Respir J* 2003; 21:74–81.
61. Spencer S, Calverley PMA, Burge PS, Jones PW. Impact of preventing exacerbations on deterioration of health status in COPD. *Eur Respir J* 2004; 23:1–5.
62. Man DCW, Polkey MI, Donaldson N et al. Community pulmonary rehabilitation after hospitalization for acute exacerbations of chronic obstructive pulmonary disease: randomised controlled study. *Br Med J* 2004; 329:1209.

10

COPD caused by occupational exposure

J. R. Balmes, D. Nowak

BACKGROUND

Smoking is clearly the major preventable cause of chronic obstructive pulmonary disease (COPD), but because this disease is so prevalent, the reduction of other preventable risk factors can have a major impact on reducing disease burden.

There are approximately 16 million people in the USA who have been diagnosed with COPD, and many more people who have abnormal lung function consistent with the diagnosis but who currently have minimal or no symptoms [1]. COPD is the fourth leading cause of death worldwide and accounts for over 100 000 deaths per year in the USA alone [2, 3].

In 1990, the World Health Organization (WHO) estimated the standardized mortality rate of COPD to be 50 in 100 000 in males and 20 per 100 000 in females in European countries. Thus, approximately 200 000–300 000 people die each year in Europe because of COPD. In Europe, it is estimated that around 4–6% of the adult population suffer from clinically relevant COPD [4, 5].

Thus, the burden of COPD is high. If occupational factors contribute substantially to the overall risk of COPD, exposure to these risk factors is preventable.

CASE REPORT

A 55-year-old ironworker sees his primary physician because he 'failed' a respirator fitness evaluation when applying for a new job on a construction site because his FEV_1 was <70% of predicted and his FEV_1/FVC was <0.70. He has never smoked and has no history of allergies, asthma, or other pulmonary disease. He has been welding for ~30 years in confined spaces with limited ventilation conditions. His physician repeats spirometry and finds similar results. The physician refers the patient for an evaluation regarding whether it is safe for him to continue welding. When seen, the patient complains of mild dyspnoea on heavy exertion, but insists that he is able to do his job as a welder. He denies wheezing, but does admit to a mostly non-productive cough while working. He has had several episodes of persistent productive cough annually for the past several years for which he has been treated with antibiotics. His physical examination and chest radiograph are unremarkable except that he is overweight. His pulmonary function tests show the following results: FEV_1 = 67% of predicted; FVC = 78% of predicted; FEV_1/FVC = 0.68; the expiratory flow-volume curve has decreased flows at low lung volumes; RV/TLC is increased consistent with air trapping; the DLCO is normal.

John R. Balmes, MD, Professor, University of California San Francisco, Division of Occupational and Environmental Medicine, San Francisco General Hospital, San Francisco, California, USA

Dennis Nowak, MD, Director, Institute and Outpatient Clinics for Occupational and Environmental Medicine, Ludwig-Maximilians-University, Munich, Germany

© Atlas Medical Publishing Ltd 2007

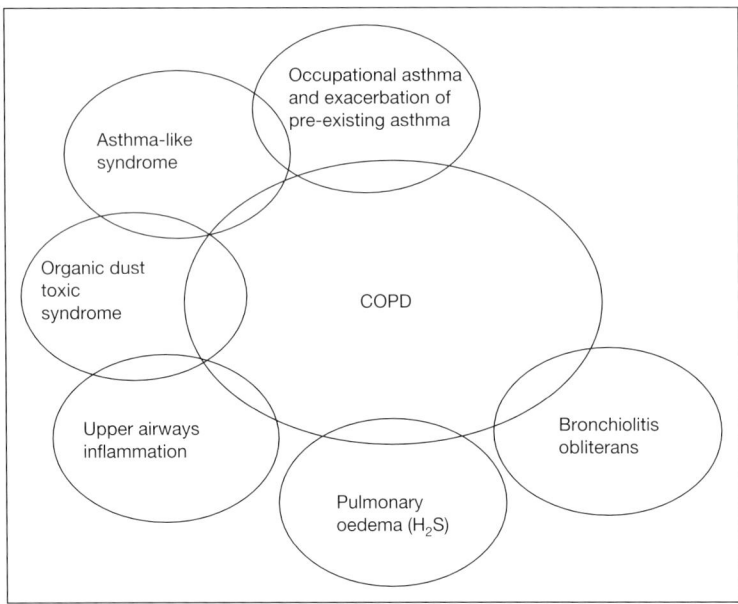

Figure 10.1 Scheme showing how occupational COPD may overlap clinically with other conditions.

The patient was diagnosed with moderate (stage IIA according to GOLD) COPD, which is most likely due to his occupational exposure to welding fumes. The initial recommendations for management of his disease were for him to try long-acting inhaled bronchodilator medication plus a short-acting bronchodilator for symptomatic relief, and to wear appropriate respiratory protective gear while welding. Because it is unlikely that welding will result in an acute, life-threatening exacerbation of his COPD, it was felt that he could return to welding if it is practical for him to wear a cartridge respirator. However, because of concerns about the progression of his COPD with continued welding, even with respiratory protective gear, it was also recommended that he should undergo annual monitoring of his pulmonary function.

DISCUSSION

COPD is defined as a disease state characterized by the presence of airflow limitation that is not fully reversible. The airflow limitation is usually both progressive and associated with an abnormal inflammatory response of the lungs to noxious particles or gases [6]. COPD can result from chronic bronchitis accompanied by hypersecretion of mucus and/or emphysema characterized by destruction of alveolar walls. COPD does not have a clinical subcategory that is clearly identified as occupational, largely because the condition develops slowly and, given that the airflow obstruction is chronic, does not reverse when exposure is discontinued. Thus, a clinical diagnosis of occupationally-related COPD is rarely made by clinicians. Figure 10.1 presents a scheme showing how occupational COPD may clinically overlap with other conditions.

The identification of COPD caused by occupational exposures typically rests either on obtaining a history of prior occupational asthma, or on knowledge of the epidemiological literature (e.g. chronic bronchitis after many years of work as an underground coal miner or emphysema in a battery factory worker exposed to cadmium fumes). Epidemiologically, identification of occupationally-related COPD is based on observing excess occurrence of COPD among exposed workers.

Some work-related obstructive airway disorders may be classified as COPD, but do not neatly fit into this category. For example, work-related variable airway limitation may occur with occupational exposure to organic dusts such as cotton (i.e. byssinosis), flax, hemp, jute, sisal, and various grains. Such organic dust-induced airway disease is sometimes classified as an asthma-like disorder [6], but both chronic bronchitis (by clinical definition) and poorly reversible airflow limitation can develop with chronic exposure. Bronchiolitis obliterans and irritant-induced asthma are two other conditions that may overlap clinically with work-related COPD.

OCCUPATIONAL EXPOSURES AND COPD

Epidemiology

While there is consensus that cigarette smoking is a specific cause of COPD, most of the data on which this is based come from longitudinal epidemiological studies in which a dose–response relationship between the amount smoked and the decline in ventilatory function has been observed for the population studied. This effect has consistently been confined to a minority of smokers, however, and it is still not possible to predict based on smoking exposure alone which individual smokers will develop chronic bronchitis, emphysema, or both. Thus, a genetic component to the risk of COPD from cigarette smoking is strongly suspected. Cigarette smoke is analogous to a mixed inhalational exposure at a workplace, i.e. a complex mixture of particles and gases. Epidemiological studies of the effects of cigarette smoke have not attempted to determine the specific aetiological role of any of its over 400 constituents. The airway dysfunction that has been clearly associated with cigarette smoking may, therefore, be a non-specific response to inhaled irritants in predisposed individuals.

The term 'nuisance dust' is frequently used to characterize exposures generally thought to be without adverse health effects. There is abundant evidence to demonstrate that this is an inappropriate term. Although there is no *a priori* biological reason to believe that a similar response to inhaled workplace irritants should not occur, it has been somewhat more difficult to demonstrate an association between occupational exposures and COPD in epidemiological studies. This may be due to several factors:

1. COPD is multifactorial in aetiology with critical (and mostly unknown) host as well as non-occupational environmental determinants of risk.
2. Unlike workers with pneumoconioses, individuals with COPD due to occupational exposures cannot be distinguished from those with the disease due to other causes.
3. Many workers with COPD have concurrent exposure to cigarette smoke (direct and/or second-hand) and workplace irritants.
4. Exposed workers at baseline tend to have better overall health and higher ventilatory function than the general population, the so-called 'healthy worker effect'.
5. Workforce studies are often limited to a 'survivor' population due to an inability to assess or follow workers who leave their jobs, thereby underestimating the chronic effects of occupational exposures.

Despite the difficulties listed above, an increasingly impressive body of literature demonstrating that specific occupational exposures contribute to the development of COPD has accumulated over the past two decades [7–17]. Table 10.1 lists the agents associated with work-related COPD.

Longitudinal studies of the effects of occupational exposures have been performed in coal miners [18–21], hard-rock miners [10, 22], tunnel workers [23], concrete-manufacturing

Table 10.1 Some agents causing chronic bronchitis

Minerals
Coal
Asbestos
Man-made vitreous fibres
Oil mist
Portland cement
Silica
Silicates

Metals
Osmium
Vanadium
Steel dust

Organic dusts
Cotton
Grain
Wood

Chemicals/gases/fumes
Ammonia
Firefighting
Cadmium
Isocyanates
Sulphur dioxide
Welding fumes
Environmental tobacco smoke

workers [24], and in a cohort of non-mining industrial workers in Paris [25]. As Becklake has pointed out, a consistent feature of these studies is a roughly comparable magnitude of effect for moderate smoking and occupational exposures [26]. For example, in UK coal miners, the excess annual loss of FEV_1 attributable to average exposure in mines was 8 ml/year after accounting for age and smoking, compared to 11 ml/year attributable to smoking after accounting for age and dust exposure [22]. For US coal miners, the data were remarkably similar at 7 and 9 ml/year, respectively [23]. In Parisian workers exposed to a variety of potential respiratory irritants, the findings were again similar, with 8 ml/year excess loss attributable to occupational exposure and 11 ml/year attributable to smoking [25].

A number of longitudinal studies have also been published in farming populations. Farmers are exposed to high levels of irritant gases and organic dusts, which include grain dusts, aeroallergens, endotoxins, insect antigens, β-1,3-glucans, fungi, and mycotoxins. Endotoxin and β-1,3-glucans especially are thought to mediate macrophage activity and, therefore, may induce neutrophilic inflammation of the respiratory tract [26]. Among more than 6000 randomly selected animal farmers in Europe, the prevalence of bringing up phlegm in winter was significantly higher than in the general population [27]. In French dairy farmers vs. non-farming controls, farming was associated with an accelerated decline in FEV_1/FVC [28, 29]. In grain farmers, excess annual decline in FEV_1 was 16 ml over control subjects, and in swine confinement workers, excess annual decline was 26 ml [30]. The increased loss in FEV_1 among swine farmers was associated with the use of disinfectants (an additional 43 ml/year) [31] and with endotoxin exposure (an extra decline of 19 ml/year with an increase in endotoxin by a factor of two) [32].

Acute obstructive changes in response to occupational exposures to organic and inorganic dusts, diisocyanates, and irritant gases appear to predict subsequent chronic (i.e. fixed) airflow limitation [33].

Perhaps, the strongest evidence implicating occupational exposures in the pathogenesis of COPD comes from community-based studies. Although these studies were typically not designed to examine the relationship of occupational exposures to COPD, they nonetheless yielded evidence of such a relationship. A major advantage of community-based studies is that the problem of survivor bias is largely avoided. Community-based studies from China, France, Italy, The Netherlands, New Zealand, Norway, Poland, Spain, and the USA have demonstrated increased relative risks (RR) for respiratory symptoms and/or chronic airflow limitation consistent with COPD [34–44] as well as for excess annual declines in FEV_1 associated with occupational exposure to dusts, gases, and fumes [34, 40, 41]. Because the predictor variable used in these studies, self-reported 'occupational exposure to dusts, gases, and/or fumes' is only a crude index of exposure, one would expect that these studies would be biased towards the null hypothesis (i.e. finding no effect of occupational exposures). The fact that these studies show a consistent association provides strong evidence that the observed effect is real.

Mechanistic information

Experimental studies have demonstrated that several agents known to be associated with clinically-defined chronic bronchitis in humans (e.g. endotoxin, mineral dusts, sulphur dioxide, and vanadium) are capable of inducing pathologically-defined chronic bronchitis in animal models [45–48]. The list of agents that can cause emphysema in animals includes several for which there is also epidemiological evidence in exposed occupational cohorts, such as cadmium, coal, endotoxin, and silica [49].

A severe deficiency of α_1-antitrypsin (protease inhibitor phenotype Z [PI*Z]) remains the only genetic factor that has clearly been associated with COPD in humans. This phenotype, which can be inherited as an autosomal recessive trait, affects only a small percentage of the general population (approximately 1 in 3000 in the US) and is responsible for a correspondingly small fraction of the total burden of COPD. While exposure to tobacco smoke is the major environmental risk factor for PI*Z individuals, occupational exposure to dusts, gases, fumes, and/or smoke has been shown to increase the risk of chronic cough, lower FEV_1, and lower FEV_1/FVC independent of personal tobacco use [50, 51].

Because the primary enzyme inhibited by α_1-antitrypsin is neutrophil elastase, this enzyme and the neutrophil have long been considered the major players in the development of emphysema. This view is rapidly changing, however, as data about other proteases and cells have emerged in recent years. Now that chronic exposure to cigarette smoke has been convincingly shown to produce emphysema in mice [52], genetic manipulation has already yielded new mechanistic information. The finding that a murine knockout model lacking macrophage metalloelastase (MME) is resistant to the development of cigarette smoke-induced emphysema has created great interest in this enzyme and in the potential importance of other proteases [53–55].

The occupationally relevant agents that can cause emphysema in animals (cadmium, coal, endotoxin, and silica) all cause the centrilobular form of the disease rather than the panacinar form that is associated with α_1-antitrypsin deficiency, so mechanisms other than uninhibited neutrophil elastase activity are likely operative [56]. The recent evidence about MME suggests a potential mechanism by which inhaled dusts or fumes could cause emphysema since macrophages have a primary role in the clearance of these materials from the terminal airways and alveoli.

OCCUPATIONALLY-RELATED COPD

Diagnosis

The clinician must be aware of the potential occupational aetiologies for obstructive airway disease and consider them in every patient with COPD. Identifying occupational risk factors at the individual level is important for prevention of disease before it is advanced and for modifying disability risk once disease is established [52]. In addition, the clinician has a critical role in case identification for the purposes of public health surveillance and appropriate work-related insurance compensation.

The key tool for identifying work-related factors that may be contributing to a patient's COPD is the occupational exposure history. A proper occupational history consists of a chronological list of all jobs, including job title, a description of the job activities, potential toxins at each job, and an assessment of the extent and duration of exposure. The length of time exposed to the agent, the use of personal protective equipment such as respirators, and a description of the ventilation and overall hygiene of the workplace are helpful in attempting to quantify exposure from the patient's history. Photos from the patient's workplaces may be helpful. Measurements of dust concentrations are frequently available. If the suspected occupational agents allow for biomonitoring (e.g. in welders or workers occupationally exposed to environmental tobacco smoke), these data may reflect individual exposure even more precisely. When documenting the patient's history, it is very important to list spirometric indices over time in a table in order to calculate the longitudinal decline, otherwise, subjects starting with e.g. an FEV_1 of 110% predicted will not be detectable as being at risk for COPD until their lung function falls below average levels. A decline from 110% predicted to 100% predicted, however, may be a sensitive indicator of increased risk.

Management and prevention

The treating clinician should attempt to understand the patient's occupational exposures and whether they have been adequately trained in the dangers of these exposures and how to avoid them. Effective clinical management requires efforts to reduce exposures as well as treatment with appropriate medications. Appropriate strategies to reduce exposures to respiratory tract irritants, in order of decreasing efficacy, include:

- Elimination (e.g. substitute alternate materials).
- Engineering controls (e.g. exhaust ventilation or process enclosure).
- Administrative controls (e.g. transfer to another job or change in work practices).
- Personal protective equipment (e.g. masks or respirators).

Guidelines for the identification and management of individuals with work-related asthma were recently published and are relevant to work-related COPD [57]. There are some data to support the efficacy of specific interventions. For example, elimination of exposure was associated with improvement in the health of already-diagnosed cases of work-related asthma in a plant where use of diisocyanates was halted [58]. Benefit has also been realized by having sick workers transfer to unexposed jobs [59]. Unlike workers with sensitizer-induced asthma, workers with irritant-induced asthma or COPD may continue to work in their usual jobs if their exposure to the inciting agent is diminished *via* proper engineering controls or respiratory protective equipment if engineering controls are not feasible. However, the effective use of personal protective equipment requires that the appropriate equipment be selected, properly fit-tested, maintained, and worn when there is potential for exposure (Figure 10.2). The failure to properly carry out any one of these essential tasks may cause failure of personal protective equipment to prevent exposure so that it is not surprising that data regarding the efficacy of such equipment are equivocal. For example, workers with asthmatic symptoms or abnormal spirometry at an aluminium plant showed improvements in peak expiratory flow rate (PEFR), but not symptoms, with use of a powered air-purifying respirator compared to disposable masks [60].

Prevention must be the primary tool for decreasing the incidence of, morbidity and disability from work-related COPD, which can become a severely disabling disease. Prevention must

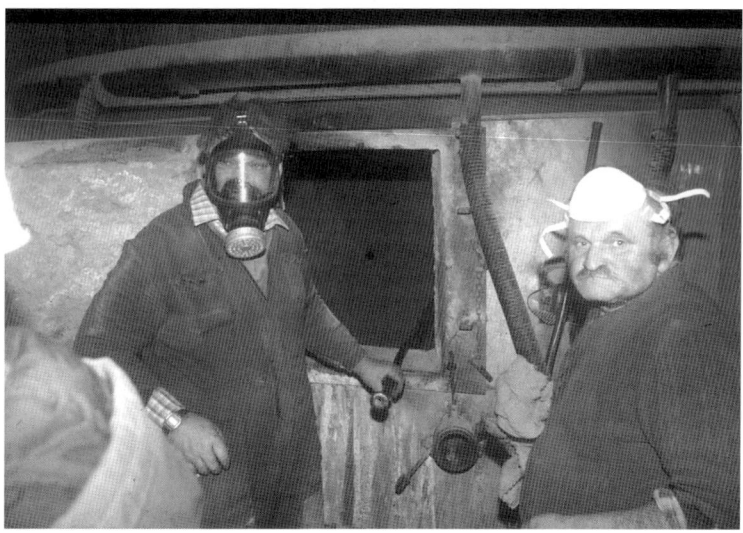

Figure 10.2 An example of personal protective equipment being worn by an individual with work-related asthma.

involve cooperation between employers, workers and their representatives, regulators, and medical personnel [57, 58]. The goal of primary prevention is to prevent occupational exposure. Primary prevention strategies involve the same hierarchy of exposure controls (elimination, engineering controls, administrative controls, personal protective equipment) as described for management of work-related asthma and COPD due to irritant exposures. Secondary prevention detects COPD early so that its duration and severity can be minimized. Tertiary prevention applies to individuals who have already been diagnosed with work-related COPD. It includes institution of appropriate healthcare and an effort to prevent permanent disease by early removal from, or reduction of, exposure [57, 58]. Worker education and training in work processes, safety equipment and procedures may also be of benefit in the prevention of COPD.

Another important component in the prevention of irritant-induced COPD is surveillance for these diseases in the workplace. Surveillance programmes are a type of secondary prevention, in that their principal goal is the early detection of disease. In making an earlier diagnosis, morbidity and disability can be prevented *via* timely intervention. Any diagnosis of irritant-induced COPD must be considered a sentinel event; other exposed workers are at risk and need to be identified promptly [61, 62].

A general approach to surveillance programmes includes medical screening of co-workers as well as exposure monitoring [61, 62]. For medical surveillance of COPD, short symptom questionnaires can be administered annually that include items such as improvement in respiratory symptoms on weekends and holidays [58, 61, 62]. In addition, spirometry can be performed on an annual basis and compared to baseline spirometric testing at the time of starting the job. Review of PEFR records over several weeks can also detect workers at risk for developing irritant-induced COPD. Industrial hygienists can perform environmental monitoring to ensure that appropriate engineering controls are in place to protect worker safety. Reviewing and updating lists of agents used at a given workplace should be performed on a periodic basis, to identify possible respiratory tract irritants.

Occupational contribution to the burden of COPD

An *ad hoc* committee of the American Thoracic Society (ATS) has reviewed population-based studies in which associations between occupational factors and COPD have been reported in order to assess the contribution of occupational exposures to the overall burden of this disease [63]. For COPD, a population-attributable risk (PAR) of approximately 15–20% was estimated to be due to occupational factors. Ten papers that were reviewed had sufficient data to calculate a PAR; several of the papers presented data supporting a >20% PAR for respiratory symptoms and lung function impairment due to work-related factors. Several recent papers published since the completion of the ATS statement provide further evidence in support of a major contribution of occupational exposures to the burden of COPD.

Hnizdo *et al.* [64] from the National Institute for Occupational Safety and Health used data collected in the US population-based Third National Health and Nutrition Examination Survey (NHANES) on over 9800 subjects to estimate the PAR for COPD (defined by a decreased FEV_1/FVC) due to work. The analysis was adjusted for multiple factors including smoking history. The industries with increased risk include rubber, plastics, and leather manufacturing; utilities; building services; textile manufacturing; the armed forces; food products manufacturing; chemical, petroleum, and coal manufacturing; and construction. The PAR for COPD due to work was estimated at 19% overall and 31% among never-smokers.

A second US population-based study conducted by Trupin and coworkers [65] obtained survey information on over 2000 subjects. Occupational exposures were associated with increased risk of COPD (self-reported physician diagnosis of either chronic bronchitis or emphysema) after adjustment for smoking history and demographic variables. The PAR for COPD due to these exposures was 20%; it was 31% for a narrower definition of COPD (excluding chronic bronchitis). In this study, the PAR for combined current and former smoking was 56%. Smoking and occupational exposures to dusts, gases, and/or fumes had greater than additive effects.

A third study from Sweden was designed to determine whether occupational exposure to dust, fumes, or gases, especially among never-smokers, increased the mortality from COPD [66]. A cohort of over 317 000 Swedish male construction workers was followed from 1971 to 1999. Exposure to inorganic dusts, gases and irritant chemicals, fumes, and wood dusts was based on a job-exposure matrix. An internal control group with 'unexposed' construction workers was used, and the analyses were adjusted for age and smoking. There was a statistically significant increased mortality from COPD among those with any airborne exposure (RR = 1.12). In a Poisson regression model, including smoking, age and the four major exposure groups listed above, exposure to inorganic dust was associated with an increased risk, especially among never-smokers. The fraction of COPD among the exposed attributable to any airborne exposure was estimated as 10.7% overall and 52.6% among never-smokers. Thus, occupational exposure among construction workers increases mortality due to COPD, even among never-smokers.

A conservative estimate of the annual costs of work-related COPD disease is nearly $5 billion in the USA alone [67]. Based on the estimated PAR due to occupational exposures for COPD (15–20%), strategies designed to prevent occupationally-induced obstructive airways disease should receive high priority in the global efforts to reduce disease burden [3, 68, 69].

SUMMARY

Although prevention must be the primary tool for decreasing the incidence of morbidity and disability from work-related COPD, there are still many workers affected by COPD. Clinicians should therefore be aware that in some cases COPD is not determined by smoking, or *only* by the smoking habit, but may be due to occupational exposure.

An increasingly impressive body of literature has accumulated over the past two decades demonstrating that specific occupational exposures contribute to the development of COPD. Pinpointing cases where COPD is due to occupational exposure typically rests on a good knowledge of the epidemiological literature (e.g. chronic bronchitis may occur after years of work as an underground coal miner; emphysema may be a consequence of working in a battery factory exposed to cadmium fumes) in association with obtaining a full medical and occupational history of the patient.

Experimental studies have demonstrated that several agents known to be associated with clinically-defined chronic bronchitis in humans (e.g. endotoxin, mineral dusts, sulphur dioxide, and vanadium) are capable of inducing pathologically-defined chronic bronchitis in animal models. The list of agents that can cause emphysema in animals includes several for which there is also epidemiological evidence in exposed occupational cohorts, such as cadmium, coal, endotoxin and silica.

The clinician should be aware of the potential occupational aetiologies for obstructive airways disease and consider these carefully in each patient with COPD. Identifying occupational risk factors at the individual level is important for the prevention of disease before it is advanced and for modifying disability risk once disease is established.

REFERENCES

1. National Heart Lung and Blood Institute. Morbidity and mortality: 1998 chart book on cardiovascular, lung and blood diseases. National Institute of Health, Hyattsville, MD, 1998.
2. Mannino DM, Brown C, Giovino GA. Obstructive lung disease deaths in the United States from 1979 through 1993: an analysis using multiple-cause mortality data. *Am J Respir Crit Care Med* 1997; 156:814–818.
3. Global Initiative for Chronic Obstructive Lung Disease. Workshop Report, Global Strategy for Diagnosis, Management, and Prevention of COPD: 2005 Update. www.goldcopd.org.
4. European Respiratory Society: European Lung White Book. The Charlesworth Group, Huddersfield, 2003.
5. Nowak D, Berger K, Lippert B, Kilgert K, Caeser M, Sandtmann R. Epidemiology and health economics of COPD across Europe: a critical analysis. *Treat Respir Med* 2005; 4:381–395.
6. Bernstein IL, Chan-Yeung M, Malo J-L, Bernstein DI. Definition and classification of asthma. In: Bernstein IL, Chan-Yeung M, Malo J-L, Bernstein DI (eds). *Asthma in the Workplace*, 2nd edition. Marcel Dekker, New York, 1999, pp 1–4.
7. Hendrick DJ. Occupation and chronic obstructive pulmonary disease. *Thorax* 1996; 51:947–955.
8. Viegi G, Scognamiglio A, Baldacci S, Pistelli F, Carozzi L. Epidemiology of chronic obstructive pulmonary disease (COPD). *Respiration* 2001; 68:4–19.
9. Coggon D, Taylor AN. Coal mining and chronic obstructive pulmonary disease: a review of the evidence. *Thorax* 1998; 53:398–407.
10. Hnizdo E, Baskind E, Sluis-Cremer GK. Combined effect of silica dust exposure and tobacco smoking on the prevalence of respiratory impairments among gold miners. *Scand J Work Environ Health* 1990; 16:411–422.
11. Nakadate T, Aizawa Y, Yagami T, Zheg Y-Q, Kotani M, Ishiwata K. Change in obstructive pulmonary function as a result of cumulative exposure to welding fumes as determined by magnetopneumography in Japanese arc welders. *Occup Environ Med* 1998; 55:673–677.
12. Davison AG, Fayers PM, Newman-Taylor AJ et al. Cadmium fume inhalation and emphysema. *Lancet* 1988; 1:663–667.
13. Irslinger GB, Visser PJ, Spangenberg PAL. Asthma and chronic bronchitis in vanadium workers. *Am J Ind Med* 1999; 35:366–374.
14. Becklake MR, Goldman HI, Bosman AR, Freed CC. The long-term effects of exposure to nitrous fumes. *Am Rev Tuberc Pulm Dis* 1957; 76:398–409.
15. Piirila PL, Nordman H, Korhonen OS, Winblad I. A thirteen-year follow-up of respiratory effects of acute exposure to sulfur dioxide. *Scand J Work Environ Health* 1996; 22:191–196.
16. Becklake MR. Chronic airflow limitation: its relationship to work in dusty occupations. *Chest* 1985; 88:606–617.

17. Becklake MR. Occupational exposures: evidence for a causal association with chronic obstructive pulmonary disease. *Am Rev Respir Dis* 1989; 140:S85–S91.
18. Love RG, Miller BG. Longitudinal study of lung function in coalminers. *Thorax* 1982; 37:193–197.
19. Attfield MD. Longitudinal decline in FEV1 in United States coalminers. *Thorax* 1985; 40:132–137.
20. Attfield MD, Hodus TK. Pulmonary function of US coalminers related to dust exposure estimates. *Am Rev Respir Dis* 1992; 145:605–609.
21. Seixas NS, Robins TG, Attfield MD, Moulton LH. Longitudinal and cross-sectional analyses of coal mine dust and pulmonary function in new miners. *Br J Ind Med* 1993; 50:929–937.
22. Holman CDJ, Psaila-Savona P, Roberts M, McNulty JC. Determinants of chronic bronchitis and lung dysfunction in Western Australian gold miners. *Br J Ind Med* 1987; 44:810–818.
23. Ulvestad B, Bakke B, Eduard W, Kongerud J, Lund MB. Cumulative exposure to dust causes accelerated decline in lung function in tunnel workers. *Occup Environ Med* 2001; 58:663–669.
24. Meijer E, Kromhoult H, Heederik D. Respiratory effects of exposure to low levels of concrete dust containing crystalline silica. *Am J Ind Med* 2001; 40:133–140.
25. Kauffmann F, Drouet D, Lellouch J, Brille D. Occupational exposure and 12 year spirometric changes among Paris area workers. *Br J Ind Med* 1982; 39:221–232.
26. Radon K, Nowak D. Farming. In: Hendrick DJ, Burge PS, Beckett WS, Churg A (eds). *Occupational Disorders of the Lung – Recognition, Management, and Prevention*. W.B. Saunders – Harcourt Publishers, London, 2002, pp 427–437.
27. Radon K, Danuser B, Iversen M et al. Respiratory symptoms in European animal farmers. *Eur Respir J* 2001; 17:747–754.
28. Dalphin JC, Maheu MF, Dussaucy A et al. Six year longitudinal study of respiratory function in dairy farmers in the Doubs province. *Eur Respir J* 1998; 11:1287–1293.
29. Chaudemanche H, Monnet E, Westeel V et al. Respiratory status in dairy farmers in France; cross sectional and longitudinal analyses. *Occup Environ Med* 2003; 60:858–863.
30. Senthilselvan A, Dosman JA, Kirychuk SP et al. Accelerated lung function decline in swine confinement workers. *Chest* 1997; 111:1733–1741.
31. Vogelzang PF, van der Gulden JW, Folgering H, van Schayck CP. Longitudinal changes in lung function associated with aspects of swine-confinement exposure. *J Occup Environ Med* 1998; 40:1048–1052.
32. Vogelzang PF, van der Gulden JW, Folgering H et al. Endotoxin exposure as a major determinant of lung function decline in pig farmers. *Am J Respir Crit Care Med* 1998; 157:15–16.
33. Becklake MR. Relationship of acute obstructive airway change to chronic (fixed) obstruction. *Thorax* 1995; 50:516–521.
34. Xu X, Christiani DC, Dockery DW, Wang L. Exposure-response relationships between occupational exposures and chronic respiratory illness: a community-based study. *Am Rev Respir Dis* 1992; 146:413–418.
35. Viegi G, Prediletto R, Paoletti P et al. Respiratory effects of occupational exposure in a general population sample in North Italy. *Am Rev Respir Dis* 1991; 143:510–515.
36. Krzyzanowski M, Kauffmann F. The relation of respiratory symptoms and ventilatory function to moderate occupational exposure in a general population. Results from the French PAARC study of 16000 adults. *Int J Epidemiol* 1988; 17:397–406.
37. Post WK, Heederik D, Kromhout H, Kromhout D. Occupational exposures estimated by a population specific job exposure matrix and 25 year incidence rate of chronic nonspecific lung disease (CNSLD): the Zutphen Study. *Eur Respir J* 1994; 7:1048–1055.
38. Fishwick D, Bradshaw LM, D'Souza W et al. Chronic bronchitis, shortness of breath, and airway obstruction by occupation in New Zealand. *Am J Respir Crit Care Med* 1997; 156:1440–1446.
39. Bakke P, Eide GE, Hanoa R, Gulsvik A. Occupational dust or gas exposure and prevalence of respiratory symptoms and asthma in a general population. *Eur Respir J* 1991; 4:273–278.
40. Humerfelt S, Gulsvik A, Skjaerven R et al. Decline in FEV_1 and airflow limitation related to occupational exposures in men of an urban community. *Eur Respir J* 1993; 6:1095–1103.
41. Krzyzanowski M, Jedrychowski W, Wysocki M. Factors associated with the change in ventilatory function and the development of chronic obstructive pulmonary disease in a 13-year follow-up of the Cracow study. *Am Rev Respir Dis* 1986; 134:1011–1019.
42. Sunyer J, Kogevinas M, Kromhout H et al. Pulmonary ventilatory defects and occupational exposures in a population-based study in Spain. *Am J Respir Crit Care Med* 1998; 157:512–517.
43. Lebowitz MD. Occupational exposures in relation to symptomatology and lung function in a community population. *Environ Res* 1977; 14:59–67.

44. Korn RJ, Dockery DW, Speizer FE, Ware JH, Ferris BG. Occupational exposures and chronic respiratory symptoms. A population-based study. *Am Rev Respir Dis* 1987; 136:298–304.
45. Shore S, Kobzik L, Long NC et al. Increased airway responsiveness to inhaled methacholine in a rat model of chronic bronchitis. *Am J Respir Crit Care Med* 1995; 151:1931–1938.
46. Churg A, Hobson J, Wright J. Functional and morphologic comparison of silica- and elastase-induced airflow obstruction. *Exp Lung Res* 1989; 15:813–822.
47. Bonner JC, Rice AB, Moomaw CR, Mogan DL. Airway fibrosis in rats induced by vanadium pentoxide. *Am J Physiol (Lung Cell Mol Physiol)* 2000; 278:L209–L216.
48. Harkema JR, Hotchkiss JA. Ozone- and endotoxin-induced mucous metaplasia in rat airway epithelium: novel animal models to study toxicant-induced epithelil transformation in airways. *Toxicol Lett* 1993; 68:251–263.
49. Shapiro SD. Animal models for COPD. *Chest* 2000; 117:223S–227S.
50. Putulainen E, Tornling G, Erickson S. Effect of age and occupational exposure to airway irritants on lung function in nonsmoking individuals with severe α1-antitrypsin deficiency (PiZZ). *Thorax* 1997; 52:244–248.
51. Mayer AS, Stoller JK, Bucher-Bartelson B, Ruttenber AJ, Sandhaus RA, Newman LS. Occupational exposure risks in individuals with PI*Z α1-Antitrypsin deficiency. *Am J Respir Crit Care Med* 2000; 162:553–558.
52. Petty TL, Weinmann GG. Building a national strategy for the prevention and management of and research in chronic obstructive pulmonary disease: National Heart, Lung, and Blood Institute workshop summary. *JAMA* 1997; 277:246–253.
53. Hautamaki RD, Kobayashi DK, Senior RM, Shapiro SD. Macrophage elastase is required for cigarette smoke-induced emphysema in mice. *Science* 1997; 277:2002–2004.
54. Finlay GA, O'Driscoll LR, Russell KJ et al. Matrix metalloproteinase expression and production by alveolar macrophages in emphysema. *Am J Respir Crit Care Med* 1997; 156:240–247.
55. Ohnishi K, Takagi M, Kurokawa Y, Satomi S, Konttinen YT. Matrix metalloproteinase-mediated extracellular matrix protein degradation in human pulmonary emphysema. *Lab Invest* 1998; 78:1077–1087.
56. Snider GL. Collagen vs elastin in pathogenesis of emphysema; cellular origin of elastases; bronchiolitis vs emphysema as a cause of airflow obstruction. *Chest* 2000; 117:244S–246S.
57. Friedman-Jimenez G, Beckett WS, Szeinuk J, Petsonk EL. Clinical evaluation, management, and prevention of work-related asthma. *Am J Ind Med* 2000; 37:121–141.
58. Venables KM. Prevention of occupational asthma. *Eur Respir J* 1994; 7:768–778.
59. Gannon PFG, Weir DC, Robertson AS, Burge PS. Health, employment, and financial outcomes in workers with occupational asthma. *Br Med J* 1993; 50:491–496.
60. Daroowalla F, Kaufman J, Nelson N, Sama S, Kennedy S, Barnhart S. New bronchial responsiveness and asthma symptoms in a cohort of aluminum potroom workers. *Am J Respir Crit Care Med* 1998; 157(pt 2):A882.
61. Tarlo SM, Boulet L-P, Cartier A et al. Canadian Thoracic Society guidelines for occupational asthma. *Can Respir J* 1998; 5:289–300.
62. Balmes JR. Surveillance for occupational asthma. *Occup Med* 1991; 6:101–110.
63. Balmes J, Becklake M, Blanc P et al. Occupational contribution to the burden of airway disease (an official statement of the American Thoracic Society). *Am J Respir Crit Care Med* 2003; 167:787–797.
64. Hnizdo E, Sullivan PA, Bang KM, Wagner G. Association between chronic obstructive pulmonary disease and employment by industry and occupation in the U.S. population: a study of data from the Third National Health and Nutrition Examination Survey. *Am J Epidemiol* 2002; 156:738–746.
65. Trupin L, Earnest G, San Pedro M et al. The occupational burden of chronic obstructive pulmonary disease. *Eur Respir J* 2003; 22:462–469.
66. Bergdahl IA, Toren K, Eriksson K et al. Increased mortality in COPD among construction workers exposed to inorganic dust. *Eur Respir J* 2004; 23:402–406.
67. Leigh JP, Romano PS, Schenker MB, Kreiss K. Costs of occupational chronic obstructive pulmonary disease and asthma. *Chest* 2002; 121:264–272.
68. Meldrum M, Rawbone R, Curran AD, Fishwick D. The role of occupation in the development of chronic obstructive pulmonary disease (COPD). *Occup Environ Med* 2005; 62:212–214.
69. Christiani DC. Occupation and COPD. *Occup Environ Med* 2005; 62:215.

11

Body mass index as a prognostic factor in COPD

B. R. Celli

BACKGROUND

The American Thoracic and the European Respiratory Societies [1] have recently defined chronic obstructive pulmonary disease (COPD) as a preventable and treatable disease state characterized by airflow limitation that is not fully reversible.

This airflow limitation is usually progressive and is associated with an abnormal inflammatory response of the lungs to noxious particles or gases, primarily caused by cigarette smoking. In some areas of the world where biomass fuel is used as a source of energy primarily for cooking, persons exposed to the particles can develop airflow obstruction that is indistinguishable from that characteristic of COPD.

Although COPD primarily affects the lungs, it also produces significant systemic consequences that are very important because their presence is associated with significant morbidity and mortality and also because some of them are amenable to therapy. Indeed, oxygen therapy, an intervention that does not reverse airflow limitation, has been shown to prolong survival [2, 3]. This old observation is extremely important as it shows that the progressive course of COPD can be altered without having to necessarily alter lung function.

The most frequent systemic manifestations of COPD include:

- Weight loss and malnutrition;
- Osteoporosis;
- Depression;
- Peripheral muscle dysfunction;
- Anaemia;
- Different degrees of heart failure.

Of these, weight loss and malnutrition are the best known and the manifestations most closely associated with a poor prognosis.

Weight loss is a phenomenon that has long been recognized in the clinical course of COPD patients, having first been described in association with emphysema in the late nineteenth century [4]. Attempts to describe different COPD classifications retained body weight as an important discriminator [5]. In the 1960s, several studies reported that low body weight and weight loss are negative predictive factors of survival in COPD [6]. At that time, weight loss was considered to be an integral part of the clinical picture of chronic bronchitis, without adequate analysis of the underlying mechanisms or related functional consequences: nutritional

---

Bartolome R. Celli, MD, Professor of Medicine, Tufts University, Chief Pulmonary, Critical Care and Sleep Medicine, Caritas St Elizabeth's Medical Center Boston, Massachusetts, USA

© Atlas Medical Publishing Ltd 2007

depletion was considered as an inevitable and irreversible terminal event related to the severity of airflow obstruction. It was even hypothesized that weight loss was an adaptive mechanism to decrease oxygen consumption in these patients with advanced COPD.

As our knowledge about the course of COPD has expanded, it has become very clear that the goals of therapy now include therapeutic measures aimed at reversing some of the systemic manifestations. Increased attention has thus been given to all of the manifestations of COPD, with weight loss and malnutrition being 'attractive' manifestations, as they can be measured, studied and also treated. The following case presents the course of a patient with COPD who was evaluated at our institution. The management of this patient typifies the problems facing clinicians when attempting to define simple solutions to a complex problem and describes the surprising effect of an unrelated therapy.

CASE REPORT

A 64-year-old woman, S.W., smoked one pack of cigarettes per day from age 17 to age 59 years. She had begun to experience dyspnoea at age 57, and was diagnosed with COPD at age 59. Although she stopped smoking, her dyspnoea continued to progress (at first appearing only with moderate effort). Over the past year, however, she had become unable to walk up one flight of stairs, and the dyspnoea occurred during activities of daily living (washing, bathing, and dressing). She began to limit her exercise, and used a nephew's wheelchair when she went out. She began to use low-flow oxygen at age 62.

The physical examination showed her to have a resting tachycardia of 92 bpm, a respiratory rate of 24 breaths/min with accessory muscle use, normal blood pressure and she was afebrile. Her weight was 51 kg and she was 1.68 m tall. Her body mass index (BMI) was calculated at 18 kg/m^2. She had a barrel-chested shape, looked thin and had retractions of the intercostal spaces during inspiration. Even though she had no frank paradoxical breathing, there was some asynchrony between thorax and abdomen during deep, fast manoeuvres. There were distant breath sounds and mild wheezes on exhalation. The abdomen was soft, with no visceromegaly. There was no oedema, clubbing or cyanosis.

A routine chest radiograph revealed a right upper lobe nodule measuring 2 cm, which had not appeared in an X-ray taken 2 years earlier. Computerized tomography (CT) confirmed the nodule. There were no mediastinal nodes. The same scan confirmed severe hyperinflation and demonstrated the presence of inhomogeneous changes that were more prominent in the upper lobes. A positron emission tomography scan showed positive uptake in the mass without any uptake outside of the area.

Laboratory examinations were within normal limits, including cardiac echocardiogram. Physiological evaluation showed severe airflow obstruction, with a FVC of 2.05 l and a FEV_1 of 0.52 l after bronchodilators (25% of predicted). The residual volume determined by plethysmography showed severe air trapping with a value 260% of predicted. The 6-minute walking distance was 120 m, and maximal oxygen uptake in a progressive cardiopulmonary exercise test was 11 ml/kg/min. The Modified Medical Research Council (MMRC) dyspnoea scale was 3. The working diagnosis was that of a neoplasm, very likely malignant, in the right upper lobe.

By conventional criteria the patient was inoperable, because her FEV_1 was very low (26% of predicted). Nevertheless, we explained to her that we could remove the nodule using recently developed lung volume reduction surgery (LVRS) but that she would need to undergo a preoperative comprehensive pulmonary rehabilitation programme as she was very malnourished and deconditioned. Even though she understood that poor functional capacity (as expressed by the 6-minute walking test) generally predicts poor outcome with this procedure, she wanted to be treated 'aggressively' and was willing to 'do anything' to qualify for the procedure.

She began an intense pulmonary rehabilitation programme that included lower-extremity exercise at 70% of the determined VO_2 max and upper-extremity unsupported exercise. To aid in the post-operative period, we instructed her in deep-breathing exercises and in assisted cough. The programme included daily sessions as an in-patient, and ended with 3 weeks of out-patient training for a total of 20 sessions.

As part of her programme we involved the nutritionist, who recommended more frequent meals of smaller volumes (the patient referred to dyspnoea immediately after meals) and the addition of extra calories in the form of high caloric value shakes. Over the month of therapy, she gained 2 kg and became more fit. Re-testing revealed less dyspnoea with exercise, and she was able to walk 285 m over 6 min. Her peak oxygen uptake had risen to 13 ml/kg/min.

She underwent LVRS with resection of the nodule, which confirmed the diagnosis of adenocarcinoma of the lung. She recovered in the acute ward of St. Elizabeth's Medical Centre for 8 days, and was discharged to a rehabilitation facility to continue the programme while a small persistent leak (drained with a Heimlich tube) closed. After the leak closed on the 16th day after surgery, she went home. After 8 months, the mass has not recurred.

The patient is still dyspnoeic, but no longer uses a wheelchair. She has not required hospitalization, and her oxygen requirements have decreased by 0.5 l/min. She walks daily, and her last 6-minute walking distance was 268 m. In addition, her weight has increased to 57 kg, 6 kg more than on her initial evaluation.

DISCUSSION

Until very recently, this woman would have been deemed inoperable and so severely afflicted by her malnutrition that she would have been left receiving symptomatic comfort care. Her evaluation showed that she was not only malnourished but also severely deconditioned, manifestations that are often related and amenable to therapy. Furthermore, the advent of LVRS opened a window to a more aggressive approach to treatment that we can learn much from. Patients with COPD can be helped even in the most advanced cases, where a comprehensive approach can have a profound impact.

MALNUTRITION AND PHENOTYPE

It has been classically described that there are two contrasting types of patients with chronic airways obstruction based on clinical criteria and body weight: the *'pink puffer'* and the *'blue bloater'* [5]. The pink puffer, the emphysematous patient, is more breathless, with marked hyperinflation, thin in appearance with major weight loss. The blue bloater has more severe central cyanosis and is frequently obese.

The relationship between nutritional status and COPD subtypes was well described by Openbrier *et al*. [7], who demonstrated that patients with emphysema are somatically depleted in comparison with patients with chronic bronchitis. These data seem to indicate that weight loss and nutritional depletion are particularly problematic in those patients with impaired diffusing capacity. Using HRCT, Engelen *et al*. [8] analysed body weight and body composition in COPD patients, and subdivided them into an emphysematous group and a bronchitis group based on HRCT. Body weight and BMI, as well as fat-free mass (FFM), and fat mass (FM), were significantly lower in emphysematous patients compared to the bronchitis group. Thus, we have known for a while that patients with an emphysematous phenotype (as represented by our patient) are prone to develop malnutrition. It is interesting that the HRCT data confirmed what was suspected clinically.

FUNCTIONAL PERFORMANCE AND HEALTH STATUS

Dyspnoea and exercise intolerance are prominent symptoms in COPD patients. In addition to airflow limitation and impaired diffusing capacity, it is accepted that respiratory and skeletal muscle weakness are important determinants of these symptoms [9, 10]. Muscle dysfunction is highly related to muscle wasting [11]. BMI can therefore be considered as an indicator of functional disability. Underweight patients with COPD have impaired respiratory muscle strength [12–14].

Several studies have shown that a reduction in percent ideal body weight or BMI results in decreased maximal aerobic capacity [15, 16]. Indeed, reduced BMI has an independent negative effect on muscle aerobic capacity in COPD patients, as manifested by a decrease in maximal oxygen consumption, a reduction in the lactate threshold and a slowing of oxygen uptake kinetics [17]. Positive outcomes on peak exercise parameters, as well as on walking distance, have been reported by nutritional intervention in depleted COPD patients [18]. We cannot claim conclusively that the improvement observed in our patient related primarily to the nutritional intervention, but it is likely that the change in dietary habits, coupled with the comprehensive rehabilitation programme did improve her muscle function and exercise capacity.

The functional consequences of being underweight and particularly of protein mass depletion are also reflected in a decreased health status as measured by the St. George's Respiratory Questionnaire [19].

HEALTHCARE UTILIZATION

There is growing evidence in the literature that nutritional depletion in COPD is related to a high utilization of health resources. Vitacca *et al.* [20] reported that basal body weight, the decline in FEV_1 and the rate of deterioration of arterial blood gases were related to admissions to intensive care services. Kessler *et al.* [21] reported that the risk of being hospitalized with COPD was significantly increased in patients with a low BMI, patients with a limited 6-minute walking distance and patients with haemodynamic compromize. Nutritional depletion also increased the risk of early non-elective re-admissions in patients previously admitted for an exacerbation [22]. A prospective cohort study of patients admitted to hospital for exacerbations of COPD described that survival time after was independently related to severity of illness, BMI, age, prior functional status, PaO_2, FIO_2, congestive heart failure, serum albumin and the presence of cor pulmonale [23].

In patients with emphysema undergoing LVRS, such as our patient, a deficient nutritional status identifiable by BMI was observed in approximately 50% of patients. This impaired nutritional status was associated with increasing morbidity following LVRS, manifested by prolonged ventilatory support and increased hospital length of stay [24]. In patients receiving lung transplantation, those with BMIs lower than the 25th percentile, or <80% of the predicted weight for a certain height, and/or those patients with lean body mass depletion had a worse survival rate [25, 26].

BMI AND COPD RELATED MORTALITY

Vandenbergh *et al.* [6] reported a significant association between weight loss and survival in patients with COPD: 5-year mortality was 50% in those losing weight, compared with only 20% in weight-stable patients with COPD. Several retrospective studies using different COPD populations have also provided evidence for a relationship between low BMI and mortality, independent of FEV_1 [27]. In COPD patients randomly allocated to long-term oxygen therapy (LTOT) or medical treatment, Gorecka *et al.* [28] found that BMI was a significant predictor of survival, independent of FEV_1. In a cohort of more than 4000 patients treated with LTOT, Chailleux *et al.* [27] reported that low body weight was an independent risk factor for mortality: the 5-year survival rates were 24%, 34%, 44% and 59%, respectively, for patients with BMIs <20, 20–24, 25–29 and ≥30. The best prognosis was observed in overweight and obese COPD patients on LTOT. In another study, weight gain after nutritional supplementation was also related to decreased mortality independent of FEV_1, resting arterial blood gases, smoking, age and gender [29]. The Danish population study,

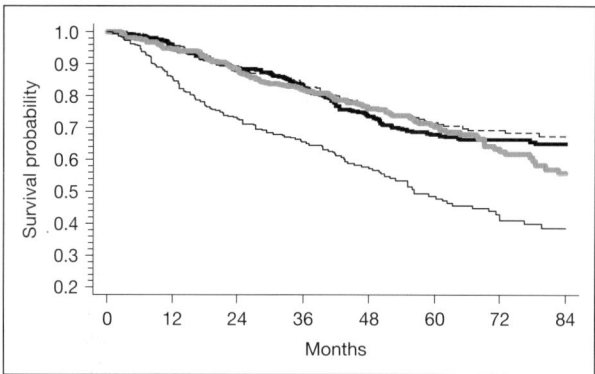

Figure 11.1 Kaplan-Meier survival plot of 1467 patients with COPD followed for close to 8 years divided by quartiles. The dashed line represents BMI >29, the grey line BMI ≥25 but ≤29, the thick black line BMI ≥21 but <25 and the thin black line BMI <21.

including more than 2000 subjects and a 17-year follow-up, confirmed these noted associations between body weight and mortality risk. Using normal weight subjects (BMI = 20–24.9 kg/m^2) as a reference, the relative risk of death, adjusted for smoking, chronic mucus hypersecretion, FEV_1 and gender was significantly increased in underweight subjects but decreased in overweight and even obese subjects with airflow obstruction. A similar but weaker association was observed in subjects with mild and moderate disease. The specific relationship between FFM and mortality was reported by Marquis et al. [30], demonstrating that mid-thigh muscle cross-sectional area obtained by CT scan and FEV_1 were found to be the only significant predictors of mortality.

In a prospective study lasting over 5 years, we also showed that in patients with a wide range of airflow obstruction, the BMI was an independent predictor of survival [31]. The BMI (B) together with the degree of airflow obstruction (O), level of dyspnoea (D) measured with the Modified Medical Research Council scale and exercise performance as determined by the 6-min walk distance (E) allowed us to develop a multidimensional index, the BODE index, which proved to be a better predictor of mortality than the FEV_1.

The patient in the case report outlined in this chapter had a BODE index of 9. After pulmonary rehabilitation and nutrition, her BODE score improved to 7 as her distance walked improved and her MMRC scale also improved. Interestingly, her BODE further decreased to 5 after LVRS. She continues to live 2 years after her resection.

We have continued to follow the patients in the BODE cohort and have extended our observations for almost 8 years. Figure 11.1 corresponds to the Kaplan-Meier survival plots according to the BMI in this large population of 1467 patients. It is evident that this simple way to characterize patients with COPD is very useful for the clinician as it is readily obtainable.

REASONS FOR WEIGHT LOSS

Weight loss, particularly loss of FM, occurs if energy expenditure exceeds dietary intake. Muscle wasting is a consequence of an imbalance between the synthesis and breakdown of protein. Several studies have provided evidence for involvement of systemic inflammation in the pathogenesis of tissue depletion in patients with COPD [32–34]. Systemic inflammation may modify energy homoeostasis partly by interaction between cytokines and leptin metabolism [35, 36]. Leptin is synthesized by adipose tissue and is the afferent hormonal signal to the brain regulating FM. Disturbances in the tightly regulated equilibrium between protein synthesis and breakdown can also be induced by systemic inflammation, at least by activation of the ATP-dependent ubiquitin–proteasome pathway [37]. Muscle wasting may also be the result of a decreased number of fibres, resulting from changes in the regulation of skeletal muscle regeneration or activation of apoptotic pathways [38]. New insights into the regulation of the processes of atrophy and hypertrophy could provide opportunities for the modulation of these processes in the future [39].

On the other hand, the patient in our case report had a significant increase in body weight after her surgery. It is very hard to ascribe the changes to alterations in the inflammatory cytokines thought to be involved in the genesis of malnutrition in patients with COPD. It is interesting that weight gain is frequently reported after successful lung volume reduction. Perhaps the decreased work of breathing associated with the beneficial effects of this procedure, or the capacity to eat without being bothered by dyspnoea (a fact described by our patient after surgery), or a combination of all of these mechanisms, are responsible for the beneficial effect observed in our patient.

SUMMARY

What is quite clear is that it is possible to improve patients' outcome without having to necessarily improve lung function *per se*. In the patient presented in our case report, pulmonary rehabilitation resulted in a significant improvement in function and dyspnoea. This, coupled with nutritional support, also improved her weight and BMI. The rehabilitation programme resulted in a better outcome for LVRS and this in turn further improved her health as it allowed additional functional improvement and enabled the resection of an otherwise fatal lung tumour.

REFERENCES

1. Celli BR, MacNee W. Standards for the diagnosis and treatment of COPD. *Eur Respir J* 2004; 23:932–946.
2. Report of the Medical Research Council Working Party. Long-term domiciliary oxygen therapy in chronic hypoxic cor pulmonale complicating chronic bronchitis and emphysema. *Lancet* 1981; 1:681–685.
3. Nocturnal Oxygen Therapy Trial Group. Continuous or nocturnal oxygen therapy in hypoxemic chronic obstructive lung disease. *Ann Intern Med* 1980; 93:391–398.
4. Fowler J, Godlee R. *Emphysema of the Lungs*. Longmans, Green and Co, London, 1898, p 171.
5. Filley GF, Beckwitt HJ, Reeves JT, Mitchell RS. Chronic obstructive bronchopulmonary disease. II. Oxygen transport in two clinical types. *Am J Med* 1968; 44:26–38.
6. Vandenbergh E, Van de Woestijne KP, Gyselen A. Weight changes in the terminal stages of chronic obstructive pulmonary disease. Relation to respiratory function and prognosis. *Am Rev Respir Dis* 1967; 95:556–566.
7. Openbrier DR, Irwin MM, Rogers RM *et al*. Nutritional status and lung function in patients with emphysema and chronic bronchitis. *Chest* 1983; 83:17–22.
8. Engelen MP, Schols AM, Lamers RJ, Wouters EF. Different patterns of chronic tissue wasting among patients with chronic obstructive pulmonary disease. *Clin Nutr* 1999; 18:275–280.
9. Gosker HR, Engelen MP, van Mameren H *et al*. Muscle fiber type IIX atrophy is involved in the loss of fat-free mass in chronic obstructive pulmonary disease. *Am J Clin Nutr* 2002; 76:113–119.
10. Gosselink R, Troosters T, Decramer M. Peripheral muscle weakness contributes to exercise limitation in COPD. *Am J Respir Crit Care Med* 1996; 153:976–980.
11. Baarends EM, Schols AM, Mostert R, Wouters EF. Peak exercise response in relation to tissue depletion in patients with chronic obstructive pulmonary disease. *Eur Respir J* 1997; 10:2807–2813.
12. Engelen MP, Schols AM, Baken WC, Wesseling GJ, Wouters EF. Nutritional depletion in relation to respiratory and peripheral skeletal muscle function in out-patients with COPD. *Eur Respir J* 1994; 7:1793–1797.
13. Arora NS, Rochester DF. Respiratory muscle strength and maximal voluntary ventilation in undernourished patients. *Am Rev Respir Dis* 1982; 126:5–8.

14. Sahebjami H, Sathianpitayakul E. Influence of body weight on the severity of dyspnea in chronic obstructive pulmonary disease. *Am J Respir Crit Care Med* 2000; 161:886–890.
15. Palange P, Forte S, Felli A, Galassetti P, Serra P, Carlone S. Nutritional state and exercise tolerance in patients with COPD. *Chest* 1995; 107:1206–1212.
16. Schols AM, Mostert R, Soeters PB, Greve LH, Wouters EF. Nutritional state and exercise performance in patients with chronic obstructive lung disease. *Thorax* 1989; 44:937–941.
17. Palange P, Forte S, Onorati P et al. Effect of reduced body weight on muscle aerobic capacity in patients with COPD. *Chest* 1998; 114:12–18.
18. Efthimiou J, Fleming J, Gomes C, Spiro SG. The effect of supplementary oral nutrition in poorly nourished patients with chronic obstructive pulmonary disease. *Am Rev Respir Dis* 1988; 137:1075–1082.
19. Shoup R, Dalsky G, Warner S et al. Body composition and health-related quality of life in patients with obstructive airways disease. *Eur Respir J* 1997; 10:1576–1580.
20. Vitacca M, Foglio K, Scalvini S, Marangoni S, Quadri A, Ambrosino N. Time course of pulmonary function before admission into ICU. A two-year retrospective study of COLD patients with hypercapnia. *Chest* 1992; 102:1737–1741.
21. Kessler R, Faller M, Fourgaut G, Mennecier B, Weitzenblum E. Predictive factors of hospitalization for acute exacerbation in a series of 64 patients with chronic obstructive pulmonary disease. *Am J Respir Crit Care Med* 1999; 159:158–164.
22. Pouw EM, Ten Velde GP, Croonen BH, Kester AD, Schols AM, Wouters EF. Early non-elective readmission for chronic obstructive pulmonary disease is associated with weight loss. *Clin Nutr* 2000; 19:95–99.
23. Connors AF Jr, Dawson NV, Thomas C et al. Outcomes following acute exacerbation of severe chronic obstructive lung disease. The SUPPORT investigators (Study to Understand Prognoses and Preferences for Outcomes and Risks of Treatments). *Am J Respir Crit Care Med* 1996; 154:959–967.
24. Mazolewski P, Turner JF, Baker M, Kurtz T, Little AG. The impact of nutritional status on the outcome of lung volume reduction surgery: a prospective study. *Chest* 1999; 116:693–696.
25. Sharples L, Hathaway T, Dennis C, Caine N, Higenbottam T, Wallwork J. Prognosis of patients with cystic fibrosis awaiting heart and lung transplantation. *J Heart Lung Transplant* 1993; 12:669–674.
26. Plochl W, Pezawas L, Artemiou O, Grimm M, Klepetko W, Hiesmayr M. Nutritional status, ICU duration and ICU mortality in lung transplant recipients. *Intensive Care Med* 1996; 22:1179–1185.
27. Chailleux E, Laaban JP, Veale D. Prognostic value of nutritional depletion in patients with COPD treated by long-term oxygen therapy: data from the ANTADIR observatory. *Chest* 2003; 123:1460–1466.
28. Gorecka D, Gorzelak K, Sliwinski P, Tobiasz M, Zielinski J. Effect of long-term oxygen therapy on survival in patients with chronic obstructive pulmonary disease with moderate hypoxaemia. *Thorax* 1997; 52:674–679.
29. Schols AM, Slangen J, Volovics L, Wouters EF. Weight loss is a reversible factor in the prognosis of chronic obstructive pulmonary disease. *Am J Respir Crit Care Med* 1998; 157:1791–1797.
30. Marquis K, Debigare R, Lacasse Y et al. Midthigh muscle cross-sectional area is a better predictor of mortality than body mass index in patients with chronic obstructive pulmonary disease. *Am J Respir Crit Care Med* 2002; 166:809–813.
31. Celli BR, Cote CG, Marin JM et al. The body mass index, airflow obstruction, dyspnea and exercise capacity index in chronic obstructive pulmonary disease. *N Engl J Med* 2004; 350:1005–1012.
32. Schols AM, Buurman WA, Staal van den Brekel AJ, Dentener MA, Wouters EF. Evidence for a relation between metabolic derangements and increased levels of inflammatory mediators in a subgroup of patients with chronic obstructive pulmonary disease. *Thorax* 1996; 51:819–824.
33. De Godoy I, Donahoe M, Calhoun WJ, Mancino J, Rogers RM. Elevated TNF-alpha production by peripheral blood monocytes of weight-losing COPD patients. *Am J Respir Crit Care Med* 1996; 153:633–663.
34. Francia M, Barbier D, Mege JL, Orehek J. Tumor necrosis factor alpha levels and weight loss in chronic obstructive pulmonary disease. *Am J Respir Crit Care Med* 1994; 150:1453–1455.
35. Schols AM, Creutzberg EC, Buurman WA, Campeld LA, Saris WH, Wouters EF. Plasma leptin is related to proinflamatory status and dietary intake in patients with chronic obstructive pulmonary disease. *Am J Respir Crit Care Med* 1999; 160:1220–1226.
36. Takabatake N, Nakamura H, Abe S et al. Circulating leptin in patients with chronic obstructive pulmonary disease. *Am J Respir Crit Care Med* 1999; 159:1215–1219.
37. Fagoe RT, Goldberg AL. What do we really know about the ubiquitin-proteasome pathway in muscle atrophy? *Curr Opin Clin Nutr Metab Care* 2001; 4:183–190.

38. Agustí AG, Sauleda J, Miralles C et al. Skeletal muscle apoptosis and weight loss in chronic obstructive pulmonary disease. *Am J Respir Crit Care Med* 2002; 166:485–489.
39. Glass DJ. Signalling pathways that mediate skeletal muscle hypertrophy and atrophy. *Nat Cell Biol* 2003; 5:87–90.

12

Multiple vertebral fractures in a COPD patient on long-term inhaled corticosteroids

F. De Benedetto, A. Spacone

BACKGROUND

Osteoporosis is a systemic skeletal disease characterized by low bone tissue, reduced bone strength and increased fracture risk. Bone strength depends on bone density and bone quality. Bone mass density (BMD), expressed as grams of mineral per area or volume, is frequently used as a proxy measure for bone strength. Osteoporosis is a major complication of long-term corticosteroid administration. The use of this drug is common for the long-term management of a variety of inflammatory disorders, rheumatic diseases, pulmonary disorders, and organ transplants [1]. For patients with chronic lung disease, osteoporosis is a serious health problem associated with pain, loss of independence and increased mortality [2]. Advanced age, oxidative stress, hypogonadism, limited activity, poor nutrition status, cigarette smoking, long-term corticosteroid use and systematic inflammation may all contribute to osteoporosis in these patients [3–5].

Long-term oral and inhaled glucocorticoid (GC) therapy is commonly prescribed with excellent results in patients with asthma, although for long-term oral or inhaled GCs there is no clear evidence for their use as conventional therapy in chronic obstructive pulmonary disease (COPD) and patients with this disease who use GCs may be at risk for osteoporosis. Some studies have demonstrated that inhaled GCs may significantly improve pulmonary function and may be helpful in those COPD patients who present an asthmatic component [6]. Chronic therapy with GCs is important to control the inflammatory process in asthma, but the development of osteoporosis secondary to chronic GC therapy is of increasing concern and the risk may be greater than commonly perceived [7, 8]. In fact, previous small, cross-sectional studies have shown an association between chronic systemic corticosteroid use and lower BMD, especially in areas with trabecular bone content [9]. In patients treated with oral GCs for >1 year, 86% demonstrated a decrease of BMD at either the hip or lumbar spine. The decreases in BMD were dose-related and observed in 80% of high-dose, 71% of medium-dose and 33% of low-dose patients [10]. Recent evidence has suggested that dosage of prednisone as low as 6.0 mg/day for >6 months will increase the risk of bone loss and fracture, with the greatest rate of bone loss occurring within the first 6 months [11]. For the inhaled GCs, findings in the literature are controversial because of confounding variables such as prior or current use of oral GC therapy, study design, population sample size and vast differences in doses. Herrala *et al.* [12] examined the BMD of post-menopausal asthmatic female patients receiving beclomethasone dipropionate (1000 µg/day for 1 year) and

---

Fernando De Benedetto, MD, Director, Department of Pneumology, San Camillo De Lellis Hospital, Chieti, Italy
Antonella Spacone, MD, Department of Pneumology, San Camillo De Lellis Hospital, Chieti, Italy

© Atlas Medical Publishing Ltd 2007

showed that there were no effects on BMD in the lumbar spine or proximal femur. The Lung Health Study showed that after 3 years of using an inhaled corticosteroid (triamcinolone), patients with COPD had significantly lower BMD than the controls [13]. It is clear that inhaled GCs have been associated with a lower risk of bone loss as compared with oral, however some studies suggest that higher doses of inhaled GC therapy may also be associated with an increased risk of bone loss.

The threshold dose for adverse effects on bone metabolism may be distinct for each inhaled corticosteroid. Some long-term studies suggest that dosages of <800–1200 µg/day beclomethasone, <800–1000 µg/day budesonide, <750 µg/day fluticasone and <1000 µg/day flunisonide may have limited or no effect on bone metabolism during treatment [1].

It has been widely demonstrated that a clear relationship exists between COPD itself and osteoporosis [4, 5, 14] and it is also a well-known fact that in patients with chronic lung disease, such as COPD, malnutrition is sometimes present: in these studies, weight loss and the nutritional depletion status may be directly involved in the pathogenesis of low BMD. The reason why a malnourished state is observed in COPD patients associated with decreased BMD is not yet clear. Some recent studies have speculated that COPD is a disease that not only involves the lungs but also causes a systematic inflammatory response and pro-inflammatory cytokines such as tumour necrosis factor alpha (TNFα) may cause peripheral muscle dysfunction and malnutrition [15]. TNFα is also known as a potent inhibitor of bone collagen synthesis and a stimulator of osteoclastic bone re-absorption, suggesting that a systemic inflammatory response and increased production of TNFα may cause weight loss as well as bone loss in COPD patients. As in systemic inflammation, the loss of fat-free mass (FFM) may have an association with loss of bone with similar relationships reported in other chronic diseases with depletion of FFM [16, 17]. In fact, Bolton et al. [18] showed a direct relationship between FFM and BMD and between the loss of BMD and severity of COPD. In the context of COPD the losses from these two protein-rich body compartments may be linked by common mechanisms leading to proteolysis, which adds to the primary impacts of the lung disease leading to a loss of skeletal muscle mass, excess bone loss and progressive disability.

Finally, it is well-known that osteoporosis and vertebral fractures can have important consequences on lung function. Vertebral fracture is one of the main causes of back pain and functional disability; it also causes spinal kyphosis and a loss of the normal lumbar lordosis through a decrease in vertebral body height and a limitation of spinal motion. Kyphosis secondary to osteoporosis-related vertebral fractures may have a significant adverse effect on lung functions [19]. The fractures of the hip and wrist do not directly affect lung function, but they can cause substantial morbidity and mortality [20].

CASE REPORT

A 68-year-old woman with a 10-year history of COPD reported for her annual pneumological visit. She told her physician that she had, some weeks before, had an acute back pain that progressively led to chronic pain, severe dyspnoea and muscular weakness, with a consequent lack of activities and exercise. She was afebrile and showed no other signs of systemic infection. The increase in pain has been gradual but, in the last few days, it had reduced the patient to a sedentary lifestyle. She had never used alcohol or smoked cigarettes in the past. The first diagnosis of COPD dated back 10 years and in the last 5 years she had noticed a progression of her illness, so she began pharmacological therapy with bronchodilators and higher doses of inhaled corticosteroids (budesonide 800 µg/day). In addition, her body weight was gradually decreasing (by about 4 kg in the last 2 years) and this weight loss had increased in the last few weeks with a progressive reduction of peripheral muscle strength. In the last 2 years she had had frequent exacerbations treated with oral GCs for long periods. She went into menopause at 52 years of age and she did not receive

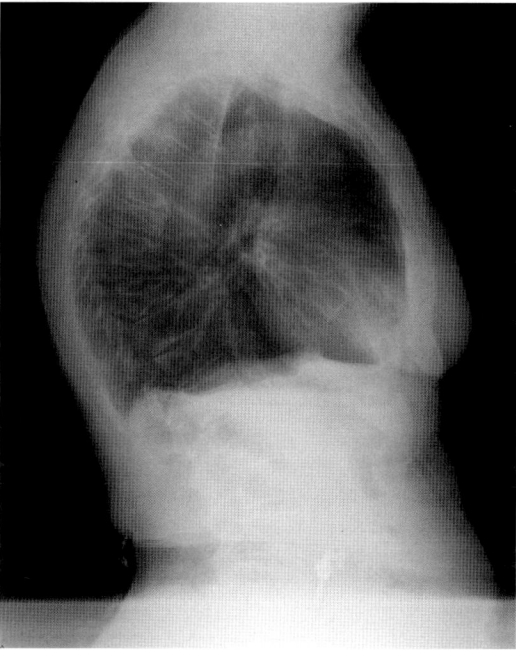

Figure 12.1 Radiograph of the patient: lateral projection showed multiple vertebral fractures with hyperkyphosis.

post-menopausal hormone replacement therapy. The patient's mother died of natural causes and in life she had not had particular problems, with two sisters who were both in good health. The patient had a long history of arterial hypertension treated with drugs for 10 years. Some weeks before her annual visit to the physician, she had a small trauma resulting from the load caused by muscle contraction.

BASIC DIAGNOSTIC ASSESSMENT

During a general medical examination the patient showed a thoracic kyphosis with problems at deambulation and a significant reduction of muscular mass especially in the peripheral district. Body weight was 55 kg and height was 1.68 m (body mass index [BMI] = 19.5 kg/m^2). A thoracic examination showed pain on deep palpitation in several vertebral levels and a reduction of vesicular murmur. No signs of exacerbation were observed. Cardiac and abdominal examinations gave normal results. She had a chest radiograph that showed a thoracic hyperinflation, but the lateral projection showed multiple vertebral fractures with hyperkyphosis (Figure 12.1). Digital radiological morphometry (Figure 12.2) showed a decrease of vertebral bodies >15% (T6, T8, T10, T12).

A specimen of arterial blood showed PaO$_2$ = 65 mmHg, PaCO$_2$ = 40.2 mmHg, pH = 7.412 and SatO$_2$ = 92% and lung function testing showed a severe pulmonary obstruction (FEV$_1$ = 35% of predicted value; FEV$_1$/FVC = 38%). In addition, laboratory tests performed at home showed normal values for liver, kidney and thyroid function, ESR, urine analysis, serum electrolytes, serum protein electrophoreses. The Mantoux test was negative. On the basis of the patient's history, the physician made a neurological examination including the cranial nerves, motor and sensory components, coordination, and reflexes. The straight leg raise was negative and neurological examination was normal. To complete the diagnosis a

Name of patient	L.S.	Date of birth	XX/XX/19XX

Measures of vertebral abnormalities

	Wedge	Biconcave	Fractures
T1	–	–	–
T2	–	–	–
T3	–	–	–
T4	–	–	–
T5	4.39	1.53	7.91
T6	15.15	3.99	0.00
T7	14.25	18.47	13.08
T8	23.13	28.13	11.26
T10	32.21	42.24	18.73
T11	9.32	6.87	0.00
T12	19.03	7.45	3.26

The exam shows decrease of vertebral bodies superior to 15% (T6, T8, T10, T12)

Figure 12.2 Digital radiological morphometry.

bone-density measurement was made to evaluate the degree of osteoporosis and, due to the low BMI, measurement of body composition was performed to provide a means of estimating protein calorie malnutrition, if present. In fact, the measurement of body weight alone is not fully appropriate and does not allow the evaluation of the real nutritional status [21]. Other techniques that can evaluate body composition, such as bioelectrical impedance analysis demonstrated a marked lean body mass loss expressed by decreased body cellular mass and phase angle. The diagnosis of osteoporosis was performed by dual-energy X-ray absorptiometry (DEXA) on the basis of BMD of the spine. The density of lumbar vertebrae L1 through L4, both as a percentage of the mean value for young adults and as a T-score has indicated osteoporosis. The World Health Organization operationally defines osteoporosis as a BMD 2.5 standard deviations (SDs) below the young normal adult mean (T-score ≤ -2.5; Table 12.1) [22]. In Figure 12.3, the values of DEXA examination in our patient are reported and are significant for severe osteoporosis.

DIFFERENTIAL DIAGNOSIS

This kind of fracture is often the result of metastatic disease of primary cancer affecting the lung, the breast, Kaposi's sarcoma, multiple myeloma and tuberculosis spondylitis or osteomyelitis secondary to infection. Clinical history and laboratory tests may exclude these causes. Our patient had fractures secondary to osteoporosis; she showed important risk factors due to the long-term use of inhaled corticosteroids, used to treat COPD and age. It is well-known that osteoporosis is generally present in women who have a precocious menopause without the use of hormone replacement therapy and with a familiar predisposition. As the last condition was excluded on the basis of the clinical history of the patient, the long-term therapy with inhaled corticosteroids seems to be the principal factor responsible for this fracturative event.

Table 12.1 World Health Organization criteria for diagnosis of osteoporosis based on BMD

Classification	BMD*	T-score
Normal	within 1 SD of reference mean*	>−1
Osteopenia	>1 SD but >2.5 SD below reference mean	between −1 and −2.5
Osteoporosis	>2.5 SD below reference mean	<−2.5

*Reference mean based on normal values for a young adult.

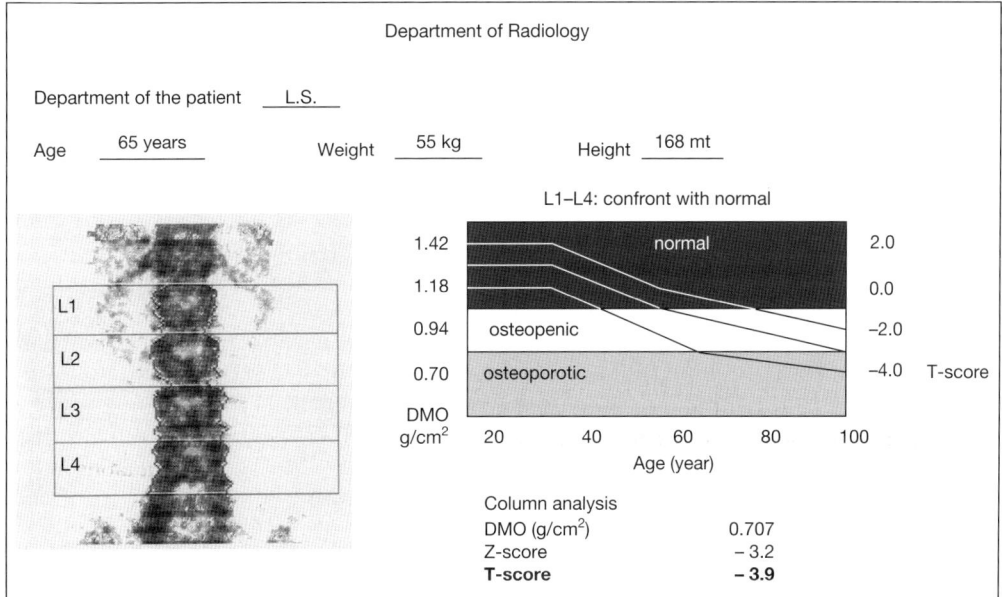

Figure 12.3 T-score indicative of severe osteoporosis.

TREATMENT

The medical treatment of patients with multiple vertebral fractures should focus on:

1. Confirmation of the early pharmacological treatment of the respiratory disease.
2. Management of acute fractures addressing both pain relief and rehabilitation. In the absence of instability or neurological involvement, the emphasis of medical treatment should be on pain relief with bed rest, appropriate analgesics and orthopaedic support.
3. Assessment and treatment of the underlying osteoporosis. BMD measurement should be performed in subjects presenting with a fracture. In this patient, dietary or supplemental calcium (1 g/day) and vitamin D intake should be optimized.
4. Bisphosphonates (risedronate at dose of 35 mg/week).
5. Calcitonin injection at a dose of 200 IU/day is helpful to reduce the pain of acute fractures, but after some days the patient presented with flushing and nausea, so these injections were interrupted.

After 4 months, although the functional lung status was stable, the patient perceived a notable improvement in her general health, with increasing mobilization.

A carefully supervised rehabilitation program should be initiated, after 3 or 4 months following the fracturative event, with muscle strengthening, training, aerobic, weight bearing and resistance exercise.

DISCUSSION

The case reported clearly shows the presence of multiple vertebral fractures secondary to osteoporosis induced by long-term GC treatment. The risk factors include being in an abusive state (alcohol or tobacco use), presence of oestrogen deficiency (early menopause or bilateral ovariectomy), familiar susceptibility, history of fractures in adulthood, low body weight or the chronic use of some drugs (e.g. GCs) [3–5]. A previous study suggested that patients receiving either oral or inhaled GC therapy are at risk for bone loss regardless of age, ethnicity, gender, or other risk factors for non-GC-induced osteoporosis [23]. This drug promotes enhanced osteoclastic activity and it also decreases osteoblastogenesis in the bone marrow, suppresses osteoblast function and increases osteoblast apoptosis. The result is a decrease in both bone remodelling and the osteoclastic signals required for osteoclastogenesis. Also, GCs (in particular oral corticosteroids) reduce the production of gonadal hormones by acting on the pituitary gland, gonads and adrenal glands *via* a negative feedback effect on the hypothalamic–pituitary–gonadal axis. Since sex hormones are important regulators of bone metabolism, inhibition of their synthesis and release through the long-term use of GCs is an important factor contributing to the development of osteoporosis [24].

Unfortunately, design issues limit the value of many studies investigating the relationship between osteoporosis and inhaled corticosteroids. Our patient received high-dose inhaled corticosteroids for a long period; van Staa and colleagues, in a retrospective review of a large UK primary care database, found a dose-related increase in relative rates of non-vertebral, hip and vertebral fractures in inhaled GC users. The significant effect in the patient was that of receiving >700 µg/day of inhaled corticosteroids; however, when the relationship between inhaled corticosteroid use and fractures was adjusted for bronchodilator therapy, the effect was no longer significant. This suggested that it was the underlying lung disease and not simply the use of inhaled corticosteroids that accounted for the increased fracture rates [25]. The presence of COPD can influence the development of osteoporosis, as also seen in previous studies [4, 5]. COPD patients may lose body weight and muscle mass when the disease progresses. Exercise limitation and immobility from both loss of muscle mass and dyspnoea may contribute to osteoporosis. A systematic inflammatory response in COPD patients, demonstrated by circulating levels of some cytokines, such as TNFα and possibly hypoxaemia, may play a role in both weight loss and stimulation of bone re-absorption [15]. An important advance in understanding the correlation between inflammation and osteoporosis has been the recent identification of receptor activator of nuclear factor κB (RANK), a receptor found on the surface of precursor osteoclasts. Its ligand is expressed by osteoblasts, T cells and macrophages. In the presence of macrophage colony-stimulating factor (M-CSF), RANK-L binds RANK, resulting in both osteoclastogenesis and the suppression of normal osteclast apoptosis. Osteoprogesterin is a receptor that neutralizes RANK-L, so inhibiting osteoclastogenesis. Inflammatory mediators, such as TNFα and interleukin-6 may affect bone dynamics by stimulating RANK-L and M-CSF expression and decreasing osteoprogesterin expression [26].

Our patient is therefore clearly at risk: she used corticosteroids to treat her disease and she was suffering from a chronic disease with chronic inflammation.

In general, women are at greatest risk. The prevalent rate for these fractures increases steadily with age, ranging from 20% for 50-year-old women to 65% for older women. Most

Table 12.2 Complications with vertebral fractures

Prolonged inactivity
Increased osteoporosis
Progressive muscle weakness
Loss of independence
Kyphosis and loss of height
Prolonged pain
Crowding of internal organs
Respiratory decrease – atelectasis, pneumonia

vertebral fractures are not associated with severe trauma. Our patient, as reported in the clinical history, reported a minimal trauma some weeks before the observation and many patients remain undiagnosed even in the presence of symptoms such as back pain and increased kyphosis, as in the case of our patient. A neurological examination was fundamental in order to exclude the presence of spinal cord damage or neural deficits, even if minor fractures do not usually result in associated neurological involvement and are considered mechanically stable. Patients with multiple vertebral fractures can develop thoracic kyphosis and lumbar lordosis as vertebral height is lost and the rib cage presses down on the pelvis, reducing thoracic and abdominal space. In severe cases, this results in impaired pulmonary function, a protuberant abdomen and, because of compressed abdominal organs, early satiety and weight loss (as in the case of our patient). Complications due to compression fracture are summarized in Table 12.2.

The physical examination can reveal tenderness directly over fractures and an increased kyphosis, as in our patient.

The diagnosis can be confirmed if plain radiographs show the classic wedge deformity correlating with the area of tenderness found on physical examination. Frontal and lateral plain radiographs are the initial imaging study obtained for a suspected compression fracture. In Italy, if an X-ray shows a decrease in vertebral height by $\geq 15\%$, it is considered positive for fractures secondary to osteoporosis (according to American guidelines, this decrease must be 20%). These fractures can occur anywhere from the occiput to the sacrum, but they most commonly occur at the lumbodorsal junction (T8–T12 and L4), as in our case. Computed tomography (CT) and magnetic resonance imaging (MRI) are helpful for identifying a fracture that is not well-visualized on plain film, for distinguishing a compression fracture from a burst fracture and for further evaluation of a complex fracture. CT can also reveal a narrowing of the spinal canal. MRI is recommended when patients have suspected spinal cord compression or other neurological symptoms.

An assessment of BMI (in our case BMI was $19.5 \, kg/m^2$) is the easiest mode of nutritional screening, even if it is not complete. Our patient presented with a body weight loss that had occurred particularly in recent years, associated with her chronic lung disease; this condition had increased during the last few weeks after the presence of back pain. To complete the study of the patient, we analysed the body compartments with bioelectrical impedance. The relationship between FFM and BMD in COPD patients has been previously described; our patient showed a marked lean body mass loss that not only could have contributed to the development of osteoporosis, but may also have increased the inactivity and chronic pain presented by the patient. Assessment of BMI and particularly FFM can be very helpful in understanding peripheral and respiratory muscle weakness, exercise capacity and reduced health status [18]. In a previous study, we described the systemic effects of COPD: in particular, weight loss is often accompanied by peripheral muscle dysfunction and weakness, which markedly contribute to exercise limitation and impaired quality of life [27]. After the first period in which bed rest is fundamental, analgesics and orthopaedic support are important to begin a specific rehabilitation. In fact, in many patients, severe pain and limited activity persist for up to 3 months. As the acute fracture pain subsides, many patients continue to experience mechanical pain, which limits standing or walking time. A carefully supervised rehabilitation programme designed to strengthen the spinal extensor musculature is therefore fundamental; this programme should be initiated a few months (3 or 4) after the acute trauma. Our patient took this advice.

BMD (preferably in the lumbar spine or femoral neck) should be determined periodically in all patients receiving or expecting to receive long-term GC therapy. Patients who have received ≥7.5 mg/day oral prednisone or ≥1.0 mg/day inhaled steroids for >6 months are clearly at risk for bone loss [28] and dual X-ray absorptiometry for the assessment of BMD should be advised. BMD analysis might also be prudent in our patient who presented with important risk factors (body weight loss, back pain, kyphosis, recent fractures). Preferably, BMD should be measured *before* or shortly after the initiation of long-term GC treatment: unfortunately this was not the case with our patient.

Although chronic GC therapy clearly reduces morbidity and mortality, GCs must be used prudently in the light of their numerous side-effects. For certain inhaled corticosteroids, which are not adequately cleared by hepatic metabolism, the risk of osteoporosis may be further decreased with the use of spacer devices and a mouth rinse after inhalation. Our patient should have begun therapy to prevent the development of osteoporosis and should continue therapy for COPD (bronchodilators and inhaled corticosteroids).

In fact, the American College of Rheumatology recommends starting therapy with bisphosphonates, calcium and vitamin D; these drugs must be used during the whole time in which the patient receives GC treatment. Bisophosphonate therapy is associated with significant increases in spine BMD and a significant reduction in osteoporotic fractures. As described in other studies, the absence of hypercalciuria should be determined. As regards hormone replacement therapy, there is no evidence that it reduces the risk of osteoporotic fractures in COPD patients [29].

SUMMARY

In summary, although the mechanisms that link osteoporosis (and hence secondary fracturative events) and inhaled GC long-term therapy as reported in previous studies, are not yet fully understood, our case report tries to explain this relationship. Nevertheless, experience has shown that it is of paramount importance to treat the chronic inflammation that is present in COPD because this clearly seems to represent the best way of influencing the development of osteoporosis.

REFERENCES

1. Goldstein JL, Fallon JJ, Harning R. Chronic glucocorticoid therapy-induced osteoporosis in patients with obstructive lung disease. *Chest* 1999; 116:1733–1749.
2. Myers AH, Robinson EG, Van Natta ML *et al*. Hip fractures among elderly: factors associated with in-hospital mortality. *Am J Epidemiol* 1991; 134:1128–1137.
3. Forli L, Halse J, Haug E *et al*. Vitamin D deficiency, bone mineral density and weight in patients advanced pulmonary disease. *J Intern Med* 2004; 256:56–62.
4. Iqbal F, Michaelson J, Thaler L *et al*. Declining bone mass in men with chronic pulmonary disease: contribution of glucocorticoid treatment, body mass index and gonadal function. *Chest* 1999; 116:1616–1624.
5. McEvoy CE, Ensrud KE, Bender E *et al*. Association between corticosteroid use and vertebral fractures in older men with chronic obstructive pulmonary disease. *Am J Respir Crit Care Med* 1998; 157:704–709.
6. Weiner P, Weiner M, Rabner M *et al*. The response to inhaled and oral steroids in patients with stable chronic obstructive pulmonary disease. *J Intern Med* 1999; 245:83–89.
7. Barnes N. Relative safety and efficacy of inhaled corticosteroids. *J Allergy Clin Immunol* 1998; 101:460S–464S.

8. Woodcock A. Effects of inhaled corticosteroids on bone density and metabolism. *J Allergy Clin Immunol* 1998; 101:S456–S459.
9. Seeman EH, Wagner K, Offord R *et al*. Differential effects of endocrine dysfunction on the axial and appendicular skeleton. *J Clin Invest* 1982; 69:1302–1309.
10. Reddy BM, Villar ME, Silverman BA *et al*. Osteoporosis among adult asthma patients receiving chronic corticosteroid therapy. *J Allergy Clin Immunol* 1998; 101:290–294.
11. Pearce G, Ryan PFJ, Delmas PD *et al*. The deleterious effects of low-dose corticosteroids on bone density in patients with polymyalgia rheumatica. *Br J Rheumatol* 1998; 37:292–299.
12. Herrala J, Puolijoki H, Impivaara O *et al*. Bone mineral density in asthmatic women on high-dose inhaled beclomethasone dipropionate. *Bone* 1994; 15:621–623.
13. The Lung Health Study Research Group. Effect of inhaled triamcinolone on the decline in pulmonary function in chronic obstructive pulmonary disease. *N Engl J Med* 2000; 343:1902–1909.
14. Katsura H, Kida K. A comparison of bone mineral density in elderly female patients with COPD and bronchial asthma. *Chest* 2002; 122:1949–1955.
15. Wouters EF. Nutrition and metabolism in COPD. *Chest* 2000; 117 (suppl):274S–280S.
16. Espat NJ, Moldawer LL, Copeland EM. Cytokine-mediated alterations in host metabolism prevent nutritional repletion in cachectic cancer patients. *J Surg Oncol* 1995; 58:77–82.
17. Anker SD, Clark AL, Teixeira MM *et al*. Loss of bone mineral in patients with cachexia due to chronic heart failure. *Am J Cardiol* 1999; 83:612–615.
18. Bolton CE, Ionescu AA, Kathleen MS *et al*. Associated loss of fat free mass and bone mineral density in chronic obstructive pulmonary disease. *Am J Respir Crit Care Med* 2004; 170:1286–1293.
19. Nevitt MC, Ettinger B, Black DM *et al*. The association of radiographically detected vertebral fractures with back pain and function: a prospective study. *Ann Intern Med* 1998; 128:793–800.
20. Myers Er, Wilson SE. Biomechanics of osteoporosis and vertebral fracture. *Spine* 1997; 22:25S–31S.
21. De Benedetto F, Del Ponte A, Marinari S *et al*. In COPD patients body weight excess can mask lean tissue depletion: a simple method of estimation. *Monaldi Arch Chest Dis* 2000; 55:273–278.
22. World Health Organization. Assessment of fracture risk and its application to screening for postmenopausal osteoporosis: report of a WHO Study Group. *World Health Organ Tech Rep Ser* 1994; 843:1–129.
23. Ledford D, Apter A, Brenner AM *et al*. Osteoporosis in the corticosteroid-treated patient with asthma. *J Allergy Clin Immunol* 1998; 102:353–362.
24. Manolagas SC. Birth and death of bone cells; basic regulatory mechanisms and implications for the pathogenesis and treatment of osteoporosis. *Endocr Rev* 2000; 21:115–137.
25. Lane NE. An update on glucorticoid-induced osteoporosis. *Rheum Dis Clin North Am* 2001; 27:235–253.
26. Gluck O, Colice G. Recognizing and treating glucocorticoid-induced osteoporosis in patients with pulmonary disease. *Chest* 2004; 125:1859–1876.
27. Decramer M, De Benedetto F, Del Ponte A *et al*. Systemic effects of COPD. *Respir Med* 2005; 99 (supplB):S3–S10.
28. Van Staa TP, Leufkens HG, Cooper C. Use of inhaled corticosteroids and risk of fractures. *J Bone Miner Res* 2001; 16:581–588.
29. Recommendations for the prevention and treatment of glucocorticoid-induced osteoporosis: American College of Rheumatology Task Force on Osteoporosis Guidelines. *Arthritis Rheum* 1996; 39:1791–1801.

13

Managing acute respiratory failure during exacerbation of COPD

A. Torres, M. Ferrer, S. Nava

BACKGROUND

Patients with advanced chronic obstructive pulmonary disease (COPD) and severe exacerbation of their disease often exhibit acute respiratory failure (ARF). Although many definitions of acute exacerbation of COPD exist and many studies dealing with this clinical condition poorly describe their inclusion criteria, most published definitions embrace some combination of three clinical findings: worsening of dyspnoea, increase in sputum purulence, and increase in sputum volume [1]. Clinicians should be aware that other conditions such as heart failure and pulmonary embolism can mimic an acute exacerbation. Among others, the causes of COPD exacerbation include bacterial or viral infections, failure to follow the treatment, consumption of sedatives, inappropriate oxygen therapy, thoracic trauma, vertebral fracture, pneumothorax, pulmonary thromboembolic disease, cardiac failure, anaemia, poor nutritional status, active tobacco consumption and atmospheric pollution. Unlike the staging systems for stable COPD [2–5], there are no standardized and validated systems to assess the severity of an acute exacerbation. The most commonly used system is based on these and other symptoms. Patients with type 1 (severe) exacerbations have all three of the above symptoms, those with type 2 (moderate) exacerbations have two of the three symptoms, and those with type 3 (mild) exacerbations have at least one of these symptoms, as well as one of the following clinical criteria: a recent upper respiratory tract infection, fever without another apparent cause, or increased wheezing, cough or respiratory or heart rate [6].

Patients with COPD exacerbation may require hospital admission when the symptoms of increased dyspnoea, cough or phlegm production are accompanied by lack of response to the treatment of the exacerbation, inability to feed or sleep caused by dyspnoea, inability to comply with the treatment at home, progressive or prolonged symptoms, altered mental status, worsening of hypoxaemia, new or progressive hypercapnia, the presence of new signs or worsening of previous signs of cor pulmonare, as well as any intercurrent process that deteriorates pulmonary function. The ability to identify patients at high risk for relapse, defined as a return visit to an emergency department within 14 days of initial presentation, should improve decisions about hospital admissions and follow-up appointments. Several studies have confirmed what most clinicians know intuitively, that patients who have lower baseline

---

Antoni Torres, MD, PhD, Pneumology Service, Institute and Clinic of the Thorax, IDIBAPS, Faculty of Medicine, University of Barcelona, Barcelona, Spain

Miguel Ferrer, MD, PhD, Pneumology Service, Institute and Clinic of the Thorax, IDIBAPS, Faculty of Medicine, University of Barcelona, Barcelona, Spain

Stefano Nava, MD, Respiratory Intensive Care Unit, 'Salvatore Maugeri' Foundation IRCCS, Institute of Care and Research, Scientific Institute of Pavia, Pavia, Italy

© Atlas Medical Publishing Ltd 2007

forced expiratory volume in the first second of the forced expiration manoeuvre (FEV_1), low arterial O_2 tension (PaO_2), high arterial CO_2 tension ($PaCO_2$), low arterial pH, and who receive more bronchodilator treatments while in the emergency department are more likely to relapse within 14 days of the initial presentation. However, none of the predictive models performs satisfactorily enough to justify uniform use in clinical practice [1, 7].

The criteria of severity of COPD exacerbations include severe dyspnoea not responding to the treatment initiated in the emergency room, confusion or decreased consciousness, clinical signs suggestive of respiratory muscle fatigue and/or increased work of breathing, such as the use of respiratory accessory muscles, paradoxical motion of the abdomen, or retraction of the intercostal spaces, inability to expectorate, severe tachypnoea, assessed by a respiratory rate persistently higher than 35 breaths/min, severe hypoxaemia, assessed by $PaO_2 < 35$ mmHg despite appropriate oxygen therapy, and severe or progressive hypercapnia with respiratory acidosis, assessed by arterial pH < 7.30–7.35.

In addition to the pharmacological treatment, which includes inhaled bronchodilators, corticosteroids, and antibiotics, supporting measures for ARF are needed. There is ample evidence that oxygen therapy provides important benefits to in-patients with COPD exacerbation and hypoxaemia. The goal of oxygen therapy is to prevent tissue hypoxia by maintaining arterial oxygen saturation (SaO_2) at >90% or $PaO_2 > 60$ mmHg. The choice of delivery devices depends on the patient's oxygen requirement, efficacy of the device, reliability, ease of therapeutic application and patient acceptance. The main delivery devices include nasal cannula and Venturi mask. Arterial blood gases (ABG) should be monitored for PaO_2, $PaCO_2$ and pH after initiation of oxygen therapy, as well as upon switching delivery devices. In this case, SaO_2 as measured by pulse oximetry monitoring for trending and adjusting oxygen settings may be acceptable. The major concern with the administration of this therapy is the risk of developing new or worsening hypercapnia and respiratory acidosis. Several observational studies have shown that oxygen administration at concentrations ranging from 24 to 28% in patients with COPD exacerbation resulted in hypercapnia in the majority of them [8–11]. If CO_2 retention occurs, patients should be monitored for development of acidaemia and, in this case, mechanical ventilatory support should be considered.

Mechanical ventilation, either 'invasive' or 'non-invasive', is not a therapy but a form of life support until the underlying cause of ARF is reversed with medical therapy [12–14]. Non-invasive ventilation (NIV) should be offered to patients with COPD exacerbations when, after optimal medical therapy and oxygenation, respiratory acidosis (pH < 7.36) and/or excessive breathlessness persist. All patients considered for mechanical ventilation should have their ABG measured. If arterial pH is <7.30, NIV should be delivered under controlled environments such as intermediate care units and/or high-dependency units. If arterial pH is <7.25, NIV should be administered in the intensive care unit (ICU) and intubation should be readily available. In the first hours, NIV requires the same level of assistance as conventional mechanical ventilation. Patients meeting exclusion criteria should be considered for immediate intubation and ICU admission.

The combination of some continuous positive airway pressure (CPAP) and pressure support ventilation (PSV) provides the most effective mode of NIV. The pathophysiological rationale for the combined application of CPAP and PSV is explained by the fact that, in patients with advanced COPD and underlying lung hyperinflation, bronchospasm, mucus production and airway inflammation increases air trapping and airway resistance. The consequence is diaphragm flattening with associated muscle weakness, and increased intrinsic positive end-expiratory pressure (PEEP) and elastic recoil with associated increase of dyspnoea and work of breathing. Muscle weakness and increased work of breathing are the mechanisms for the development of ventilatory muscle fatigue and a rapid and shallow pattern of breathing. Although this type of breathing pattern is effective in decreasing the work of breathing and dyspnoea, it also causes decreased ventilation and respiratory acidosis due to acute hypercapnia or worsening of previous hypercapnia. NIV with PSV may reduce the work of breathing because of the inspiratory support, and the addition of CPAP offers an additional reduction of the work of breathing due to a counterbalance of the intrinsic PEEP [15]. The consequence of this is the development of a slower and deeper breathing pattern without major modifications of the pulmonary ventilation–perfusion relationships, with increased ventilation and improved hypercapnia and respiratory acidosis [16].

NIV fails when the patient either needs intubation or dies because intubation is not performed for ethical reasons (e.g. patient's non-consent, oldest age, terminal condition) or because it is not available. Intubation should be considered in patients with the following:

1. Evidence of NIV failure, such as worsening of ABG and/or pH in 1–2 h following NIV implementation, with severe acidosis (pH < 7.25) and hypercapnia ($PaCO_2$ > 60 mmHg).
2. Lack of improvement in ABG and/or pH after 4 h [17].
3. Life-threatening hypoxaemia.
4. Persistent tachypnoea > 35 breaths/min.
5. Other complications, such as metabolic abnormalities, sepsis, pneumonia, pulmonary embolism, barotrauma, or massive pleural effusion [18].

CASE REPORT

DAY 1

At 9.52 pm, a 69-year-old male, a former heavy smoker with a history of COPD was admitted to the emergency room because of a 24-h history of worsened dyspnoea and increased purulence and volume of phlegm. The physical examination revealed tachycardia (heart rate = 118 beats/min) and generalized decreased breath sounds with crackles. Indeed the patient showed a moderate bilateral effusion of the ankles. Body temperature was abnormal (37.8°C) and laboratory results were as follows:

- White blood cells = $11.32 \times 10^6/l$
- Red blood cells = $533 \times 10^6/l$
- Haemoglobin = 13.5 mg/dl

Chest radiography showed hyperinflation and no acute infiltrates, while electrocardiography revealed signs of cor pulmonare. Respiratory rate was 27 breaths/min and dyspnoea score was quantified as grade 4 of the Borg scale. ABG breathing room air were: pH = 7.32, PaO_2 = 58.4 mmHg, $PaCO_2$ = 51.1 mmHg with HCO_3^- = 32.5 mEq/l. After oxygen administration with an FiO_2 of 28% with a Venturi mask it was: pH = 7.33, PaO_2 = 67.1 mmHg, $PaCO_2$ = 53.4 mmHg with HCO_3^- = 32.9 mEq/l. Medical treatment was started in the emergency room and included: amoxycillin 1 g every 12 h, nebulized salbutamol 2.5 mg and ipratropium 1.5 mg three times a day and furosemide 20 mg i.v. Oxygen therapy at low flow (2 l/min) with a nasal cannula was also prescribed for 18 h a day.

After 3 h of monitoring, the patient was transferred to the medical ward at the fourth floor.

DAY 2

The morning after, the clinical condition was satisfactory, the patient was feeling better and in a good mood since it was his birthday, and the physical examination revealed a reduction in breathing frequency (20 breaths/min), heart rate (88 beats/min) and dyspnoea (2 on the Borg scale). Body temperature was still abnormal (i.e. 37.5°C). Discharge from the unit was scheduled for the following morning. At 7.35 pm, immediately after dinner the patient suddenly suffered from increased dyspnoea (Borg scale = 5) and respiratory rate (26 breaths/min), malaise and headache. He was perfectly lucid and attributed his symptoms to having eaten a piece of cake that relatives had brought him from outside too fast. The ABG performed at the oxygen flow of 2 l/min was: pH = 7.28, PaO_2 = 62.1 mmHg, $PaCO_2$ = 61.4 mmHg with HCO_3^- = 34.4 mEq/l. The attending physician delayed any clinical decision to the night-time doctor on duty. At 8.45 pm, it was decided to increase the dose of salbutamol to 3.5 mg and that of ipratropium to 3.0 mg and administer 40 mg of methylprednisolone i.v. every 12 h. At 11.30 pm the subjective conditions, including dyspnoea, improved and ABG at the same oxygen flow showed: pH = 7.29, PaO_2 = 62.8 mmHg, $PaCO_2$ = 59.9 mmHg with HCO_3^- = 35.6 mEq/l.

DAY 3

At 8.05 am, the nurse found the patient supine in bed with significant labial and nail cyanosis. His respiratory rate was reported to be 'superficial' with 10 breaths/min and heart rate was increased to 136 beats/min. Inward inspiratory movements of the abdomen were also observed. It was not possible to quantify the degree of dyspnoea since the patient was semi-conscious and lethargic, although arousable and able to follow simple commands (i.e. Kelly score = 3) [19]. The ABG performed with an oxygen flow of 2 l/min showed: pH = 7.18, PaO_2 = 46.8 mmHg, $PaCO_2$ = 93.9 mmHg with HCO_3^- = 31.6 mEq/l. A brief trial of NIV in pressure support mode was attempted for 15 min, and then the intensivist was called. On her arrival, the patient was gasping for air and unconscious, so that he was immediately intubated and transferred to the ICU at the ground floor, where he was sedated and ventilated in volume assist/control mode with a tidal volume of 7 ml/kg, a breathing frequency of 14 breaths/min and a FiO_2 of 35%.

DAY 4

The patient was switched to the pressure support mode with the following parameters: inspiratory pressure of 17 cmH_2O, continuous expiratory pressure of 4 cmH_2O and FiO_2 of 33%. The ABG performed at 1 pm showed a moderate hypercapnia ($PaCO_2$ = 51.5 mmHg) with a normal PaO_2.

DAYS 5–6

The inspiratory support was gradually decreased to 12 cmH_2O and the vital parameters during mechanical ventilation, including ABG, were within the normal range.

DAY 7

The patient was extubated and spent the following 48 h on NIV, delivered intermittently (3 h in every 5).

DAY 9

The patient was discharged from the ICU breathing spontaneously with the following ABG in air: pH = 7.38, PaO_2 = 63.8 mmHg, $PaCO_2$ = 43.9 mmHg with HCO_3^- = 34.4 mEq/l.

DISCUSSION

The optimal strategy of treatment for a patient with an acute exacerbation of COPD involves diagnostic assessment and use of medical therapy that includes the use of bronchodilators, systemic corticosteroids and antibiotics, when needed. Unfortunately when ARF ensues, as in the case presented, the overall rate of failure of medical management ranges between 27% [17] and 74% [18] in about 50%, so that half of these patients may need to be mechanically ventilated, as in the case described above.

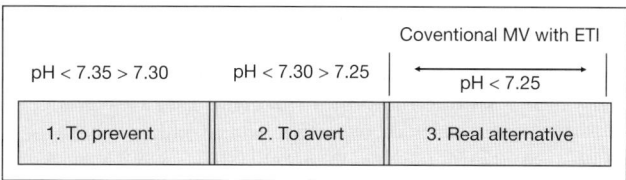

Figure 13.1 Acute exacerbation of COPD – timing of NIV application: 1. To prevent the occurrence of impending ARF; 2. To avert the need for endotracheal intubation; 3. As an alternative to invasive ventilation.

Patients affected by severe ARF have been traditionally treated by endotracheal intubation and mechanical ventilation to correct life-threatening hypoxaemia and/or acute progressive respiratory acidosis, while reducing dyspnoea and inspiratory effort [20]. Although conventional invasive mechanical ventilation is a life-saving procedure, endotracheal intubation is the most important risk factor for nosocomial pneumonia [14] and may damage the tracheal mucosa [13]; furthermore, it increases patient discomfort and the need for sedatives.

NIV is nowadays widely recognized as a valid means to avoid intubation and its associated side-effects and complications in patients with ARF [12, 21, 22]. Unlike conventional invasive ventilation, NIV preserves airway defence mechanisms, speech, and swallowing; furthermore, NIV affords greater flexibility in applying and removing the ventilatory assistance [14].

The success of NIV depends on several factors, such as the type of ARF (hypoxaemic or hypercapnic), the underlying disease, the location of treatment, and the experience of the care team [12]. Time is also important, both in terms of the moment at which NIV is applied and its total duration (i.e. the number of days of NIV and the daily hours of use). The timing of NIV use is still a matter of debate, since on one side a too-early application may signify an excessive human and financial burden (in the light of similar clinical results obtained with standard therapy) and, on the other side, when used in a very severe stage of ARF, it may unduly delay the time of intubation.

In this case, NIV may have been used at different moments as illustrated in Figure 13.1 to prevent the occurrence of impending ARF, i.e. (1) at the moment of emergency room admission (day 1); (2) at an early stage, when respiratory failure is already established (day 2), to avert the need for endotracheal intubation; and (3) as an alternative to invasive ventilation at a more advanced stage of ARF (day 3).

DAY 1 – EMERGENCY ROOM ADMISSION

The patients who benefit most from NIV are those with acute respiratory acidosis caused by an exacerbation of COPD [12]. Although pH is by far the most important determinant for deciding whether to institute NIV, other clinical indicators such as the severity of the dyspnoea, tachypnoea, and the use of accessory muscles are also considered in the selection of patients for NIV [12], which has the potential to prevent further clinical deterioration by increasing alveolar ventilation [16] and reducing inspiratory effort [15].

A pH of 7.32 may be considered the landmark of mild respiratory acidosis, so that the use of NIV in this early stage of ARF remains controversial. For example, one randomized trial found that adding NIV to standard treatment in hypercapnic COPD patients admitted to a respiratory ward with very mild ARF did not produce further advantages; the success rate, however, was 100% for both NIV and standard treatment [23]. Moreover, a recent systematic review [24] concluded that, unlike patients with severe exacerbation and established acidosis, patients with extremely mild ARF do not benefit from NIV. On the other hand, in a large multicentre trial including mild-to-moderate acidotic COPD patients (initial pH ≤ 7.35 and ≥ 7.25) admitted to a medical ward, Plant et al. [17] found that the rate of failure was lower with NIV than with standard therapy alone; subgroup analysis showed that NIV improved the outcome of patients whose pH at enrolment was ≥7.30, while rate of failure and mortality did not differ between the two treatment groups among patients whose enrolment pH was <7.30. These findings suggest that more severely ill patients need a higher dependency setting with a more favourable nurse-to-patient ratio and a higher level of monitoring [25].

DAY 2

A pH of 7.28 is roughly similar to the mean value at enrolment of the randomized controlled trials published in the literature [17, 18, 26–31] that have shown that the addition of NIV to medical treatment relieves dyspnoea [17, 26], improves vital signs and gas exchange [17, 18, 26], prevents endotracheal intubation [17, 18, 27], reduces complications [18, 31], lowers mortality [17, 18], and shortens the time spent in hospital [18, 28–30]. Brochard et al. [18], however, found that the benefits of NIV over standard treatment vanished when only those patients in whom treatment failed and who required intubation were considered; in particular, after adjustment for intubation, there was no difference in mortality.

With few exceptions [17, 18], the above cited clinical trials were underpowered, so heavy use has been made in the last few years of systematic reviews and meta-analyses [22, 24, 32–35]. By analysing pooled results from different trials, these studies confirmed that the addition of NIV to standard therapy decreases the need for endotracheal intubation [22, 24, 32, 34, 35], reduces complications [22, 35], lowers mortality rate [22, 24, 32, 34, 35], shortens the time spent in hospital [22, 24, 35] and reduces costs [33] in patients with acute hypercapnic respiratory failure secondary to an exacerbation of COPD.

Notwithstanding a general consensus on the value of NIV resulting from this large body of evidence [12, 13], some aspects still deserve consideration. For example, the more acidotic the patient is, the higher the likelihood of NIV failure. Although the need for intubation is reduced remarkably by NIV, it is not entirely abolished, so it is definitely advisable to manage patients with more severe ARF straight away in the ICU, where endotracheal intubation can be rapidly performed if necessary, and move those patients who deteriorate or do not improve despite NIV to the ICU [36–39].

Considering the strong evidence of efficacy, the relatively few hours of daily use and, compared to other applications, the fairly low rate of failure, NIV is probably the best approach to avoid intubation in patients with mild-to-moderate ARF secondary to COPD in those units that are willing to implement this strategy.

DAY 3

As discussed above, the early use of NIV in COPD patients with respiratory acidosis and impending respiratory muscle failure is effective in preventing further clinical deterioration and avoiding endotracheal intubation. However, as in this case, because of the delay in receiving medical evaluation and appropriate treatment, some patients may worsen so much that mechanical ventilation becomes mandatory. However, if endotracheal intubation in such patients is not strictly required because of gasping for air, unconsciousness or the need to protect the airway, NIV might still be advantageous compared to invasive ventilation.

There is only one randomized controlled trial that compared NIV with invasive ventilation in COPD patients with severe ARF in whom ventilatory support was deemed necessary [40]. Twenty-three and 26 patients were randomized to receive NIV and conventional invasive ventilation, respectively. The average pH on study entry was 7.20 for both groups, indicating that these patients had more severe ARF than those enrolled in the clinical trials in which NIV was used at an earlier stage. In the NIV group, treatment failed in 12 patients (52%), who were thus intubated to receive invasive mechanical ventilation. The authors found no significant differences between the two groups in ICU and hospital mortality, overall complications, duration of mechanical ventilation, and ICU stay. The patients in the NIV group had a lower rate of sepsis and septic shock and showed a trend toward a lower incidence of nosocomial pneumonia during their time in the ICU. In addition, at a 12-month follow-up, the rate of hospital re-admissions and the number of patients on long-term oxygen therapy were lower in the NIV group. Unfortunately, because of the relatively small number of patients included, this study was exposed to the risk of a type II error and, in addition, it was not possible to perform a *post hoc* analysis to assess whether or not the patients in whom NIV failed were harmed by delayed intubation and invasive ventilation.

These results were confirmed by a subsequent case–controlled clinical trial including 64 consecutive COPD patients with severe ARF caused by exacerbation or community-acquired pneumonia [41]. Data from these patients were prospectively collected and compared with those from a tightly matched historical control group taken from a large database of COPD patients treated in the same ICU with conventional invasive ventilation during the previous 2 years. The average pH of the patients and controls on entry into the study was 7.18. NIV failed in 40 patients (62%), who were intubated. The mortality rate, duration of mechanical ventilation, time spent in the ICU and duration of post-ICU hospitalization were similar in the two groups; however, patients in the NIV group had fewer complications and showed a trend toward a lower probability of remaining on mechanical ventilation after 30 days. Apart from confirming the results obtained by Conti *et al.* [40], the large sample of patients and high rate of NIV failures allowed a subgroup analysis that showed that the outcomes of the 40 patients in whom NIV failed and of the 64 controls were no different, while the 24 patients in whom NIV was successful had better outcomes.

In both the aforementioned studies, NIV was used in an ICU and the study protocols had predefined criteria for NIV failure which led in all cases to a prompt intubation, when required. Unlike the clinical trials in which NIV was used to avoid intubation and was then intermittently applied for relatively few hours [17, 18, 26, 27], in these two studies patients received almost continuous ventilatory support, at least for the first 24–48 h. This might account for approximately 40% of patients in whom NIV failed because of mask intolerance and discomfort, as reported by Squadrone *et al.* [41].

SUMMARY

In conclusion, in patients with COPD deemed severe enough to require ventilatory support, the use of NIV at a more advanced stage of ARF is more likely to fail. A NIV trial before proceeding to intubation and invasive ventilation does not, however, harm the patient and may be cautiously attempted, closely monitoring the patient in an ICU and avoiding excessive delay of intubation, if required.

ACKNOWLEDGEMENT

This work was supported by Red GIRA-ISCIII-03/063, Red Respira-ISCIII-RTIC-03/11, and 2005 SGR 00822.

REFERENCES

1. McCrory DC, Brown C, Gelfand SE, Bach PB. Management of acute exacerbations of COPD: a summary and appraisal of published evidence. *Chest* 2001; 119:1190–1209.
2. Siafakas NM, Vermeire P, Pride NB *et al*. Optimal assessment and management of chronic obstructive pulmonary disease (COPD). The European Respiratory Society Task Force. *Eur Respir J* 1995; 8:1398–1420.

3. American Thoracic Society. Standards for the diagnosis and care of patients with chronic obstructive pulmonary disease. *Am J Respir Crit Care Med* 1995; 152(pt 2):S77–S121.
4. The COPD Guidelines Group of the Standards of Care Committee of the BTS. BTS guidelines for the management of chronic obstructive pulmonary disease. *Thorax* 1997; 52(suppl 5):S1–S28.
5. Celli BR, MacNee W. Standards for the diagnosis and treatment of patients with COPD: a summary of the ATS/ERS position paper. *Eur Respir J* 2004; 23:932–946.
6. Anthonisen NR, Manfreda J, Warren CPW, Hershfield ES, Harding GKM, Nelson NA. Antibiotic therapy in exacerbations of chronic obstructive pulmonary disease. *Ann Intern Med* 1987; 106:196–204.
7. Murata GH, Gorby MS, Kapsner CO, Chick TW, Halperin AK. A multivariate model for the prediction of relapse after outpatient treatment of decompensated chronic obstructive pulmonary disease. *Arch Intern Med* 1992; 152:73–77.
8. Bedon GA, Block AJ, Ball WC Jr. The '28 percent' Venturi mask in obstructive airway disease. *Arch Intern Med* 1970; 125:106–113.
9. Bone RC, Pierce AK, Johnson RL Jr. Controlled oxygen administration in acute respiratory failure in chronic obstructive pulmonary disease: a reappraisal. *Am J Med* 1978; 65:896–902.
10. Eldridge F, Gherman C. Studies of oxygen administration in respiratory failure. *Ann Intern Med* 1968; 68:569–578.
11. Warrell DA, Edwards RH, Godfrey S, Jones NL. Effect of controlled oxygen therapy on arterial blood gases in acute respiratory failure. *Br Med J* 1970; 1:452–455.
12. International Consensus Conferences in Intensive Care Medicine. Noninvasive positive pressure ventilation in acute respiratory failure. *Am J Respir Crit Care Med* 2001; 163:283–291.
13. British Thoracic Society Standards of Care Committee. Non-invasive ventilation in acute respiratory failure. *Thorax* 2002; 57:192–211.
14. Mehta S, Hill NS. Noninvasive ventilation (State of the Art). *Am J Respir Crit Care Med* 2001; 163: 540–577.
15. Appendini L, Patessio A, Zanaboni S et al. Physiologic effects of positive end-expiratory pressure and mask pressure support during exacerbations of chronic obstructive pulmonary disease. *Am J Respir Crit Care Med* 1994; 149:1069–1076.
16. Diaz O, Iglesia R, Ferrer M et al. Effects of noninvasive ventilation on pulmonary gas exchange and hemodynamics during acute hypercapnic exacerbations of chronic obstructive pulmonary disease. *Am J Respir Crit Care Med* 1997; 156:1840–1845.
17. Plant PK, Owen JL, Elliott MW. Early use of non-invasive ventilation for acute exacerbations of chronic obstructive pulmonary disease on general respiratory wards: a multicentre randomised controlled trial. *Lancet* 2000; 355:1931–1935.
18. Brochard L, Mancebo J, Wysocki M et al. Noninvasive ventilation for acute exacerbations of chronic obstructive pulmonary disease. *N Engl J Med* 1995; 333:817–822.
19. Kelly BJ, Matthay MA. Prevalence and severity of neurologic dysfunction in critically ill patients. Influence on need for continued mechanical ventilation. *Chest* 1993; 104:1818–1824.
20. Tobin MJ. Advances in mechanical ventilation. *N Engl J Med* 2001; 344:1986–1996.
21. Girou E, Brun-Buisson C, Taille S, Lemaire F, Brochard L. Secular trends in nosocomial infections and mortality associated with noninvasive ventilation in patients with exacerbation of COPD and pulmonary edema. *JAMA* 2003; 290:2985–2991.
22. Lightowler JV, Wedzicha JA, Elliott MW, Ram FS. Non-invasive positive pressure ventilation to treat respiratory failure resulting from exacerbations of chronic obstructive pulmonary disease: Cochrane systematic review and meta-analysis. *Br Med J* 2003; 326:185–189.
23. Barbe F, Togores B, Rubi M, Pons S, Maimo A, Agusti AG. Noninvasive ventilatory support does not facilitate recovery from acute respiratory failure in chronic obstructive pulmonary disease. *Eur Respir J* 1996; 9:1240–1245.
24. Keenan SP, Sinuff T, Cook DJ, Hill NS. Which patients with acute exacerbation of chronic obstructive pulmonary disease benefit from noninvasive positive-pressure ventilation? A systematic review of the literature. *Ann Intern Med* 2003; 138:861–870.
25. Elliott MW, Confalonieri M, Nava S. Where to perform noninvasive ventilation? *Eur Respir J* 2002; 19:1159–1166.
26. Bott J, Carroll M, Conway J et al. Randomised controlled trial of nasal ventilation in acute ventilatory failure due to chronic obstructive pulmonary disease. *Lancet* 1993; 341:1555–1557.
27. Kramer N, Meyer T, Meharg J, Cece R, Hill N. Randomized, prospective trial of noninvasive positive pressure ventilation in acute respiratory failure. *Am J Respir Crit Care Med* 1995; 151:1799–1806.

28. Celikel T, Sungur M, Ceyhan B, Karakurt S. Comparison of noninvasive positive pressure ventilation with standard medical therapy in hypercapnic acute respiratory failure. *Chest* 1998; 114:1636–1642.
29. Avdeev SN, Tret'iakov AV, Grigor'iants RA, Kutsenko MA, Chuchalin AG. Study of the use of noninvasive ventilation of the lungs in acute respiratory insufficiency due exacerbation of chronic obstructive pulmonary disease. Anesteziol Reanimatol 1998; 45–51.
30. Dikensoy O, Ikidag B, Filiz A, Bayram N. Comparison of non-invasive ventilation and standard medical therapy in acute hypercapnic respiratory failure: a randomised controlled study at a tertiary health centre in SE Turkey. *Int J Clin Pract* 2002; 56:85–88.
31. Thys F, Roeseler J, Reynaert M, Liistro G, Rodenstein DO. Noninvasive ventilation for acute respiratory failure: a prospective randomised placebo-controlled trial. *Eur Respir J* 2002; 20:545–555.
32. Keenan S, Kernerman P, Cook DJ, Martin C, McCormack D, Sibbald W. Effect of noninvasive positive pressure ventilation on mortality in patients admitted with acute respiratory failure: a meta-analysis. *Crit Care Med* 1997; 25:1685–1692.
33. Keenan SP, Gregor J, Sibbald WJ, Cook D, Gafni A. Noninvasive positive pressure ventilation in the setting of severe, acute exacerbations of chronic obstructive pulmonary disease: more effective and less expensive. *Crit Care Med* 2000; 28:2094–2102.
34. Peter JV, Moran JL, Phillips-Hughes J, Warn D. Noninvasive ventilation in acute respiratory failure-a meta-analysis update. *Crit Care Med* 2002; 30:555–562.
35. Ram FS, Picot J, Lightowler J, Wedzicha JA. Non-invasive positive pressure ventilation for treatment of respiratory failure due to exacerbations of chronic obstructive pulmonary disease. *Cochrane Database Syst Rev* 2004; CD004104.
36. Ambrosino N, Foglio K, Rubini F, Clini E, Nava S, Vitacca M. Non-invasive mechanical ventilation in acute respiratory failure due to chronic obstructive pulmonary disease: correlates for success. *Thorax* 1995; 50:755–757.
37. Soo Hoo GW, Santiago S, Williams J. Nasal mechanical ventilation for hypercapnic respiratory failure in chronic obstructive pulmonary disease: determinants of success and failure. *Crit Care Med* 1994; 27:417–434.
38. Anton A, Guell R, Gomez J et al. Predicting the result of noninvasive ventilation in severe acute exacerbations of patients with chronic airflow limitation. *Chest* 2000; 117:828–833.
39. Carlucci A, Richard JC, Wysocki M, Lepage E, Brochard L. Noninvasive versus conventional mechanical ventilation. An epidemiologic survey. *Am J Respir Crit Care Med* 2001; 163:874–880.
40. Conti G, Antonelli M, Navalesi P et al. Noninvasive vs. conventional mechanical ventilation in patients with chronic obstructive pulmonary disease after failure of medical treatment in the ward: a randomized trial. *Intensive Care Med* 2002; 28:1701–1707.
41. Squadrone E, Frigerio P, Fogliati C et al. Noninvasive vs invasive ventilation in COPD patients with severe acute respiratory failure deemed to require ventilatory assistance. *Intensive Care Med* 2004; 30: 1303–1310.

14

Difficult weaning in a COPD patient with acute respiratory failure after use of benzodiazepines

C. Girault, N. Ambrosino

BACKGROUND

Endotracheal mechanical ventilation (ETMV) involves nearly 10% of patients with chronic obstructive pulmonary disease (COPD) admitted to the intensive care unit (ICU) for acute respiratory failure (ARF) management [1]. Apart from the known risks of intubation, prolonged ETMV increases morbidity and mortality of patients [2]. Among numerous complications, ETMV leads to difficulties of weaning and extubation, particularly in COPD patients [3], increasing the duration of ETMV and subsequent risks. Weaning from ETMV appears easy and rapid in 75% of cases, however almost 25% of patients experience weaning difficulties, 4% of whom will be considered as 'unweanable' with conventional techniques [4, 5]. In fact, weaning difficulties could reach up to 70% of mechanically ventilated COPD patients [3]. Although closely related to application modalities of weaning techniques, the time devoted to difficult weaning may therefore reach up to 41% of the total ETMV duration, and as high as 60% in COPD patients [6]. Therefore, COPD patients represent a population at risk of weaning or extubation failure, exposed to ventilator dependency resulting in a non-negligible impact on morbidity, mortality and cost of care. A reduction in the duration of ETMV, and weaning in particular, should be a constant routine daily concern of the ICU physician, specifically in this patient population.

From a pathophysiological basis, COPD is characterized by an obstructive ventilatory disorder, a consequence of bronchoconstriction, inflammation and hypersecretion involving small and large airways, responsible for an increase of airways resistance. Particularly in the case of emphysema, there is also a decrease in the elastic recoil forces of the lungs responsible for an expiratory alveolar collapse with an increase in functional residual capacity (FRC). These two phenomena, i.e. increase of airways resistance and lost of the elastic recoil forces of the lungs, lead to morphological changes of the thorax placing the respiratory muscles, particularly the diaphragm, in a poor functional geometrical configuration [7, 8]. At a more advanced stage, these two characteristics may impair alveolar emptying during the expiratory phase, thus inducing an increase in end-expiratory lung volume above FRC. This pulmonary dynamic hyperinflation is associated with an intrinsic positive end-expiratory pressure (PEEPi) with thoracic distension, responsible for an impairment in lung volumes and bronchial flow rates [9]. These different mechanisms (i.e. increase of airways resistance, decrease of elastic recoil forces and pulmonary dynamic hyperinflation with PEEPi) finally

---

Christophe Girault, MD, Medical Intensive Care Physician, Medical Intensive Care Department and GRHV Research Group, Rouen University Hospital Charles Nicolle, Rouen, France
Nicolino Ambrosino, MD, Pulmonologist, Pulmonary Unit, Cardiothoracic Department, University Hospital Pisa, Pisa, Italy

© Atlas Medical Publishing Ltd 2007

lead to heterogeneous ventilation–perfusion relationships [10] and increased respiratory muscle workload [11]. During spontaneous breathing (SB), these pathophysiological conditions expose the COPD patient to hypoxaemia, respiratory muscle dysfunction with alveolar hypoventilation and cardio-circulatory consequences, primarily pulmonary hypertension, particularly during acute exacerbations [12]. During ETMV, the increase of airways resistance induces a heterogeneous partitioning of the insufflated tidal volume. The pulmonary dynamic hyperinflation could also be significantly increased due to the positive airway pressure (PAP), particularly in cases of inadequate ventilator settings [13, 14]. The main respiratory consequences will therefore be a decrease of the respiratory compliance, risk of baro-volutrauma and gas exchange impairment [9, 13, 14]. From a cardio-circulatory perspective, pulmonary dynamic hyperinflation in ventilated COPD patients may increase right ventricular (RV) dysfunction associated with underlying pulmonary hypertension. This is due to the increase in RV afterload related to an increase of lung volumes and a decrease in venous return related to an increase of intrathoracic pressures. Pulmonary hypertension also increases left ventricular (LV) afterload and the RV–LV inter-dependency. Therefore, these cardio-circulatory consequences may subsequently lead to a drop in cardiac output with systemic arterial hypotension [15]. To minimize these deleterious respiratory and haemodynamic effects, it is therefore useful and necessary to optimize ventilator settings in ventilated COPD patients [13, 14].

Weaning from ETMV, or 'de-ventilation', is in fact defined by the progressive transition from ETMV to SB, i.e. the withdrawal or discontinuation process from ETMV, and should be clearly distinguished from extubation, even if weaning success must meet both conditions [16]. Although weaning and extubation failures appear closely related in time and development, their respective pathophysiological determinants may be potentially different (Table 14.1). Weaning from ETMV is characterized by an increased work of breathing which can be enhanced by different circumstances, particularly in severe COPD patients. Apart from psychological factors and quality of pulmonary gas exchange, impairment of the respiratory muscle performance represents the main pathophysiological determinant of weaning failure. This respiratory muscle dysfunction is due to the imbalance between capacity to generate sufficient strength and efficient gas exchange, and the ventilatory workload imposed on respiratory muscles (Table 14.1). In cases of weaning failure in COPD patients, the

Table 14.1 Main pathophysiological determinants of weaning/extubation failure

Weaning
Pulmonary gas exchange impairment
Imbalance between imposed respiratory workload and muscle capacity
   Increased ventilation
   Increased elastic or resistive load
   Dynamic hyperinflation/PEEPi
Central respiratory drive impairment/diaphragmatic dysfunction
Inadequate cardio-circulatory response by LV dysfunction
   Sudden changes in LV pre and afterload conditions
   Myocardial ischaemia
Psychological factors

Extubation
LV dysfunction
Obstruction/increased upper airways resistance (oedema, inflammation . . .)
Bronchial hypersecretion/swallowing disorders
Diaphragmatic paralysis/dysfunction
Hypoxaemia/atelectasis
Consciousness disorders/encephalopathy

increased work of breathing appears related to an increase in pulmonary elasticity, airways resistance and PEEPi even though the central respiratory drive remains hyperstimulated [17, 18]. The consequence on breathing pattern will frequently be an increase in the respiratory rate and a decrease in tidal volume. This rapid shallow breathing may lead to hypoxaemia with frequent alveolar hypoventilation [17, 18]. The impairment of the muscle performance during weaning can be induced by several factors, i.e. inactivity during ETMV leading to muscle atrophy [8] and other factors (medications, respiratory, haemodynamic, metabolic and nutritional factors) enhancing the risk of acquired critical illness neuromyopathies (CIN) [19]. In contrast, respiratory muscle fatigue, which may be the cause or consequence of weaning difficulties, appears much more controversial [16, 20].

In addition to respiratory muscle performance, weaning or extubation failure could also be related to sudden changes in LV pre- and afterload conditions and/or occurrence of myocardial ischaemia during the transition from ETMV with PAP to SB (Table 14.1). Consequently, this can generate an acute cardiogenic pulmonary oedema, with or without a drop in cardiac output, particularly in cases of underlying or unknown cardiac disease [16, 21].

Numerous criteria, more or less complex, are capable of predicting weaning outcome [22]. However, their multiplicity and the lack of an infallible criterion certainly express the complexity of pathophysiological mechanisms that underlie the transition from ETMV to SB, as well as the difficulties of predicting the success or failure of weaning and extubation in weaker patients [23]. The value of these criteria seems to give more insight into mechanisms of discontinuation failure rather than in predicting the success or failure of the weaning process. In fact, the clinical and arterial blood gas tolerance of a SB trial (SBT) represents the most direct way of assessing the muscle workload that will be imposed after extubation and to consider permanent ventilator discontinuation [16]. However, predicting the success of extubation may be difficult as inspiratory effort can be increased following extubation, particularly by a rise in upper airways resistance [24]. Furthermore, factors affecting extubation failure (Table 14.1) appear less well-established and valuable at the bedside than those of weaning [23, 25]. Re-intubation would thus be necessary in 15–20% of cases despite the success of a SBT [24, 25]. Re-intubation can therefore increase morbidity as well as the intrahospital mortality by as much as 30–40% in reintubated patients [25, 26].

Finally, weaning from ETMV should be considered as a true challenge for ICU clinicians. In practice, they have to find the optimal compromise between the risks of an overprolonged ETMV and those of premature weaning and extubation, taking into consideration the pathophysiological characteristics of COPD patients.

CASE REPORT

A 65-year-old man was admitted to the emergency department for consciousness disorders and ARF. He was an alcoholic with systemic hypertension, diabetes mellitus, coronary artery disease with acute antero-septal myocardial infarction 2 years prior to admission, and tobacco-induced chronic bronchitis with regular tobacco use of 60 pack-years. In the previous year, he had been hospitalized twice for acute exacerbation of COPD requiring the use of non-invasive mechanical ventilation (NIV). He was discovered at home by his family, surrounded by empty boxes of medications. In the recent medical history, the family reported dyspnoea on exertion and at rest worsening for a few weeks with increased bronchial expectoration. In addition, since the death of his wife 6 months previously, he had refused medical care because of a depressive syndrome leading the family physician to prescribe psychotropic treatment. His current treatment included: inhaled combined long-acting β_2-agonists with ipratropium bromide, inhaled corticosteroids, aspirin (160 mg/day), simvastatin (40 mg/day), β-blocker (bisoprolol 10 mg/day), angiotensin convertase inhibitor (perindopril 4 mg/day), tricyclic antidepressant (clomipramine 75 mg/day), benzodiazepines (bromazepam 6 mg/day) and meprobamate (800 mg/day). The previous year, a lung function test showed a FEV_1 of 900 ml (45% of predicted value), FEV_1/FVC ratio of 40% and total lung capacity (TLC) of 9.5 l (145% of predicted value). At emergency department admission, the patient was comatose with a Glasgow coma score of 7 and no neurological sign of localization. He was tachypnoeic at 35 cycles/min, with diaphoresis, sub-clavicular and intercostal space recession. Pulmonary auscultation showed bilateral wheezing with no alveolar condensation. Clinical examination also showed arterial blood pressure of 180/90 mmHg, regular tachycardia of 140 cycles/min, transcutaneous arterial oxygenation of 90% with oxygen therapy of 10 l/min using a Venturi mask and fever of 38.5°C. There were also signs of right-sided heart failure with oedema of the lower limbs, jugular venous distension and hepato-jugular reflux. The patient was immediately mechanically ventilated after intubation by the oral route, which revealed alcoholic breath and traces of vomiting. He was then transferred to the medical ICU. The suspected diagnosis was self-acute poisoning with alcohol ingestion worsening an acute exacerbation of COPD with generalized cardio-respiratory failure and suspected aspiration pneumonia. Post-intubation chest X-ray revealed cardiomegaly (cardio-thoracic index = 0.65), thoracic distension with bilateral alveolo-interstitial infiltrates predominantly in the peri-hilar area and right lower lobe, as well as slight bilateral pleural effusion. Electrocardiogram showed sinusal tachycardia with right auricular hypertrophia, incomplete right bundle-branch block, signs of LV hypertrophia with no acute myocardial ischaemia.

Arterial blood gases on admission confirmed hypoxaemia (PaO_2 = 7 kPa or 52.5 mmHg) and decompensated respiratory acidosis (pH = 7.25, $PaCO_2$ = 9 kPa or 67.5 mmHg, HCO_3^- = 35 mmol/l). Biological data showed a positive alcoholaemia (2 g/l) and confirmed benzodiazepine poisoning (bromazepam) with a normal serum meprobamate dosage. Plasmatic troponin Ic dosage was within normal range and other biological findings only showed leucocytosis ($15 \times 10^9/mm^3$) with polycythaemia (haematocrit = 53%). Medical treatment consisted of diuretics (furosemide 80 mg i.v. × 3/day), antibiotherapy (amoxicillin-clavulanate 1 g i.v. × 3/day), and β_2-agonists (salbutamol 4 mg/h i.v.), corticosteroids (methylprednisolone 80 mg i.v./day) with sedation (midazolam 5 mg/h i.v., fentanyl 75 μg/kg/h i.v.) due to a severe bronchospasm under assist-controlled mechanical ventilation (ACV) with initial settings as follows: tidal volume = 400 ml, respiratory rate = 12 cycles/min, flow rate = 60 l/min, inspiratory/expiratory ratio = 1/5, FiO_2 = 80%, extrinsic PEEP (PEEPe) = 0 cmH_2O). Intravenous β_2-agonists were rapidly stopped due to a worsening of tachycardia with arrhythmia poorly tolerated from a haemodynamic perspective, and switched to inhaled β_2-agonists combined with ipratropium bromide (6/day). Aspiration pneumonia was subsequently confirmed based on culture of endobronchial microbiological sampling using blinded protected telescoping catheter (*Echerichia coli*: 3×10^3 cfu/ml), and after disappearance of the part of pulmonary oedema on chest X-ray.

Favourable clinical outcome at day 3, with apyrexia, weight loss of 8 kg and bronchospasm relief, presented an opportunity to consider the withdrawal of sedation. However, the patient's awakening was very agitated which indicated delirium tremens and led again to the decision to sedate the patient for a further 48 h. Awakening was then marked by a severe bronchospasm resisting intravenous β_2-agonists and corticosteroids, requiring the use of heavy sedation and myorelaxant paralysis (cisatracurium 12 mg/h i.v.) during 72 h. Finally, the patient exhibited quiet and full awakening at day 12 with low doses of neuroleptics (levopromazine 50 mg i.v./day) and benzodiazepines (chlorazepam 20 mg i.v./day). The attending physician preferred to wait for the complete stop of psychotropic treatment before considering weaning from ETMV. The first SBT using T-tube finally occurred at day 15 and the patient was extubated after 30 min with a good clinical tolerance but no arterial blood gas control. He was re-intubated 2 h later in emergency for sudden bronchospastic respiratory distress with bronchial obstruction and respiratory encephalopathy again requiring ACV with sedation and myorelaxant paralysis. Endotracheal aspirations were found to be abundant and foamy with peri-hilar infiltrates on chest X-ray with no pneumothorax.

Diuretics were prescribed and ETMV was maintained for an additional 48 h. Progressive withdrawal was then again attempted using pressure support ventilation (PSV) with PEEPe. The gradual decrease of PSV level was well-tolerated up to 10 cmH$_2$O but patient-ventilator asynchrony occurred with poor clinical tolerance as soon as the PEEPe was removed and/or the PSV level was reduced below 10 cmH$_2$O.

DISCUSSION

Dependence on mechanical ventilation following resolution of an acute respiratory illness is a major healthcare problem. As previously mentioned, approximately 75% of patients mechanically ventilated in the ICU resume SB in a few days [4, 5]. The remaining 25% suffer from difficult weaning due to a combination of unresolved primary illness or pre-existing cardio-respiratory or neuromuscular disease. Forty-one percent of the overall ICU time has been reported to be devoted to weaning with large differences between different aetiologies requiring mechanical ventilation, the process of weaning accounting for more than half of ICU stay in patients with COPD, cardiac failure or neurological problems [6]. Therefore, severe COPD often represents a high risk factor for weaning difficulties from ETMV, as reported in the case report scenario.

First of all, the recent acute exacerbation in our patient may have been precipitated, before self-acute poisoning, by the medical treatment including β-blockers and psychotropic medications. β-blockers have traditionally been considered contraindicated in COPD patients. However, compared to placebo, no adverse respiratory effects (no change in FEV$_1$ or respiratory symptoms) or impairment in the FEV$_1$ treatment response to β$_2$-agonists have been demonstrated with cardioselective β-blockers in a recent meta-analysis including 20 randomized controlled trials [27]. These results concern more severe COPD patients as well as those with a reversible obstructive component. Therefore, given their demonstrated benefit (heart failure, coronary artery disease and hypertension treatment) cardioselective β-blockers, as bisoprolol, could be routinely used in COPD patients. In contrast psychotropic drugs, mainly benzodiazepines, are generally not recommended in these SB patients due to their depressant effect on central respiratory drive and their myorelaxant effect [28].

The patient's ICU stay was marked by prolonged ETMV and sedation. Heavy and prolonged sedation with paralysis was motivated by agitation and occurrence of severe bronchospasm. These characteristics illustrate the relationship between sedation and duration of ETMV. It is now well-established that duration of ETMV, including weaning, appears closely influenced by the modality of sedation (bolus or continuous i.v. infusion), leading to the recommendation to use practice guidelines for sedation [29]. However, modalities of sedative and analgesic withdrawal, which should be included in these guidelines, are not as well-established. Although daily interruption seems to be associated with shorter duration of ETMV and ICU stay [30], it must be kept in mind that patients exposed to more than 1 week of high-dose opioid or sedative therapy may develop neuroadaptation or physiological dependence. In critically ill adult patients, rapid discontinuation of these agents could lead to withdrawal symptoms requiring further sedation and prolonging ETMV and ICU stay [31]. In high-risk patients (high doses or more than 7 days of continuous therapy), sedative and analgesic withdrawal should be progressive with doses systematically tapered to prevent withdrawal symptoms [30]. Our patient developed agitation with suspected alcohol-induced delirium tremens but sedative and analgesic withdrawal symptoms could not be formally excluded since he had received psychotropic treatment before ICU admission.

The patient was re-intubated within 2 h after extubation for bronchospastic ARF with bronchial obstruction and respiratory encephalopathy symptoms. However, upper airway obstruction may have played a role, in part, in the extubation failure of this agitated patient requiring prolonged ETMV [32]. As previously stated, numerous weaning criteria have been proposed [22]. However, none of these criteria has sufficient performance to predict the weaning process outcome, particularly in COPD patients [33]. Furthermore, these criteria are of limited use in predicting extubation failure, which may occur despite success of an SBT. Moreover, none of the extubation criteria, including the cuff-leak test, has been satisfactorily validated [23, 34]. In fact, extubation may be considered when adequate consciousness is achieved with no sedation and the patient is able to protect the airway with an effective cough. Nevertheless, in our experience, some patients may require low doses of benzodiazepines and/or neuroleptics to hinder psychological factors or physiological dependence during the weaning process, but this should be applied with particular caution in COPD patients.

Finally, after daily assessment of the weaning potential, performing an SBT should currently represent the main second step of the weaning process [16]. Either T-piece, PSV or continuous PAP may be used to perform SBT in COPD patients but more data are currently available for the first two techniques. Similar results have been obtained with these two methods [4, 5]. T-piece, best mimicking the real respiratory conditions after extubation, requires close supervision due to the disconnection from the ventilator. PSV requires a minimum level of 7 cmH$_2$O of inspiratory support to compensate for the additional resistive work of breathing caused by the endotracheal tube and ventilator circuit [35]. In COPD patients, applying PEEPe to PSV may also enhance breath triggering if significant PEEPi is suspected [9, 11, 14]. Similar results have been obtained with SBT lasting for 30–120 min, particularly with T-piece [26], but not exceeding 120 min to prevent potential diaphragmatic fatigue [20]. However, in contrast in our patient, SBT could be prolonged for 120 min in potentially difficult-to-wean patients [36]. In COPD patients, clinical criteria of SBT tolerance are similar to those of the general population (respiratory pattern, SaO$_2$, haemodynamic stability, consciousness and subjective comfort), but the SaO$_2$ threshold value of intolerance could be lowered at <85%. Although not performed in our patient, arterial blood gas control is also recommended in cases of poor clinical SBT tolerance or suspected weaning difficulties [16].

In cases of SBT or extubation failure, even though persistent respiratory system mechanical impairment is frequently involved [17], other potential causes must be researched and its reversibility considered (Table 14.1). On the basis of the patient's medical history, although bronchospastic, he seems to have been re-intubated, in part, for LV dysfunction with symptoms of acute cardiogenic pulmonary oedema. This LV dysfunction could be investigated using echocardiography or a pulmonary artery catheter [21]. Despite adequate treatment of this episode and progressive withdrawal from ETMV using partial ventilatory support, weaning difficulties persisted and should be investigated further. Our patient required heavy sedation and myorelaxant paralysis for more than 72 h, received high dose i.v. corticosteroids and underwent ACV. These factors may combine, leading to difficult, if not impossible weaning. Heavy sedation and/or myorelaxant paralysis, particularly in the initial days of critical illness, may lead to a generalized neuromyopathy [37]. Acquired CIN, a combination of neuropathy and myopathy, may develop, particularly in critically ill adult patients with sepsis and multiple organ failure and this represents a frequent cause of neuromuscular weaning failure [19, 38]. Impairment in skeletal muscle strength in the ICU could also be a consequence of electrolyte disturbances [39] or a direct effect of hypercapnia, hypoxia, malnutrition, and treatment with corticosteroids or other agents. In fact, it has been shown that even a short course of high-dose i.v. corticosteroids may be followed by generalized and respiratory muscle weakness lasting for months [40]. The use of continuous i.v. sedation, as well as that of controlled mechanical ventilation, as observed in our patient, may be associated with prolonged ETMV and with the development of selective diaphragmatic atrophy after only 48 h [30, 41]. Therefore, respiratory muscle weakness following all of the above-mentioned conditions is a major determinant of weaning or extubation failure in mechanically ventilated patients [42] and should be suspected in our patient. In practice, neuromuscular weaning or extubation failure, particularly CIN, can be predicted in the high-risk patients described above, based on clinical examination using a simple bedside muscle strength score and confirmed by peripheral electrophysiological abnormalities [19, 38].

In difficult-to-wean patients, persistent respiratory system mechanical abnormalities require the consideration of progressive withdrawal from ETMV. Once daily SBT and partial ventilatory support using a gradual decrease of PSV level seems to give similar weaning and extubation outcome [4, 5]. However, due to the imbalance between respiratory muscle performance and the ventilatory workload (Table 14.1) during transition from controlled ventilatory support (i.e. ACV) to an SBT or extubation, a gradual reduction strategy of PSV level should be preferred in difficult to wean COPD patients [16]. Furthermore, the clinician should focus on optimizing this gradual ventilatory support strategy aimed at improving respiratory muscle unloading, comfort and patient–ventilator synchrony [43]. Adjustments to ventilator settings may be based on detection of ineffective inspiratory efforts by using clinical examination as well as pressure and flow-time curves on the monitor screen of the ventilator [44]. Including the previous aims, optimization of PSV in difficult-to-wean COPD patients should consider all the following issues: use of sensitive, responsive ventilator-triggering systems [45], flow-triggering with flow patterns matched to patient demand (i.e. increased flow rate and flow-ramp) [46, 47] and adequate ventilator inspiratory and expiratory cycling to avoid air-trapping [48]; adjust level of PSV [49]; apply PEEPe in the presence of a triggering threshold load from suspected PEEPi [9, 11, 14]. In cases of weaning difficulties, particular attention should also be paid to humidification devices. Many heat and moisture exchangers are known to increase ventilatory demand, mainly due to the increase of instrumental dead-space. During SBT or gradual withdrawal with PSV, a heated humidifier should be preferred, otherwise PSV level must be increased (by 5–8 cmH$_2$O) to compensate for the additional work of breathing induced by the heat and moisture exchanger [50].

Other ventilatory support modes have been developed in an attempt to automatically wean patients by feedback from one or more ventilator-measured parameters [51]. Among these 'dual-modes', a knowledge-based system for adjusting pressure support level could be promising, as favourable results have been recently reported in a multicentre clinical study involving a heterogeneous population [52]. Primarily used to avoid ETMV, NIV has also recently been developed as a weaning technique from ETMV. In difficult-to-wean COPD patients particularly, NIV should be used as an alternative weaning technique, either systematically when the patient cannot sustain SB [53, 54] or more practically when the clinician encounters weaning difficulties with conventional methods [55]. Traditionally, tracheostomy is not considered as a weaning technique. However, tracheostomy should be considered in more difficult-to-wean patients, currently probably after NIV failure in COPD patients [55], and/or when long-term ventilatory support is highly predictable. In addition to the advantages commonly ascribed to tracheostomy (enhanced patient mobility and comfort with ability to speak and eat orally, more effective airway suctioning, decreased airway, resistance and more secure airway), although its exact timing remains highly controversial [56], it should be kept in mind that tracheostomy might accelerate the ability to transfer ventilator-dependent patients from the ICU to general wards or long-term facilities [16]. Including these aims, neuromuscular weaning failure may currently represent one of the best indications for tracheostomy which, therefore, could be proposed for our patient. In all cases, bronchodilators and respiratory physiotherapy are useful adjuvants in difficult-to-wean COPD patients.

SUMMARY

Prolonged ETMV and weaning difficulties in our patient were primarily due to the underlying severe COPD and coronary artery disease, as well as the chronic alcoholic status and depressive syndrome requiring psychotropic treatment. All these conditions have led to the use of prolonged and heavy sedation with muscle paralysis. Secondly, and subject to PSV settings used for ventilator discontinuation, weaning and extubation difficulties could probably be related to and supported by the development of an acquired CIN in this patient.

The clinician must find the optimal compromise between the risks of a prolonged ETMV and those of a premature discontinuation from the ventilator and extubation. This should be considered as soon as the patient is intubated. Once the underlying cause of ARF has been resolved, the weaning process to follow in COPD patients is similar to that of the general population but must take into account their pathophysiological characteristics. The main steps of the weaning process should therefore consider the following issues:

1. Assessment of the patient's readiness for subsequent discontinuation from ETMV.
2. Discontinuation assessment from ETMV by performing an SBT with evaluation of clinical and arterial blood gas tolerance.
3. Assessment of the ability to protect the airway for subsequent extubation.
4. Investigation of the cause and its potential reversibility if SBT has failed or in cases of subsequent extubation failure.
5. If SBT has failed, use of a comfortable, non-fatiguing and gradual weaning technique.

Due to the pathophysiological characteristics of COPD patients, the following issues should also be addressed: PSV should be used as the preferred gradual ventilatory support mode; PSV settings have to be optimized, including PEEPe adjustment; NIV currently represents a valuable weaning technique in this particular patient population and tracheostomy should be considered in long-term ventilator-dependent patients. In all cases, bronchodilators and respiratory physiotherapy are useful adjuvants in this population. Finally, all the previous conditions should ideally be implemented in weaning protocols locally adapted by ICUs, including sedation and its withdrawal, which could be developed and designed for non-physician healthcare professionals (respiratory therapists or nurses) [30, 57].

ACKNOWLEDGEMENT

The authors thank Richard Medeiros, Rouen University Hospital Medical Editor, for his expert advice in editing the manuscript.

REFERENCES

1. Esteban A, Anzueto A, Frutos F et al. Characteristics and outcomes in adult patients receiving mechanical ventilation: a 28-day international study. *JAMA* 2002; 287:345–355.
2. Pingleton SK. Complications associated with mechanical ventilation. In: Tobin MJ (ed.). *Principles and Practice of Mechanical Ventilation*. McGraw-Hill, Inc., New York, 1994, pp 775–792.
3. Vitacca M, Vianello A, Colombo D et al. Comparison of two methods for weaning patients with chronic obstructive pulmonary disease requiring mechanical ventilation for more than 15 days. *Am J Respir Crit Care Med* 2001; 164:225–230.
4. Brochard L, Rauss A, Benito S et al. Comparison of three methods of gradual withdrawal from ventilatory support during weaning from mechanical ventilation. *Am J Respir Crit Care Med* 1994; 150:896–903.
5. Esteban A, Frutos F, Tobin MJ et al. A comparison of four methods of weaning patients from mechanical ventilation. *N Engl J Med* 1995; 332:345–350.
6. Esteban A, Alia I, Ibanez J et al. Modes of mechanical ventilation and weaning. A national survey of Spanish hospitals. *Chest* 1994; 106:1188–1193.
7. Marchand E, Decramer M. Respiratory muscle function and drive in chronic obstructive pulmonary disease. *Clin Chest Med* 2000; 21:679–692.
8. Laghi F, Tobin MJ. Disorders of the respiratory muscles. *Am J Respir Crit Care Med* 2003; 168:10–48.

9. Rossi A, Polese G, Brandi G et al. Intrinsic positive end-expiratory pressure (PEEPi). *Intensive Care Med* 1995; 21:522–536.
10. Barbera JA, Roca J, Ferrer A et al. Mechanisms of worsening gas exchange during acute exacerbations of chronic obstructive pulmonary disease. *Eur Respir J* 1997; 10:1285–1291.
11. Smith TC, Marini JJ. Impact of PEEP on lung mechanics and work of breathing in severe airflow obstruction. *J Appl Physiol* 1988; 65:1488–1499.
12. Wright JL, Levy RD, Churg A. Pulmonary hypertension in chronic obstructive pulmonary disease: current theories of pathogenesis and their implications for treatment. *Thorax* 2005; 60:605–609.
13. Gladwin MT, Pierson DJ. Mechanical ventilation of the patient with severe chronic obstructive pulmonary disease. *Intensive Care Med* 1998; 24:898–910.
14. Blanch L, Bernabe F, Lucangelo U. Measurement of air trapping, intrinsic positive end-expiratory pressure, and dynamic hyperinflation in mechanically ventilated patients. *Respir Care* 2005; 50:110–123.
15. Pinsky MR. The hemodynamic consequences of mechanical ventilation: an evolving story. *Intensive Care Med* 1997; 23:493–503.
16. MacIntyre NR, Cook DJ, Ely EW Jr et al. Evidence-based guidelines for weaning and discontinuing ventilatory support. *Chest* 2001; 120:375S–395S.
17. Jubran A, Tobin MJ. Pathophysiologic basis of acute respiratory distress in patients who fail a trial of weaning from mechanical ventilation. *Am J Respir Crit Care Med* 1997; 155:905–915.
18. Purro A, Appendini L, De Gaetano A et al. Physiologic determinants of ventilator dependence in long-term mechanically ventilated patients. *Am J Respir Crit Care Med* 2000; 161:1115–1123.
19. De Jonghe B, Cook D, Sharshar T et al. Acquired neuromuscular disorders in critically ill patients: a systematic review. *Intensive Care Med* 1998; 24:1242–1250.
20. Laghi F, Cattapan SE, Jubran A et al. Is weaning failure caused by low-frequency fatigue of the diaphragm? *Am J Respir Crit Care Med* 2003; 167:120–127.
21. Richard C, Teboul JL, Archambaud F et al. Left ventricular function during weaning of patients with chronic obstructive pulmonary disease. *Intensive Care Med* 1994; 20:181–186.
22. Girault C, Defouilloy C, Richard JC et al. Weaning criteria from mechanical ventilation. *Monaldi Arch Chest Dis* 1994; 49:118–124.
23. Meade M, Guyatt G, Cook D et al. Predicting success in weaning from mechanical ventilation. *Chest* 2001; 120:400S–424S.
24. Mehta S, Nelson DL, Klinger JR et al. Prediction of postextubation work of breathing. *Crit Care Med* 2000; 28:1341–1346.
25. Epstein SK, Ciubotaru RL, Wong JB. Effect of failed extubation on the outcome of mechanical ventilation. *Chest* 1997; 112:186–192.
26. Esteban A, Alia I, Tobin MJ et al. Effect of spontaneous breathing trial duration on outcome of attempts to discontinue mechanical ventilation. *Am J Respir Crit Care Med* 1999; 159:512–518.
27. Salpeter S, Ormiston T, Salpeter E. Cardioselective beta-blockers for chronic obstructive pulmonary disease. *Cochrane Database Syst Rev* 2005; 4:CD003566.
28. Murciano D, Armengaud MH, Cramer PH et al. Acute effects of zolpidem, triazolam and flunitrazepam on arterial blood gases and control of breathing in severe COPD. *Eur Respir J* 1993; 6:625–629.
29. Jacobi J, Fraser GL, Coursin DB et al. Clinical practice guidelines for the sustained use of sedatives and analgesics in the critically ill adult. *Crit Care Med* 2002; 30:119–141.
30. Kress JP, Pohlman AS, O'Connor MF et al. Daily interruption of sedative infusion in critically ill patients undergoing mechanical ventilation. *N Engl J Med* 2000; 342:1471–1477.
31. Cammarano WB, Pittet JF, Weitz S et al. Acute withdrawal syndrome related to the administration of analgesic and sedative medications in adult intensive care unit patients. *Crit Care Med* 1998; 26:676–684.
32. Epstein SK, Ciubotaru RL. Independent effects of etiology of failure and time to reintubation on outcome for patients failing extubation. *Am J Respir Crit Care Med* 1998; 158:489–493.
33. Alvisi R, Volta CA, Righini ER et al. Predictors of weaning outcome in chronic obstructive pulmonary disease patients. *Eur Respir J* 2000; 15:656–662.
34. Engoren M. Evaluation of the cuff-leak test in a cardiac surgery population. *Chest* 1999; 116:1029–1031.
35. Brochard L, Rua F, Lorino H et al. Inspiratory pressure support compensates for the additional work of breathing caused by endotracheal tube. *Anesthesiology* 1991; 75:739–745.
36. Vallverdu I, Calaf N, Subirana M et al. Clinical characteristics, respiratory functional parameters and outcome of a two hour T-piece trial in patients weaning from mechanical ventilation. *Am J Respir Crit Care Med* 1998; 158:1855–1861.

37. Latronico N, Fenzi F, Recupero D et al. Critical illness myopathy and neuropathy. *Lancet* 1996; 347:1579–1582.
38. Hund EF, Fogel W, Krieger D et al. Critical illness polyneuropathy: clinical findings and outcomes of a frequent cause of neuromuscular weaning failure. *Crit Care Med* 1996; 24:1328–1333.
39. Agustí AG, Torres A, Estopa R et al. Hypophosphatemia as a cause of failed weaning: the importance of metabolic factors. *Crit Care Med* 1984; 12:142–143.
40. Nava S, Fracchia C, Callegari G et al. Weakness of respiratory and skeletal muscles after a short course of steroids in patients with acute lung rejection. *Eur Respir J* 2002; 20:497–499.
41. Le Bourdelles G, Viires N, Boczkowski J et al. Effects of mechanical ventilation on diaphragmatic contractile properties in rats. *Am J Respir Crit Care Med* 1994; 149:1539–1544.
42. Ambrosino N. Weaning and respiratory muscle dysfunction. The egg-chicken dilemma. *Chest* 2005; 128:481–483.
43. Jubran A, van de Graaff WB, Tobin MJ. Variability of patient-ventilator interaction with pressure support ventilation in patients with chronic obstructive pulmonary disease. *Am J Respir Crit Care Med* 1995; 152:129–136.
44. Guglielminotti J, Alzieu M, Maury E et al. Bedside detection of retained tracheobronchial secretions in patients receiving mechanical ventilation: is it time for tracheal suctioning? *Chest* 2000; 118:1095–1099.
45. Richard JC, Carlucci A, Breton L et al. Bench testing of pressure support ventilation with three different generations of ventilators. *Intensive Care Med* 2002; 28:1049–1057.
46. Aslanian P, El Atrous S, Isabey D et al. Effects of flow triggering on breathing effort during partial ventilatory support. *Am J Respir Crit Care Med* 1998; 157:135–143.
47. Bonmarchand G, Chevron V, Chopin C et al. Increased initial flow rate reduces inspiratory work of breathing during pressure support ventilation in patients with exacerbation of chronic obstructive pulmonary disease. *Intensive Care Med* 1996; 22:1147–1154.
48. Parthasarathy S, Jubran A, Tobin MJ. Cycling of inspiratory and expiratory muscle groups with the ventilator in airflow limitation. *Am J Respir Crit Care Med* 1998; 158:1471–1478.
49. Leung P, Jubran A, Tobin MJ. Comparison of assisted ventilator modes on triggering, patient effort, and dyspnea. *Am J Respir Crit Care Med* 1997; 155:1940–1948.
50. Girault C, Briel A, Hellot MF et al. Mechanical effects of airway humidification devices in difficult to wean patients. *Crit Care Med* 2003; 31:1306–1311.
51. Branson RD, MacIntyre NR. Dual-control modes of mechanical ventilation. *Respir Care* 1996; 41:294–305.
52. Lellouche F, Mancebo J, Jolliet P et al. A multicenter randomized trial of computer-driven protocolized weaning from mechanical ventilation. *Am J Respir Crit Care Med* 2006; 174:894–900.
53. Nava S, Ambrosino N, Clini E et al. Noninvasive mechanical ventilation in the weaning of patients with respiratory failure due to chronic obstructive pulmonary disease. *Ann Intern Med* 1998; 128:721–728.
54. Girault C, Daudenthun I, Chevron V et al. Noninvasive ventilation as a systematic extubation and weaning technique in acute-on-chronic respiratory failure. A prospective randomized controlled study. *Am J Respir Crit Care Med* 1999; 160:86–92.
55. Ferrer M, Esquinas A, Arancibia F et al. Non-invasive ventilation during persistent weaning failure. A randomized controlled trial. *Am J Respir Crit Care Med* 2003; 168:70–76.
56. Maziak DE, Meade MO, Todd TR. The timing of tracheotomy: a systematic review. *Chest* 1998; 114:605–609.
57. Ely EW, Meade MO, Haponik EF et al. Mechanical ventilator weaning protocols driven by nonphysician health-care professionals: evidence-based clinical practice guidelines. *Chest* 2001; 120:454S–463S.

15

Suspected exacerbation of COPD in a 56-year-old woman with atrial fibrillation

S. Ramanuja, M. D. L. Morgan

BACKGROUND

The progressive clinical course of chronic obstructive pulmonary disease (COPD) is punctuated by exacerbations. These exacerbations are characterized by transient and often unpredictable episodes of increased cough and dyspnoea. When these are accompanied by the presence of purulent sputum they are usually and correctly attributed to an infective cause. However, when people with worsening COPD are admitted to hospital, an infective cause for their exacerbation may be obvious in only about half of the patients. If the infectious nature of the exacerbation is not obvious on clinical or radiological examination then it might be necessary to consider other causes of deterioration.

Cardiac disease is an obvious alternative cause of acute or progressive dyspnoea that may coexist with COPD. In fact patients with COPD share some of the same risk factors for cardiac disease and appear to have enhanced susceptibility to ischaemic heart disease, possibly through the mechanism of inflammation. In other situations, the features of non-ischaemic cardiac disease may also be masked by the presence of COPD and go unnoticed. The following case history illustrates a situation where an additional cardiac cause of breathlessness may develop in someone who already has recognized COPD. Clearly, careful history taking and thorough examination is necessary on each emergency admission to ensure that alternative diagnoses are not overlooked.

CASE REPORT

A 56-year-old woman with a history of hypertension and COPD presented to the emergency room complaining of a 4-day history of productive cough, subjective fever and worsening dyspnoea on exertion. She had a 3-year history of dyspnoea after walking one city block, however in the past 4 days she had noted dyspnoea after walking across the room in her house. She reported chest tightness and wheezing but denied sore throat. She had smoked 1 pack daily since the age of 16 (40 pack-years). She worked as a glass blower in a factory for 20 years until retiring 1 year ago. Her medications included atenolol, albuterol, and ipratropium inhalers. She was not on home oxygen therapy. She had no allergies, and her family history was non-contributory.

On physical examination, vital signs revealed a blood pressure of 135/92 mmHg, heart rate of 130–150 beats/min, respiratory rate of 28–40 breaths/min, temperature of 37.1°C,

---

Srinivasan Ramanuja, MD, Allergy/Immunology Fellow-in-Training, Allergy/ Immunology Fellowship Training program, Department of Medicine, Division of Basic and Clinical Immunology, University of California-Irvine, California, USA

Michael D. L. Morgan, MD, FRCP, Consultant Respiratory Physician, Department of Respiratory Medicine, University Hospitals of Leicester, Glenfield Hospital, Leicester, UK

© Atlas Medical Publishing Ltd 2007

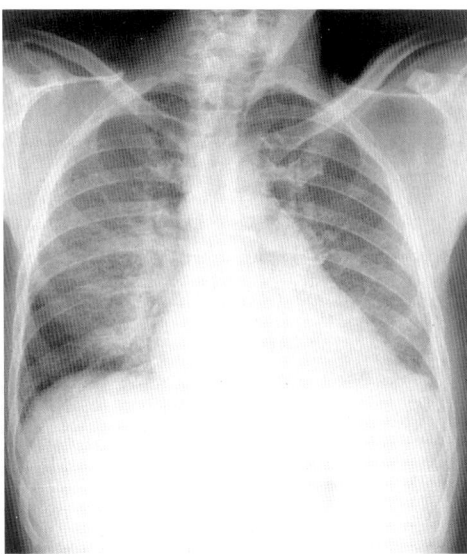

Figure 15.1 The chest radiograph shows cardiomegaly with prominent straightening of the left heart border and increased interstitial lung markings.

and oxygen saturation of 92% on 4 l/min of oxygen by nasal cannulae. She appeared thin with moderate respiratory distress, with audible wheezing and dyspnoea noted at the end of sentences. She was using accessory muscles to help with breathing. On cardiovascular examination, her rate and rhythm were tachycardic and irregularly irregular with a grade 3/6 systolic murmur heard loudest at the apex. Lung examination revealed bilateral panexpiratory wheezes and crackles. There was no cyanosis, clubbing or oedema noted on the examination of extremities. The rest of the examination was unremarkable. Pulmonary function tests from several months prior to presentation were consistent with a moderate obstructive defect (FEV_1 = 1.31 [53% predicted], FVC = 2.71 [70% predicted], FEV_1/FVC = 48%).

Laboratory findings revealed a white blood cell count of 12 200/μl with 70% neutrophils, and the haemoglobin was 12.5 g/dl. The haematocrit was 36%, and the mean corpuscular volume was 82.6 fl. Her biochemistry revealed a sodium concentration of 134 mmol/l; creatinine = 1.7 mg/dl, serum aminotransferase = 56 U/l, and serum alanine transferase = 50 U/l. The total bilirubin was 1.8 mg/dl with normal cardiac enzymes. An arterial blood gas analysis done on 4 l/min of oxygen by nasal cannulae revealed a pH of 7.54; PCO_2 = 22 mmHg (2.93 kPa); PO_2 = 80 mmHg (10.7 kPa); and bicarbonate = 22 mmol/l. Brain natriuretic peptide (BNP) was elevated at 150 pg/ml. An electrocardiogram showed atrial fibrillation with right-axis deviation and occasional premature ventricular complexes. A chest radiograph (Figure 15.1) showed cardiomegaly with prominent straightening of the left heart border and increased interstitial lung markings.

DISCUSSION

Thus far, the differential diagnosis could include the following:

- COPD exacerbation due to an lower respiratory tract infection;
- Pulmonary embolism;

- Lung cancer;
- Silicosis;
- Mitral stenosis.

INFECTIVE EXACERBATION OF COPD

Lower respiratory tract infection may initiate atrial fibrillation in the elderly. In the context of COPD this may take the form of an infective exacerbation of bronchitis or even pneumonia if there is radiographic evidence of consolidation. Not all exacerbations have an infective origin, but sputum purulence is a reliable indication of bacterial infection. Other causes of exacerbation include temperature change, pollutants or virus infection. Antibiotic treatment is indicated if symptoms develop. In most patients, the infecting organisms will be *Haemophilus influenzae*, *Streptococcus pneumoniae* or *Moraxella catarrhalis* sensitive to broad-spectrum antibiotics. Patients with COPD are also susceptible to community-acquired pneumonia with generally the same organisms as previously healthy victims. However, if they have been previously hospitalized or exposed to antibiotics, the spectrum of pathogens may change to include gram-negative organisms. The treatment of pneumonia or infective exacerbation requires antibiotics often accompanied by corticosteroids and enhanced bronchodilators. One note of caution is that treatment itself, particularly aminophylline and β-agonists may also be responsible for supraventricular arrhythmias.

PULMONARY EMBOLISM

Pulmonary embolism is a recognized cause of atrial fibrillation. Any patient admitted to hospital with acute breathlessness should have pulmonary embolus considered as a possible primary or secondary diagnosis. Obviously, this is more likely in patients where there is a high clinical index of suspicion and no alternative explanation. However, about half of recognized pulmonary emboli occur in patients who are already in the hospital. It is also estimated that up to 50% of patients with exacerbations of COPD may have clinical or subclinical pulmonary emboli. The patient with pre-existing cardiac or respiratory disease is more sensitive to the effects of a pulmonary embolus than a previously healthy person.

Making a clinical diagnosis of pulmonary embolism in the presence of pre-existing COPD may be quite difficult. A sudden deterioration in breathlessness could go unnoticed or be incorrectly attributed to infective exacerbation. The presence of pleuritic pain in the absence of features of infection or injury may help. Also the features of deep venous thrombosis or presence of other risk factors such as travel or immobility may raise suspicion. Further suspicion of pulmonary embolism may be present if there are significantly raised D-dimer levels in the absence of any other cause. Confirmation of the presence of pulmonary embolism may require a computed tomography (CT) pulmonary angiogram. The isotope V/Q scan is likely to be unhelpful in the presence of significant lung disease. Doppler ultrasound or contrast venography of the legs may also provide circumstantial evidence of thromboembolism. The treatment of pulmonary embolism with anticoagulation or thrombolysis is the same as for a patient without COPD.

LUNG CANCER

Lung cancer should be considered in any patient with COPD who develops new respiratory symptoms that cannot otherwise be explained. Atrial fibrillation is a rare but recognized complication, especially when the tumour invades the pericardium. The development of lung cancer in a smoker is usually associated with the presence of new symptoms of cough, dyspnoea, haemoptysis or chest discomfort. A change in the character of the patient's usual symptoms of COPD is especially noteworthy. A small proportion (5%) may simply present as an unexpected finding on a chest radiograph. Cigarette smoking remains the primary cause of lung cancer though some occupational exposures may be relevant. In this case silica may increase the risk. The chest radiograph in this case shows no obvious carcinoma, but tumours may not always be visible if they are central or hidden behind the cardiac silhouette. Other clinical indicators of malignancy such as finger clubbing or biochemical disturbance may be suggestive. The treatment of non-small cell lung cancer (NSCLC) is determined by the clinical and radiological staging. Obviously, this requires histological confirmation that is usually obtained by bronchoscopy and biopsy or lavage cytology. The initial staging is obtained from CT and refined if necessary by positron emission tomography (PET) scanning or mediastinoscopy. The best chance of cure in NSCLC is surgery where staging and fitness make that possible. In this case history, the FEV_1 of < 1.5 l and careful assessment of fitness would have to be made prior to surgery. In fact, surgery is unlikely to be possible in the presence of pericardial involvement unless it can be shown to be resectable or separate from the tumour. If surgical resection is not possible then radiotherapy or chemotherapy provide treatment options. Small cell lung cancer is rarely resectable and is also palliated by chemotherapy.

SILICOSIS

Silicosis is a fibrotic disease of the lungs caused by inhalation of dust containing crystalline silicon dioxide (silica) [1, 2]. Crystalline silica (most commonly quartz) stimulates alveolar macrophages and generates reactive oxygen species, which are involved in a chronic inflammation resulting in fibrosis. The most common form of silicosis is simple nodular silicosis, in which pulmonary nodules (co-centrically arranged collagen fibres, with dust-laden macrophages and lymphoid cells inside) are seen on chest radiography or CT scan. Simple nodular silicosis occurs after many years of exposure to relatively low levels of silica-containing dust, and patients with simple nodular silicosis may be asymptomatic [1]. Acute silicosis results when there is exposure to high levels of silica, and is characterized by pulmonary oedema, interstitial inflammation, and accumulation within the alveoli of proteinaceous fluid which is rich in surfactant [1]. In complicated silicosis, nodules may coalesce, and progressive massive fibrosis may develop; cavitation of the nodules may occur along with destruction of the lung parenchyma.

The present patient's occupational history (glass blower) does point to exposure to silica-containing dust, and patients with silicosis may present with dyspnoea. Additionally, silica exposure can be associated with airflow obstruction [1]. However, in this case the chest X-ray does not reveal nodules, pulmonary oedema, or fibrosis. Although the patient may have some chronic inflammation resulting from her occupational exposure to silica-containing dust, her decompensation cannot be attributed to silicosis.

MITRAL STENOSIS

Mitral stenosis, most commonly caused by rheumatic fever, is usually seen more in developing countries. However, new cases of mitral stenosis still occur in the developed world, and given the resurgence of rheumatic fever in the USA during the 1980s, there may be a recrudescence of mitral stenosis in the coming decades [3]. Manifestations of valvular dysfunction appear 10–30 years following the acute symptoms of rheumatic fever, and often the patient remains asymptomatic until she becomes pregnant or has atrial fibrillation [3, 4]. Atrial fibrillation is associated with increased morbidity and mortality in patients with mitral stenosis, and the presence of cardiac arrhythmias in association with acute COPD exacerbation should prompt investigation for any underlying cardiac conditions [4, 5].

Symptoms of dyspnoea in mitral stenosis occur when there is pulmonary vascular engorgement. Patients may present with symptoms of left-sided heart failure (due to increased left atrial pressure and reduced cardiac output) as well as right-sided heart failure

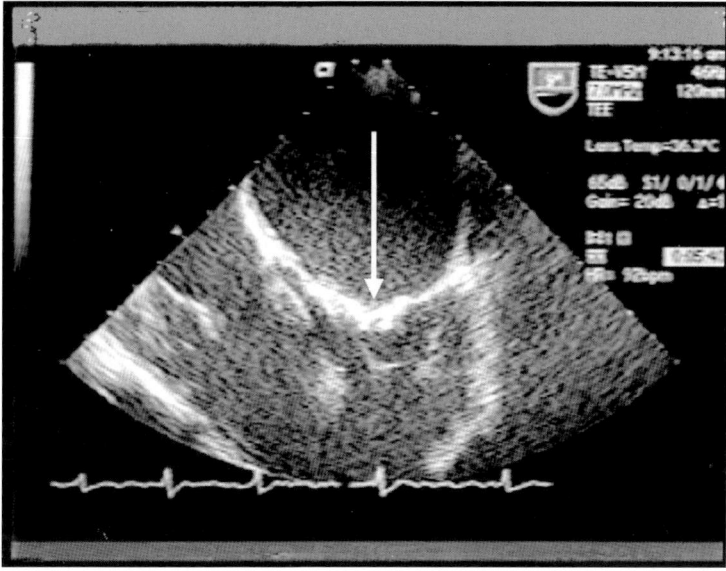

Figure 15.2 The echocardiogram demonstrates left atrial enlargement with minimal opening of a markedly fibrosed and thickened mitral valve.

due to compromised right ventricular function caused by pulmonary hypertension [4]. A diastolic murmur and opening snap may not be audible if the stenosis is severe enough to significantly decrease blood flow across the valve.

Patients with mitral stenosis may show an obstructive pattern on pulmonary function testing, due to elevated pulmonary arterial and venous pressures, which demonstrates reversibility with bronchodilators [3, 6]. Airway hyperreactivity may result from pulmonary congestion that activates sensory nerve endings in the lower airways and increases vagal tone [3, 6].

BNP is released predominantly by the ventricles (with some release from the atria) in response to myocyte stretch, and is a sensitive indicator of ventricular dysfunction and volume overload [3]. Increased left atrial pressure and increased left atrial wall stretch can cause increased atrial release of BNP in mitral stenosis, thus BNP elevation may occur when there is right ventricular dysfunction and normal left ventricular function [3, 7]. However, BNP may also be elevated in the setting of atrial fibrillation without overt heart failure, due to increased atrial production [8]. Thus, it is difficult to pinpoint the exact cause of BNP elevation in the present patient with atrial fibrillation and mitral stenosis, although the elevated BNP is noteworthy.

The present patient's chest X-ray (Figure 15.1) shows typical radiographic findings of mitral stenosis, including the enlargement of left atrium and atrial appendage with prominence of the pulmonary trunk, which causes straightening of the left heart border. Her echocardiogram (Figure 15.2) demonstrates left atrial enlargement with minimal opening of a markedly fibrosed and thickened mitral valve.

TRANSTHORACIC ECHOCARDIOGRAPHY IN COPD

Pulmonary arterial hypertension (PH) is a major cardiovascular complication of COPD [9]. Pulmonary arterial pressure is an important prognostic indicator in COPD, and dramatic elevations of pulmonary arterial pressure are observed during acute exacerbations [9]. Echocardiography is a reliable, non-invasive method of determining the presence and degree of PH in patients with COPD [9, 10]. Large studies have confirmed that echocardiographically-derived estimates correlate closely with pressures measured by catheter [9].

GENERAL TREATMENT GUIDELINES FOR ATRIAL FIBRILLATION

Anticoagulation significantly reduces the risk of stroke in patients with atrial fibrillation. Certain patients at greatest risk of stroke in whom anticoagulation is recommended include the elderly (those over 60 years of age), patients with a history of thromboembolism, diabetes mellitus, coronary artery disease, hypertension, heart failure, and thyrotoxicosis [11]. Aspirin rather than warfarin may be used in those patients who are less than 60 years old without heart disease. Aspirin may also be used in patients 60–75 years old without certain risk factors for thromboembolism (specifically heart failure, left ventricular ejection fraction <35%, and history of hypertension) [11]. Warfarin is recommended in patients older than 75 years and in those with risk factors for thromboembolism. Warfarin may also be appropriate for patients with mitral stenosis (such as our present patient), or those with prosthetic heart valves. An international normalized ratio of 2.0–3.0 is recommended [11]. For patients in whom warfarin is recommended but contraindicated or refused, aspirin may be used instead. Patients who have had an episode of atrial fibrillation lasting less than 48 h may safely undergo cardioversion without anticoagulation; for episodes lasting longer than 48 h, adequate anticoagulant therapy is warranted, both before cardioversion and for 4 weeks afterwards [11].

Rate control may be achieved by various pharmacological agents, and β-blockers and calcium-channel blockers are preferred over digoxin. Digoxin is useful in combination with other agents or when β-blockers and calcium-channel blockers are not tolerated [11]. A ventricular rate of 60–80 beats/min at rest and 90–115 beats/min during exercise is recommended.

Pharmacological agents are also used to achieve rhythm control. With the exception of β-blockers, most anti-arrhythmic drugs have a risk of serious adverse effects, and anti-arrhythmic therapy should be chosen based on the patient's underlying cardiac condition [11]. Evidence from various studies suggests that, in comparing the strategies used to treat atrial fibrillation (rate control vs. rhythm control), there is no significant difference in terms of quality of life or cardiovascular endpoints, including death [11]. Rhythm control may be preferable in highly symptomatic patients, whereas rate control may be preferred for minimally symptomatic patients or those who cannot maintain sinus rhythm. Anticoagulant therapy should be continued irrespective of the strategy used [11].

Ablation has been successful in patients with paroxysmal atrial fibrillation and those with persistent atrial fibrillation [11].

SUMMARY

This case of COPD is complicated by atrial fibrillation and demonstrates a number of features of acute decompensation. Although patients with COPD suffer exacerbations, it may be unwise to assume that the change is always due to the airways disease. Several alternative diagnoses can be considered that may both account for the acute dyspnoea and the association with atrial fibrillation. People with COPD are likely to have important co-morbid conditions particularly cardiac disease that may provide an alternative explanation for deterioration. In this case, the signs of the coincidental mitral stenosis were initially obscured and further appropriate investigation was required.

REFERENCES

1. Rimal B, Greenberg AK, Rom WN. Basic pathogenetic mechanisms in silicosis: current understanding. *Curr Opin Pulm Med* 2005; 11:169–173.
2. Fujimura N. Pathology and pathophysiology of pneumoconiosis. *Curr Opin Pulm Med* 2000; 6:140–144.
3. Ramanuja S, Mastronarde J, Dowdeswell I, Kamalesh A. A 44-year-old man with suspected exacerbation of COPD and atrial fibrillation. *Chest* 2004; 125:2340–2344.
4. Carabello BA, Crawford FA Jr. Valvular heart disease. *N Engl J Med* 1997; 337:32–41.
5. Robert G, Subramanian N, Dhar S. Significance of cardiac arrhythmias during acute exacerbation of COPD. *Chest* 2000; 118:193S–194S.
6. Nour MM, Mustafa KY, Mousa K, Abul AT, Shuhaibar H, Yousif AM. Reversible airway obstruction in rheumatic mitral valve disease. *Respirology* 1998; 3:25–31.
7. Tharaux PL, Dussaule JC, Hubert-Brierre J, Vahanian A, Acar J, Ardaillou R. Plasma atrial and brain natriuretic peptides in mitral stenosis treated by valvulotomy. *Clin Sci (Lond)* 1994; 87:671–677.
8. Inoue S, Murakami Y, Sano K et al. Atrium as a source of brain natriuretic polypeptide in patients with atrial fibrillation. *J Card Fail* 2000; 6:92–96.
9. Higham MA, Dawson D, Joshi J et al. Utility of echocardiography in assessment of pulmonary hypertension secondary to COPD. *Eur Respir J* 2001; 17:350–355.
10. Trivedi HS, Joshi MN, Gamade AR. Echocardiography and pulmonary artery pressure: correlation in chronic obstructive pulmonary disease. *J Postgrad Med* 1992; 38:24–26.
11. Page RL. Clinical practice. Newly diagnosed atrial fibrillation. *N Engl J Med* 2004; 351:2408–2416.

16

Antibiotic allergy in a COPD patient with frequent bacterial exacerbations

S. Sethi, F. Blasi

BACKGROUND

Acute exacerbations of chronic bronchitis (AECB) affect a significant proportion of the adult population worldwide and are associated with a substantial socio-economic burden. The majority of episodes of AECB are bacterial in aetiology and patients are generally treated empirically with orally administered antibacterial agents. Guidelines for the management of AECB have been developed by a number of national health authorities and international organizations, with the aim of promoting rational selection of antibacterial therapy to minimize the risk of treatment failure and subsequent hospitalization while containing the development and spread of antibacterial resistance [1–4]. Infectious agents are estimated to account for around 80% of these episodes, with the remaining 20% attributed to non-infectious causes such as inadequate medical treatment, congestive heart failure, pulmonary embolism, etc. [5]. Indeed, in a recent study that investigated the relationship between chronic obstructive pulmonary disease (COPD) exacerbations and bronchial microbial infection, higher microbial loads were associated with exacerbations and showed a statistically significant dose–response relationship [6].

Bacterial agents, including common and atypical/intracellular respiratory pathogens, are estimated to account for 50–70% of infection-related AECB episodes, and the acquisition of new strains of pathogenic bacterial species to which the patient is susceptible has been linked with AECB [7]. Non-bacterial causes of AECB include viruses (the most common being rhinovirus), which are estimated to cause 30–50% of exacerbations [8, 9]. A number of bacterial exacerbations may also be secondary to infection caused by viruses.

Choice of antibiotic treatment in AECB usually depends on a number of factors, including suspected or confirmed aetiology, clinical features and history, and local patterns of antibacterial resistance. Other relevant factors include the tolerability, convenience and cost of treatment, the ability of the antibacterial to penetrate bronchial tissue and mucus and, last but not least, low ecological risk (i.e. a low propensity to induce resistance). However, the clinical significance of *in vitro* antibacterial resistance in AECB remains a matter of debate.

A number of strategies have been put forward to minimize the development and spread of antibacterial resistance, including selection of appropriate agents based on their spectrum of activity, their pharmacokinetic and pharmacodynamic properties, and a knowledge of local resistance patterns. Some evidence derived from studies conducted in intensive care units suggests that antibacterial rotation/cycling, whereby a specific agent or class of agents is periodically withdrawn from use for a predefined time period, may also be of use in

---

Sanjay Sethi, MD, Associate Professor of Medicine, Division of Pulmonary, Critical Care and Sleep Medicine, State University of New York at Buffalo, Attending Physician, VA Western New York Healthcare System, New York, USA

Francesco Blasi, MD, PhD, Professor of Respiratory Medicine, Institute of Respiratory Diseases, University of Milan, Milan, Italy

© Atlas Medical Publishing Ltd 2007

restricting the selection pressure exerted on the microbial flora, thus reducing development of resistance [10]. However, a recent review questioned this procedure [11]. In any case, it should be noted that previous antibiotic use has been associated with an increased risk of infection with strains of antibiotic-resistant *Streptococcus pneumoniae* [12]. Therefore, even in the absence of any clear evidence in the published literature, many physicians believe that, in individual patients requiring repeated antibiotic treatment courses for AECB, rotation of antibiotics may be important in long-term management strategies.

CASE REPORT

A 71-year-old male patient with a history of COPD presents to the out-patient clinic. He has been diagnosed with COPD more than 10 years ago, and his last spirometry performed when his respiratory status was stable shows a FEV_1 of 45% predicted and a FVC of 66% predicted. He has a 35 pack-year smoking history but quit 3 years ago. Over the last year, he has had four exacerbations that were treated with different antibiotics and oral steroids. During the last episode, following amoxicillin-clavulanate treatment, he suffered from nettle rash. He also reports intolerance to levofloxacin, without any clear documentation of an allergic reaction.

Other medical history includes mild hypertension, treated with a thiazide diuretic and moderate hypercholesterolaemia for which he takes a statin. He also takes low-dose aspirin daily. He did have hepatitis 25 years ago but without sequelae, and prostatectomy for carcinoma at the age of 64 years. For his COPD, he had been prescribed regular inhaled salmeterol and oxitropium bromide. However, he uses his inhalers only when symptomatic.

In this clinic visit, he reports 3 days of increased dyspnoea, sputum volume, and a change in sputum colour from white to yellow-green. He denies fever, chills, pleuritic chest pain or haemoptysis. On examination, the patient appears distressed with a respiratory rate of 24, use of accessory muscles of respiration and prolonged expiration. Cyanosis is present and on lung examination breath sounds are diminished with expiratory rhonchi and some wheezes. Heart sounds are distant; however, no murmur is heard. There is no jugular venous distension or peripheral oedema. Pulmonary function tests (Figure 16.1a), chest X-ray (Figure 16.1b) and blood gas analysis (Figure 16.1c) are performed.

Several important clinical decisions have to be made in this patient. Should this patient be hospitalized or treated as an out-patient? Should he receive antibiotics? If yes, which antibiotic should be used, especially given his history of allergies? Should he be treated with corticosteroids? If yes, what route, dose and length of therapy are appropriate? Should he receive bronchodilators? Again, choices need to be made about agent, dose and route. Another important decision to be made is about the need for mechanical ventilation in this patient. In the subsequent sections, we will discuss the available evidence that guide our decisions regarding each of these treatment options.

ANTIBIOTICS

Should this patient receive antibiotics for the treatment of his exacerbation? The answer to this question is not clear-cut. If one were to practise evidence-based medicine, to use antibiotics in this patient we would like to have more than one randomized trial showing the superiority of antibiotics over placebo in the treatment of exacerbations. These trials would have adequate sample size, enrol only patients with well-defined COPD and control for concomitant therapy that could influence the resolution of exacerbations, e.g. systemic corticosteroids. Furthermore, one would like these trials to have clinically relevant endpoints that were uniform among the trials. Unfortunately, these criteria have not been fulfilled by any of the small number of placebo-controlled trials to date in AECB [13]. Furthermore, the advantage of using antibiotics over placebo is not consistently seen in these trials [13].

	Actual	Predicted	Percentage predicted
FVC (l)	1.95	3.80	51
FEV_1 (l)	0.78	2.92	27
FEV_1/FVC (%)	40.00	75.00	53
FEV_1/SVC (%)	37.00	70.00	52
FEF 25% (l/s)	0.67	6.95	10
FEF 50% (l/s)	0.31	4.04	8
FEF 75% (l/s)	0.11	1.36	8
FEF 25–75% (l/s)	0.25	3.05	8
FEF max (l/s)	2.92	7.76	38
Expiratory time (s)	10.48		

FEF = forced expiratory fraction; FEV_1 = forced expiratory volume in 1 second; FVC = forced vital capacity; SVC = slow vital capacity.

(a)

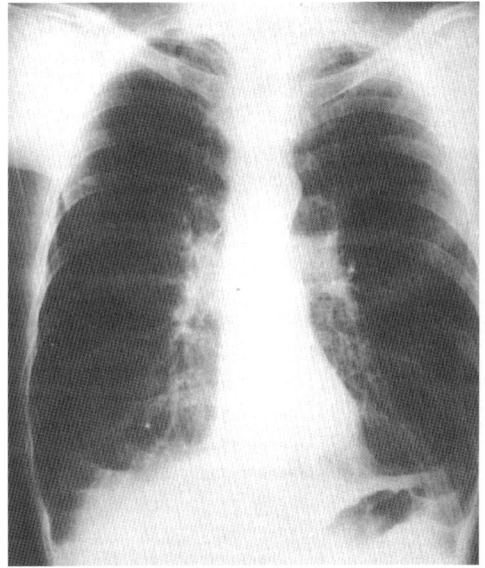
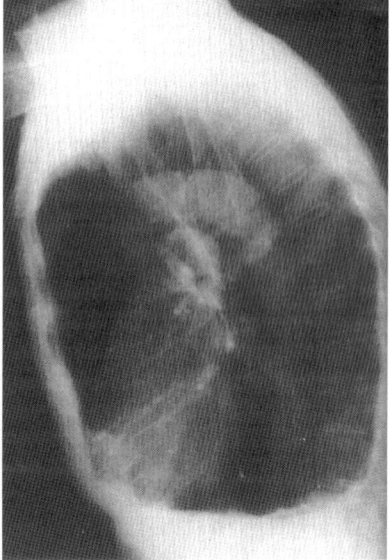

(b)

pH	7.472
PCO_2	46.4 mmHg
PO_2	49.9 mmHg
SO_2	86.7%
Hct	57.0%
Hb	19.0 g/dl
Na^+	130.8 mmol/l
BE-ECF	+10.3 mmol/l
BE-B	+9.3 mmol/l
SBC	32.6 mmol/l
HCO_3^-	34.1 mmol/l
O_2Ct	23.1 ml/dl
PO_2/FI	239.0 mmHg

(c)

Figure 16.1 (a) Pulmonary function tests, (b) chest X-ray, and (c) blood gas analysis at admission.

Differences in study design among the published placebo-controlled antibiotic trials in acute exacerbation explain their discrepant results. A closer examination of the design of these trials shows that those trials that were larger, which enrolled patients with well-defined COPD or which examined endpoints earlier were able to show a benefit with antibiotics over placebo. For example, the studies of Anthonisen et al. [14] and Allegra et al. [15] enrolled much larger numbers of exacerbation episodes, 362 and 414 respectively, and both demonstrated benefits with antibiotics. On the other hand, studies by Nicotra et al. [16] and Sachs et al. [17] which enrolled 40 and 71 patients respectively, were not able to demonstrate a difference between the antibiotics and placebo arm. Patients enrolled in these studies should be well-characterized as either COPD or chronic bronchitis, and patients with asthma and other airway disorders should be excluded. This is important because the majority of asthma exacerbations and acute bronchitis events without underlying disease are not related to bacterial infection and therefore do not benefit from antibiotics. Studies conducted by Sachs et al. [17] and Jorgensen et al. [18] are good examples of how enrolling patients with asthma or poorly characterized chronic bronchitis can affect the results. In these trials, no benefit with antibiotics was demonstrated. On the other hand, in the studies conducted by Anthonisen et al. [14] and Nouira et al. [19], patients with significant COPD were enrolled, and antibiotics were distinctly superior to placebo.

The traditional endpoint in COPD has been clinical resolution at 3 weeks after enrolment. This traditional endpoint became prevalent because it was required by regulatory agencies. However, such an endpoint has little clinical relevance. Most decisions about benefit of antibiotics are made within the first 3–5 days. Furthermore, the traditional endpoint allows spontaneous resolution to occur and mask any benefit of antibiotics that may otherwise be present in an earlier time frame [20]. Allegra et al. [15], in a bold move, decided to determine clinical success or failure at 5 days. In doing so, they found a clear benefit with antibiotics.

One unsettled issue in the use of antibiotics in exacerbations is that of the effect of concomitant therapy, specifically with corticosteroids. One would like to know whether antibiotics are beneficial in patients who receive oral corticosteroids. This question can only be answered by doing a study in which all patients receive a course of oral corticosteroids and are randomized to receive a placebo or antibiotics. However, there are several obstructions to performing such a study. Firstly, there is no data that steroids are of benefit in patients with exacerbations of COPD that are mild enough to be treated in an office setting, not requiring emergency room or hospitalization. Secondly, investigators could have ethical concerns about the safety of such studies, especially among patients with advanced COPD and exacerbations with purulent sputum. Other options for differentiating the effect of antibiotics from that of corticosteroids include a study design in which steroids are completely excluded or trials in which patients are stratified by the use of antibiotics. The first alternative implies that certain patient will get no specific treatment for the exacerbation, raising both investigator and patient concerns about safety. In the latter design, mostly sicker patients get steroids. These patients are often the ones who would benefit from antibiotics. Therefore, this can again complicate interpretation of the results.

The present case represents an exacerbation of COPD in a patient who is at risk for bacterial infection of the lower airway. In addition, failure of initial treatment of this patient could have severe consequences making requirement for intensive care and mechanical ventilation distinct possibilities. In this situation, even though one does not have the best evidence to support this practice, it would be prudent to use antibiotics in this patient.

CHOICE OF ANTIBIOTICS

There are a large variety of agents from different classes available for use in AECB. These include older agents such as pencillins, cephalosporins, tetracyclines, macrolides and amoxicillin-clavulanate that have been widely used for this disease over the last two decades. Antibiotic classes that have been relatively recently introduced include fluoroquinolones and ketolides. These antibiotics have different mechanisms of action and different spectrums of activity against the respiratory pathogens implicated in acute exacerbation.

Relatively little resistance to bacterial pathogens implicated in acute exacerbation was evident two decades ago. Therefore, choice of antibiotics was simple with most antibiotic agents providing adequate coverage. With the emergence of multi-drug resistance in *Streptococcus pneumoniae* and, β-lactamase production in *Haemophilus influenzae* and *Moraxella catarrhalis*, antibiotic choice has become more complicated [21]. Further complicating the matter is the increasing recognition that gram-negative pathogens, especially *Pseudomonas* and also *Enterobacteriaecae*, could be involved in more severely ill patients with exacerbation [22].

Ideally, antibiotic choice in exacerbations should be based on comparative trials showing clear clinical superiority of certain agents, especially those that are more active *in vitro* against respiratory pathogens and achieve better bacteriologic eradication. The literature is replete with antibiotic comparison trials. However, contrary to expectation, these trials almost uniformly show that antibiotics of different classes are of equivalent clinical efficacy. In these studies, though differences in bacteriologic eradication can be found among antibiotics, clinical efficacy is not different, with a clear disconnect between clinical and bacteriologic efficacy [20]. One interpretation of these studies is that all antibiotics are indeed equivalent in exacerbations. However, to better understand the results of these studies, one should realize that these studies are carefully designed to show equivalence rather than difference among the antibiotics tested.

More recent trials have examined non-traditional endpoints and have been able to show that respiratory fluoroquinolones, specifically, moxifloxacin in the MOSAIC trial and gemifloxacin in the GLOBE trial, were indeed superior to other agents [23, 24]. However, this should not lead us to use fluoroquinolones indiscriminately among all patients with exacerbations. Such a practice would lead to increased resistance to these valuable agents [25].

Pathogen-directed therapy in acute exacerbation would be desirable, but it is often not possible or practical. Antibiotic choice in exacerbations is often empiric and made in the absence of microbiological data. The most rational approach to the empiric choice of antibiotics is a risk-stratification approach [1, 3, 26]. In this approach, patients with exacerbation who are either likely to have a poor outcome based on underlying lung disease or comorbid conditions and/or are prone to infection with resistant pathogens are identified for more aggressive treatment with broad-spectrum agents such as the fluoroquinolones. Patients not at risk for poor outcome or resistant pathogens are treated more conservatively. This approach is outlined in Table 16.1 and Figure 16.2.

In this case, because of the severity of his underlying COPD, the patient is a complicated patient with exacerbation, and antibiotic choices would include either a fluoroquinolone or amoxicillin-clavulanate. However, antibiotic choice is even more difficult in this patient because of allergies. He has a history of penicillin allergy that would negate the use of a penicillin or a cephalosporin. It is very important to question exactly what is meant by penicillin allergy [27]. Often patients ascribe the term allergy to adverse effects. In other patients, the allergy may be relatively mild rather than a major reaction.

Table 16.1 Risk factors for poor outcome and/or for antibiotic-resistant pathogens in AECB

- \>3 exacerbations in the past 12 months
- Comorbidities (especially cardiac disease)
- Severe or very severe airflow obstruction at baseline (FEV$_1$ < 50% predicted)
- Recent (within past 3 months) systemic antibiotic use

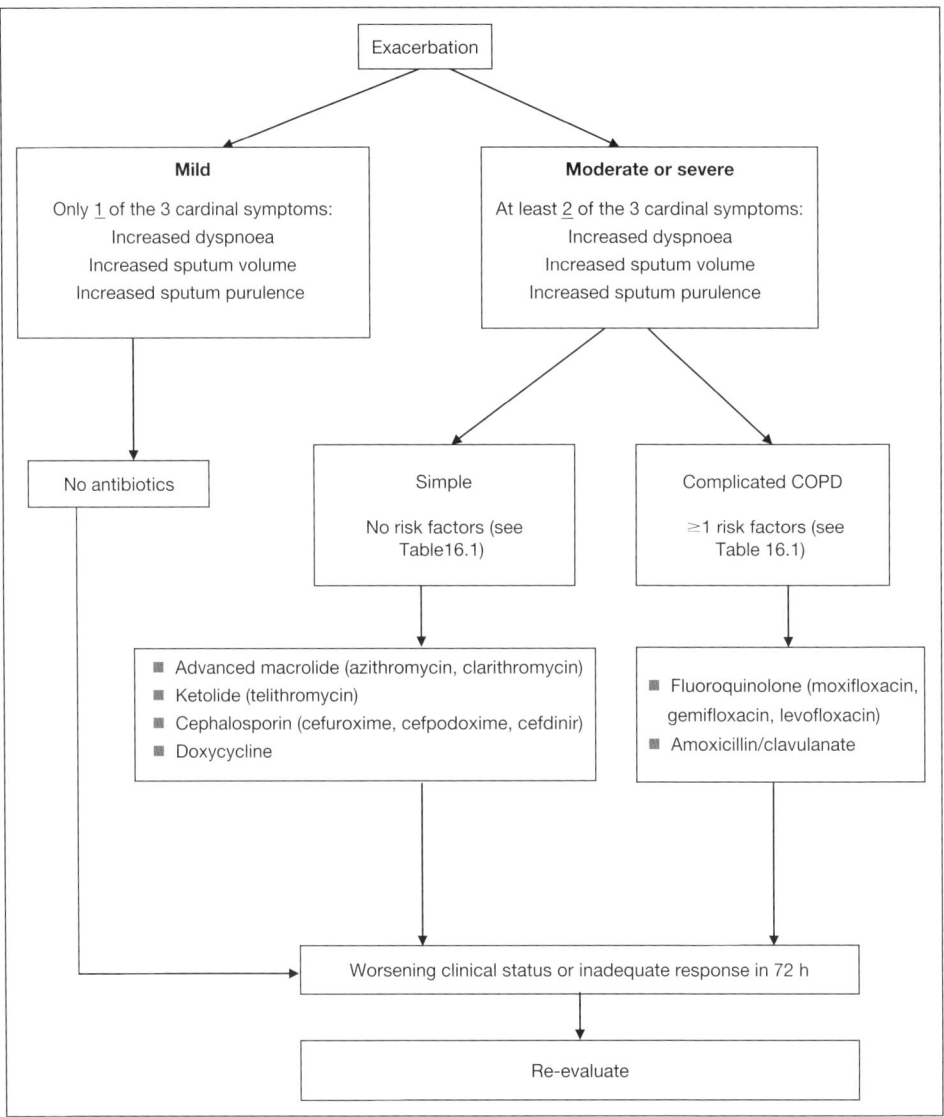

Figure 16.2 Algorithm for antibiotic selection in AECB.

How about his history of allergy to fluoroquinolones? A careful elicitation of what is meant by this allergy is important. Anaphylactic reactions to fluoroquinolones are quite uncommon. Adverse effects can differ among the fluoroquinolones and can be mistaken for allergic reactions. For instance, gatifloxacin is associated with diarrhoea and disorders of glucose homeostasis [28, 29]. Such effects may not preclude the use of other fluoroquinolones in that patient.

In this particular case, a careful elicitation of antibiotic allergy history revealed a major penicillin allergy. However, the fluoroquinolone allergy appeared to be more a case of a non-specific adverse event. In view of this additional information, a decision to use an alternative fluoroquinolone, levofloxacin, was made, with a satisfactory clinical outcome.

Table 16.2 Indications for hospital and ICU admission for exacerbations of COPD (modified from GOLD guidelines [1])

Indications for hospital admission   ■ Marked increase in symptom intensity   ■ Severe underlying COPD   ■ New physical signs such as cyanosis and peripheral oedema   ■ Failure to respond to initial medical management   ■ Significant comorbidities   ■ New cardiac arrhythmias   ■ Diagnostic uncertainty   ■ Older age   ■ Insufficient home support   *ICU admission*   ■ Severe dyspnoea unresponsive to initial emergency therapy   ■ Alteration of mental status: confusion, lethargy, coma   ■ Persistent or worsening hypoxaemia and/or severe/worsening hypercapnia and/or severe/worsening respiratory acidosis (pH < 7.25) despite supplemental oxygen and NPPV
ICU = intensive care unit; NPPV = non-invasive positive pressure ventilation

HOSPITALIZATION

A small proportion of patients with AECB are hospitalized. The decision to hospitalize has major implications, for the patient as well as for the healthcare system, and therefore should not be made lightly. No scoring systems such as the PORT score or CURB-65, which are used in community-acquired pneumonia, are available for acute exacerbations of COPD. The decision to hospitalize therefore remains more an art than an exact science.

Recent COPD guidelines have discussed criteria to consider when deciding to hospitalize and these are shown in Table 16.2 [1]. Also shown are the criteria to be considered in the decision to admit to the intensive care unit rather than treat in the medical ward. Of course, these decisions need to be tempered by the availability of local resources and the patient's wishes for intensity of care. In this particular case, based on the severity of his underlying COPD, and borderline gas exchange variables, it was prudent to hospitalize the patient.

CORTICOSTEROIDS

A number of controlled studies have shown that systemic steroid therapy may have beneficial effects in speeding up recovery from an AECB. Thompson *et al.* [30] demonstrated that out-patient (emergency room) treatment of acute COPD exacerbation with prednisone accelerates recovery of physiologic measures such as arterial oxygen tension (PaO_2), alveolar–arterial oxygen difference ($PA-aO_2$), FEV_1, and peak expiratory flow. Furthermore, in this small study, prednisone reduced the treatment failure rate and improved subjective dyspnoea [30]. In a randomized placebo-controlled trial of oral steroids in hospitalized AECB patients, post-bronchodilator FEV_1 increased more rapidly and to a greater extent and hospital stays were shorter in the corticosteroid-treated group. However, the two groups did not differ at 6-week follow-up. Therefore, the benefits in spirometric improvement seen within the first 5 days do not extend beyond hospital discharge [31].

Niewoehner *et al.* [32] have shown that treatment with systemic glucocorticoids resulted in moderate improvement in clinical outcomes among patients hospitalized for exacerbations of COPD. The maximal benefit was obtained with 2 weeks of therapy, with no additional benefit from extending therapy to 6 weeks. Hyperglycaemia of sufficient severity to warrant treatment was the most frequent complication. Sub-group analyses of the results of this study suggested that the treatment benefit may be restricted largely to patients who have previously been hospitalized because of COPD.

An important limitation of these studies is that the dose and duration of corticosteroid therapy varied widely among studies, making it virtually impossible to provide specific treatment recommendations. In any case, all the studies indicate that a short-course (10–14 days) of systemic corticosteroids is effective. Though the Niewoehner study used large doses of intravenous corticosteroids initially, subsequent studies have shown that the equivalent of 40 mg/day of oral prednisone appears to have similar effectiveness as the larger doses, and may therefore be preferred.

Steroid therapy may have additional beneficial effects. Murata et al. [33], in a retrospective study performed in an emergency room setting, demonstrated that steroid-treated individuals had a significantly reduced likelihood of relapse compared with the group not getting steroids. Seemungal et al. [34] reported that steroids prolonged the time to the next exacerbation in COPD out-patients.

The recent Canadian Thoracic Society Guidelines for COPD suggest that there is good evidence to support the use of oral or parenteral steroids for most patients with moderate to severe AECB recommending a treatment period of 5–14 days [3]. The right dose is not clearly defined but the American Thoracic Society–European Respiratory Society statement on COPD suggests a 10–14-day course of oral prednisone at 30–40 mg [4].

However, it should be taken into account that there are significant health consequences linked to the use of continuous oral corticosteroids in COPD and similar deleterious effects may occur in patients treated with frequent short courses. In patients with diabetes and risk of bone fracture these drugs should be used with caution. Determination of bone density and osteoporosis prophylaxis should be considered in patients requiring frequent courses of oral corticosteroids. Though the benefit of steroids is quite clear in patients with moderate or severe AECB, their role is unclear in patients with mild exacerbations treated in an out-patient setting. None of the placebo-controlled studies to date have included such patients.

Maltais et al. [35], in a large randomized controlled study, showed that high-dose nebulized high-potency steroids may be an alternative to oral glucocorticosteroids in the treatment of acute non-acidotic exacerbations. Both nebulized budesonide and oral prednisolone improved airflow in COPD patients with acute exacerbations when compared with placebo, though patients on the oral prednisolone tended to have larger improvements. Budesonide showed less systemic activity than prednisolone as indicated by a higher incidence of hyperglycaemia observed with prednisolone.

The patient presented above represents severe AECB and has had recurrent exacerbations. Therefore, in the case presented, a short course of steroids (prednisone 30 mg/day for 10 days) was administered.

MECHANICAL VENTILATION

Ventilatory assistance by mechanical means can be life-saving in severe AECB. According to the standards of care, institution of mechanical ventilation should be considered when, despite optimal medical therapy and oxygen administration, there is acidosis (pH < 7.35) and hypercapnia ($PaCO_2$ > 6–8 kPa (45–60 mmHg)) and respiratory frequency > 24 breaths/min [4]. Mechanical ventilation can be delivered as invasive ventilation through an endotracheal tube or non-invasive positive pressure ventilation (NPPV) through nasal or face masks using either bi-level positive airway pressure or continuous positive airway pressure.

NPPV use in acute respiratory failure has been studied in a number of uncontrolled and five randomized controlled trials, with success rates consistently of 80–85% [36]. The most common causes for acute respiratory failure in these studies were COPD exacerbation and cardiogenic pulmonary oedema. Recent studies showed a reduction in mortality using

NPPV compared to usual treatment or conventional invasive ventilation [37, 38]. Taken together, these studies provide substantial evidence that NPPV increases pH, reduces $PaCO_2$ and reduces the severity of breathlessness in the first 4 h of treatment. Furthermore, it decreases the length of hospital stay and intubation rate and, most importantly, mortality.

NPPV should be delivered in a dedicated setting with staff who have been trained in its application, who are experienced in its use and who are aware of its limitations. NPPV is not appropriate for all patients, and the main exclusion criteria are: respiratory arrest, cardiovascular instability (hypotension, arrhythmias, myocardial infarction), somnolence, impaired mental status, uncooperative patient, high aspiration risk; viscous or copious secretions, recent facial or gastro-oesophageal surgery, craniofacial trauma, fixed nasopharyngeal abnormalities, burns, and extreme obesity.

In the present case, the arterial blood gas analysis showed: pH = 7.47, PaO_2 = 46.4, $PaCO_2$ = 49.9, HCO_3^- = 34.1. Would one prescribe invasive or non-invasive mechanical ventilation in this patient?

The patient does not have respiratory acidosis. However, he appears distressed with the use of accessory muscles of respiration with prolonged expiration. Invasive ventilation was not appropriate in this patient. NPPV was considered but a decision was made to wait and see the efficacy of the initial oxygen, bronchodilator, steroid and antibiotic therapy. Strict monitoring of respiratory distress and gas exchange was instituted. The patient responded well to the initial therapy and did not require NPPV.

BRONCHODILATOR THERAPY

Are short-acting β_2-agonist and/or anticholinergic bronchodilators indicated in the treatment of dyspnoea occurring during an AECB? Few randomized controlled trials are published on the use of this therapy in the out-patient setting. More data support their use in hospitalized exacerbations, but there is no clear evidence that a combination of short-acting β_2-agonist and anticholinergic agents is better than the use of a single bronchodilator. Two emergency room studies suggest a better activity of the combination therapy than short-acting β_2-agonist alone in terms of both greater improvement of FEV_1 and shorter emergency room stays [39, 40].

No difference is reported comparing different bronchodilator delivery systems. The use of a metered-dose inhaler with a spacer compared to nebulization for bronchodilator delivery was analysed in a meta-analysis of 18 studies, showing no difference in terms of speed of recovery [41]. Patients acutely short of breath may not be able to achieve an adequate inhalation technique with metered-dose inhalers. Therefore, the choice of delivery systems should be based on the patient's ability to use these devices and often one has to resort to nebulization initially, with a switch to metered-dose inhalers with improvement in the patient's respiratory status.

Although there are data supporting the use of intravenous salbutamol in acute severe asthma, no such evidence exists for its use in COPD exacerbation. In addition, troublesome side-effects (most commonly tremor and palpitation) are more frequently seen with this route than with inhaled delivery due to the increased stimulation of extra-pulmonary β-adrenoreceptors. Similarly, continuous nebulization of salbutamol is not recommended [42]. Methylxanthines do not seem to be indicated in the treatment of dyspnoea in exacerbation of COPD unless the patient is on chronic oral therapy. The use of methylxanthines is associated with a high rate of side-effects and the possible interaction with a number of antibiotics (ciprofloxacin, clarithromycin, etc.) and other commonly used medications in these patients should be taken into account.

In this present case, the patient was hospitalized and was in acute distress. Therefore, combined therapy with short-acting β_2-agonist and anticholinergic was instituted. Initially, these medications were delivered by frequent nebulization. With improvement in the patient's respiratory status, the delivery mode was changed to metered-dose inhalers with a spacer.

SUMMARY

Appropriate treatment and prevention of exacerbations has become an integral part of chronic bronchitis and COPD management. Unfortunately, the evidence base of clinical trials in AECB, especially in mild-to-moderate episodes, is sparse and has several major deficiencies. However, this should not deter use of the appropriate multi-modality treatment of AECB. The combination of therapeutic measures discussed in this paper should improve the clinical outcome of AECB substantially, both in the short- and long-term. With the increased attention now paid to AECB as a major health problem, results from larger and better clinical trials will refine our therapeutic approach in the future.

REFERENCES

1. www.goldcopd.com. Globial initiative for obstructive lung disease [Web Page].
2. www.thoracic.org/copd. Standards for the diagnosis and management of patients with COPD. ERS/ATS Guidelines [Web Page].
3. Balter MS, La Forge J, Low DE, Mandell L, Grossman RF. Canadian guidelines for the management of acute exacerbations of chronic bronchitis. *Can Respir J* 2003; 10(suppl B):3B–32B.
4. Celli BR, MacNee W. Standards for the diagnosis and treatment of patients with COPD: a summary of the ATS/ERS position paper. *Eur Respir J* 2004; 23:932–946.
5. Sethi S. Infectious etiology of acute exacerbations of chronic bronchitis. *Chest* 2000; 117:380S–385S.
6. Rosell A, Monso E, Soler N et al. Microbiologic determinants of exacerbation in chronic obstructive pulmonary disease. *Arch Intern Med* 2005; 165:891–897.
7. Sethi S, Evans N, Grant BJB, Murphy TF. Acquisition of a new bacterial strain and occurrence of exacerbations of chronic obstructive pulmonary disease. *N Engl J Med* 2002; 347:465–471.
8. Ball P. Epidemiology and treatment of chronic bronchitis and its exacerbations. *Chest* 1995; 108:43S–52S.
9. Rohde G, Wiethege A, Borg I et al. Respiratory viruses in exacerbations of chronic obstructive pulmonary disease requiring hospitalization: a case–control study. *Thorax* 2003; 58:37–42.
10. Niederman MS. Appropriate use of antimicrobial agents: challenges and strategies for improvement. *Crit Care Med* 2003; 31:608–616.
11. Brown EM, Nathwani D. Antibiotic cycling or rotation: a systematic review of the evidence of efficacy. *J Antimicrob Chemother* 2005; 55:6–9.
12. Ruhe JJ, Hasbun R. Streptococcus pneumoniae bacteremia: duration of previous antibiotic use and association with penicillin resistance. *Clin Infect Dis* 2003; 36:1132–1138.
13. Saint S, Bent S, Vittinghoff E, Grady D. Antibiotics in chronic obstructive pulmonary disease exacerbations. A meta-analysis. *JAMA* 1995; 273:957–960.
14. Anthonisen NR, Manfreda J, Warren CPW, Hershfield ES, Harding GKM, Nelson NA. Antibiotic therapy in exacerbations of chronic obstructive pulmonary disease. *Ann Intern Med* 1987; 106:196–204.
15. Allegra L, Blasi F, de Bernardi B, Cosentini R, Tarsia P. Antibiotic treatment and baseline severity of disease in acute exacerbations of chronic bronchitis: a re-evaluation of previously published data of a placebo-controlled randomized study. *Pulm Pharmacol Ther* 2001; 14:149–155.
16. Nicotra MB, Kronenberg S. Con: Antibiotic use in exacerbations of chronic bronchitis. *Semin Respir Infect* 1993; 8:254–258.
17. Sachs APE, Koeter GH, Groenier KH, van der Waaij D, Schiphuis J, Jong BM. Changes in symptoms, peak expiratory flow, and sputum flora during treatment with antibiotics of exacerbations in patients with chronic obstructive pulmonary disease in general practice. *Thorax* 1995; 50:758–763.
18. Jorgensen AF, Coolidge J, Pedersen PA, Petersen KP, Waldorff S, Widding E. Amoxicillin in treatment of acute uncomplicated exacerbations of chronic bronchitis. A double-blind, placebo-controlled multicentre study in general practice. *Scand J Prim Health Care* 1992; 10:7–11.
19. Nouira S, Marghli S, Belghith M, Besbes L, Elatrous S, Abroug F. Once daily oral ofloxacin in chronic obstructive pulmonary disease exacerbation requiring mechanical ventilation: a randomised placebo-controlled trial. *Lancet* 2001; 358:2020–2025.

20. Sethi S. Bacteria in exacerbations of chronic obstructive pulmonary disease. Phenomenon or epiphenomenon? *Proc Am Thorac Soc* 2004; 1:109–114.
21. Sethi S, Anzueto A, Farrell DJ. Antibiotic activity of telithromycin and comparators against bacterial pathogens isolated from 3,043 patients with acute exacerbation of chronic bronchitis. *Ann Clin Microbiol Antimicrob* 2005; 4:5.
22. Soler N, Torres A, Ewig S et al. Bronchial microbial patterns in severe exacerbations of chronic obstructive pulmonary disease (COPD) requiring mechanical ventilation. *Am J Respir Crit Care Med* 1998; 157:1498–1505.
23. Wilson R, Schentag JJ, Ball P, Mandell L. A comparison of gemifloxacin and clarithromycin in acute exacerbations of chronic bronchitis and long-term clinical outcomes. *Clin Ther* 2002; 24:639–652.
24. Wilson R, Allegra L, Huchon G et al. Short-term and long-term outcomes of moxifloxacin compared to standard antibiotic treatment in acute exacerbations of chronic bronchitis. *Chest* 2004; 125:953–964.
25. Chen DK, McGeer A, de Azavedo JC, Low DE. Decreased susceptibility of *Streptococcus pneumoniae* to fluoroquinolones in Canada. Canadian Bacterial Surveillance Network. *N Engl J Med* 1999; 341:233–239.
26. Sethi S, File TM. Managing patients with recurrent acute exacerbations of chronic bronchitis: a common clinical problem. *Curr Med Res Opin* 2004; 20:1511–1521.
27. Stember RH. Prevalence of skin test reactivity in patients with convincing, vague, and unacceptable histories of penicillin allergy. *Allergy Asthma Proc* 2005; 26:59–64.
28. Frothingham R. Glucose homeostasis abnormalities associated with use of gatifloxacin. *Clin Infect Dis* 2005; 41:1269–1276.
29. Gaynes R, Rimland D, Killum E et al. Outbreak of *Clostridium difficile* infection in a long-term care facility: association with gatifloxacin use. *Clin Infect Dis* 2004; 38:640–645.
30. Thompson WH, Nielson CP, Carvalho P, Charan NB, Crowley JJ. Controlled trial of oral prednisone in outpatients with acute COPD exacerbation. *Am J Respir Crit Care Med* 1996; 154:407–412.
31. Davies L, Angus RM, Calverley PM. Oral corticosteroids in patients admitted to hospital with exacerbations of chronic obstructive pulmonary disease: a prospective randomised controlled trial. *Lancet* 1999; 354:456–460.
32. Niewoehner DE, Erbland ML, Deupree RH et al. Effect of systemic glucocorticoids on exacerbations of chronic obstructive pulmonary disease. Department of Veterans Affairs Cooperative Study Group. *N Engl J Med* 1999; 340:1941–1947.
33. Murata GH, Gorby MS, Chick TW, Halperin AK. Intravenous and oral corticosteroids for the prevention of relapse after treatment of decompensated COPD. Effect on patients with a history of multiple relapses. *Chest* 1990; 98:845–849.
34. Seemungal TAR, Donaldson GC, Bhowmik A, Jeffries DJ, Wedzicha JA. Time course and recovery of exacerbations in patients with chronic obstructive pulmonary disease. *Am J Respir Crit Care Med* 2000; 161:1608–1613.
35. Maltais F, Ostinelli J, Bourbeau J et al. Comparison of nebulized budesonide and oral prednisolone with placebo in the treatment of acute exacerbations of chronic obstructive pulmonary disease: a randomized controlled trial. *Am J Respir Crit Care Med* 2002; 165:698–703.
36. Lightowler JV, Wedzicha JA, Elliott MW, Ram FS. Non-invasive positive pressure ventilation to treat respiratory failure resulting from exacerbations of chronic obstructive pulmonary disease: Cochrane systematic review and meta-analysis. *BMJ* 2003; 326:185.
37. Conti G, Antonelli M, Navalesi P et al. Noninvasive vs. conventional mechanical ventilation in patients with chronic obstructive pulmonary disease after failure of medical treatment in the ward: a randomized trial. *Intensive Care Med* 2002; 28:1701–1707.
38. Plant PK, Owen JL, Elliott MW. Non-invasive ventilation in acute exacerbations of chronic obstructive pulmonary disease: long term survival and predictors of in-hospital outcome. *Thorax* 2001; 56:708–712.
39. Cydulka RK, Emerman CL. Effects of combined treatment with glycopyrrolate and albuterol in acute exacerbation of chronic obstructive pulmonary disease. *Ann Emerg Med* 1995; 25:470–473.
40. Shrestha M, O'Brien T, Haddox R, Gourlay HS, Reed G. Decreased duration of emergency department treatment of chronic obstructive pulmonary disease exacerbations with the addition of ipratropium bromide to beta-agonist therapy. *Ann Emerg Med* 1991; 20:1206–1209.
41. Turner MO, Patel A, Ginsburg S, FitzGerald JM. Bronchodilator delivery in acute airflow obstruction. A meta-analysis. *Arch Intern Med* 1997; 157:1736–1744.
42. Hurst JR, Wedzicha JA. Chronic obstructive pulmonary disease: the clinical management of an acute exacerbation. *Postgrad Med J* 2004; 80:497–505.

17

Tuberculosis re-exacerbation in an older smoker with COPD

L. Casali, J.-P. Zellweger

BACKGROUND

Smoking by itself is an important risk factor in the loss of healthy life for years both in low- and high-income countries, and is a direct or indirect cause of death worldwide [1]. Some reports have begun to draw the attention of epidemiologists and clinicians to the possible role of tobacco smoke in increasing the risk of latent tuberculosis (TB) infection and disease in low- and high-income countries.

CASE REPORT

A 76-year-old Swiss farmer, a heavy smoker with chronic cough and exertional dyspnoea, visited his family physician in winter 1996 because of exacerbation of cough and increase in sputum. The chest X-ray demonstrated some scarring in the right upper lobe and subpleural fibrosis in the right middle field with calcifications in the hilum (Figure 17.1). No further examination was performed. The patient improved with antibiotics and bronchodilators.

One year later, he visited the family doctor again for similar symptoms. He was still a heavy smoker with severe dyspnoea, cough and sputum. The chest X-ray was unchanged (Figure 17.2). The patient improved with symptomatic treatment and antibiotics.

A similar exacerbation occurred in 1998. This time, the chest X-ray demonstrated a slight increase in the infiltrates (Figure 17.3).

In 2000, a more severe exacerbation necessitated an emergency hospitalization. The chest X-ray demonstrated an extensive infiltrate in the right lung (Figure 17.4). A microscopic examination of the smear revealed acid-fast bacteria. The culture was positive for *Myobacterium tuberculosis*.

Diagnosis: TB in a smoker with COPD.

DISCUSSION

This case illustrates two aspects of the relationship between COPD, smoking and TB. Firstly, the fact that TB can exacerbate slowly in elderly patients and that symptoms can be misleading, particularly in smokers where the cough, sputum, dyspnoea and weight loss can be interpreted as symptoms of COPD or TB. The chest X-ray abnormalities were interpreted as being due to COPD with multiple scars of prior infectious episodes (the so-called 'dirty

---

Lucio Casali, MD, PhD, Chair of Respiratory Diseases, Faculty of Medicine and Surgery, University of Perugia, Sede di Terni, Italy

Jean-Pierre Zellweger, MD, Senior Consultant, University Medical Policlinic, Lausanne, Switzerland

© Atlas Medical Publishing Ltd 2007

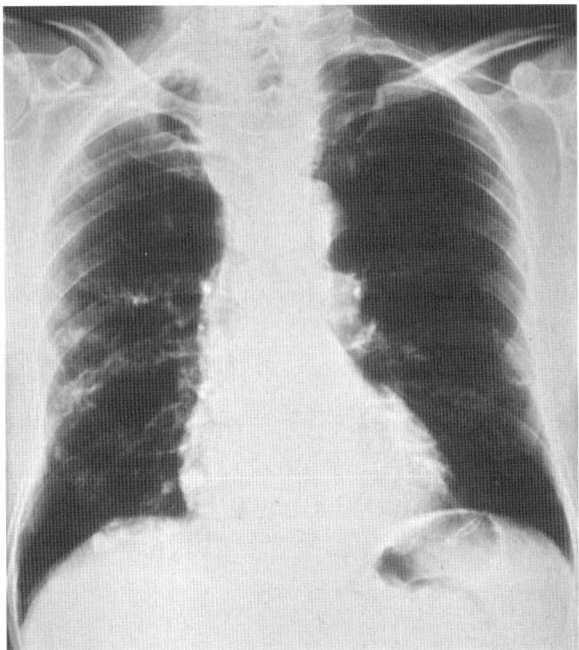

Figure 17.1 Chest X-ray in 1996.

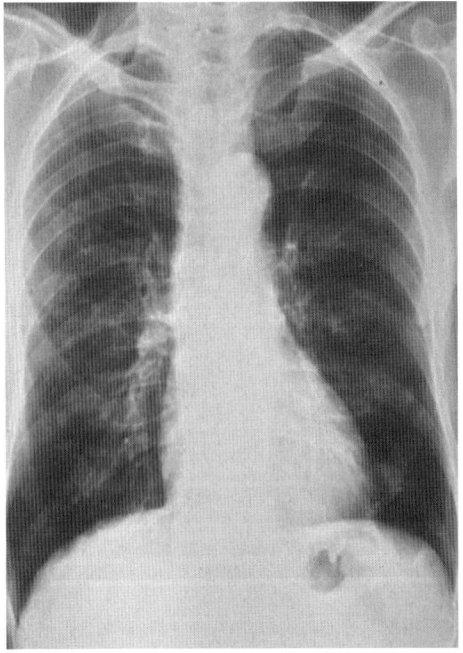

Figure 17.2 Chest X-ray in 1997.

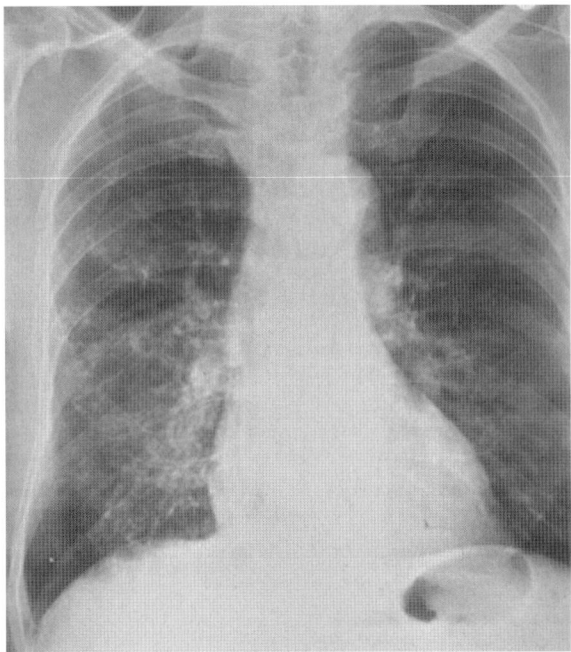

Figure 17.3 Chest X-ray in 1998.

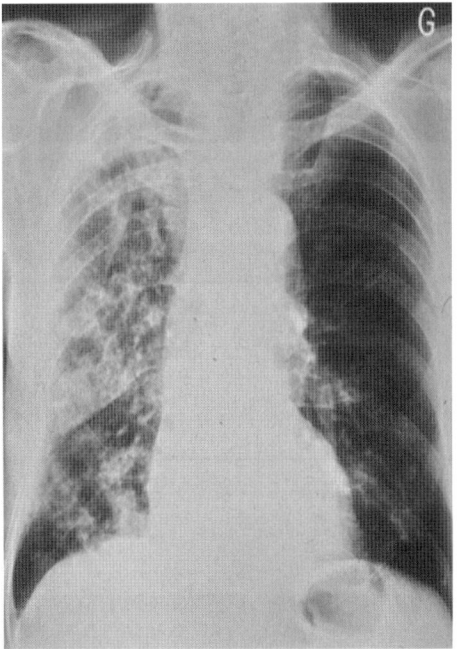

Figure 17.4 Chest X-ray in 2000: tuberculosis in right lung.

chest' of elderly smokers), whereas they corresponded more probably to fibrotic lesions of spontaneously stabilized TB. As COPD exacerbation is much more frequent than reactivation of TB in countries with a low incidence of TB, but a high prevalence of smoking, the patient received treatment for the most obvious cause of his symptoms and the diagnosis of TB was not made before the disease had evolved into a severe form, necessitating hospitalization and a more comprehensive assessment, including bacteriological examination of the sputum.

Secondly, although it cannot be proven with certainty, the fact that the patient was a heavy smoker may have played a role in the reactivation of TB. Smoking is related to TB in many ways. From the available evidence, smoking increases the risk of:

- Infection if exposed to TB.
- Reactivation if infected.
- Unfavourable outcome of TB (slow bacteriological negativation, more extensive lung destruction).
- Relapse after treatment for TB.

In children, even passive smoking increases the risk of TB infection and disease after exposure to infectious cases. Kuemmerer and Comstock [2] reported a higher percentage of positive tuberculin skin test among children exposed to the smoke of their parents than among non-exposed children. This has been confirmed by Altet et al. [3], who demonstrated a higher rate of reactivation of infection to TB among children exposed to passive smoking.

In Norway, a strong association between smoke and tuberculin skin test reactivity was demonstrated by linear regression analysis [4] and in Kuwait, Abal et al. [5] demonstrated a relationship between tobacco smoke and tuberculin reactivity with a positive dose–response relationship to the number of pack-years smoked in the controls, but not in the patients. Very recently den Boon et al. [6] compared data on smoking and tuberculin skin test in a cross-sectional study which included 2401 adult subjects in Cape Town (South Africa). A total of 1832 (76%) subjects had a positive tuberculin reaction. Among 1309 current smokers or ex-smokers, 1070 (82%) had a positive reaction (≥ 10 mm of induration) and the heavy smokers were exposed to the highest risk (unadjusted odds ratio [OR] 1.99; 95% confidence interval [CI] 1.62–2.45). A positive relationship with pack-years was observed, with those smoking more than 15 pack-years having the highest risk (adjusted odds ratio [OR] 1.90; 95% CI 1.28–2.81).

In Hong Kong, a cohort of 42 655 clients of the Elderly Health Service were followed for several years after retirement. The TB notification rates were 735, 427 and 174 per 100 000 respectively in current smokers, ex-smokers and never smokers [7]. In comparison with never smokers, current smokers had an excess risk for pulmonary TB (risk adjusted 2.87; $P < 0.001$) but not for extrapulmonary TB ($P = 0.95$). Moreover, there was a significant dose–response relationship between the level of consumption and the risk of active and culture-confirmed TB ($P < 0.05$).

A striking relationship between smoking habits and mortality from TB was demonstrated by Gajalakshmi et al. [8]. The authors carried out a case–control study of the smoking habits of 27 000 urban and 16 000 rural men who died in the Tamil state of India. They observed an impressive excess of mortality from TB in smokers (risk ratio in the urban area of 5.1 for subjects aged 25–34 years and 4.5 for subjects aged 25–69 years). In the rural area, the model of smoking appeared different as people usually smoke 'bidis' instead of cigarettes but the risk for smokers remains.

Some interesting remarks are reported by Altet-Gomez et al. [9] in their cross-sectional observational study of cases (smokers with TB) and controls (non-smokers with TB) in Catalunya. Smokers had a higher proportion of pulmonary TB (50%), cavitary lesions (90%) and positive sputum smears (40%) than non-smokers and experienced more severe lesions and a faster progression of the disease.

Cigarette smoking is associated with a variety of alterations in both the cellular and humoral immune system, and smoking may furthermore affect the mechanical defences of the respiratory tree. It seems that tobacco smoke decreases the macrophage immune response, which represents the first line of defence against bacilli through the phagocytic process [10]. The protective role of macrophages against an excessive local immune response is also impaired. The interaction between smoke and TB also leads to an increased apoptosis of macrophages [11]. On the other hand, nicotine depresses the processes of antigen presentation, impairing the correct development of the immune response [12]. Moreover, cigarette smoke can decrease the number of CD4 lymphocytes and contributes to the disruption of the cilia in the bronchial tree [13, 14] causing an impairment of mucociliary clearance. The association of these elements in elderly people, combined with other comorbidities induced by tobacco smoke, leads to an enhancement of the disease progression [15].

Widening the analysis to the action on lymphocytes, it has been demonstrated that the activity of natural killer cells in the peripheral blood is reduced in smokers when compared with that of non-smokers [16, 17]. These alterations seem to be reversible in ex-smokers [18].

Studies on bronchoalveolar lavage of smokers confirmed a marked decrease in the percentage and absolute number of CD4+ cells with an increase of CD8+, with a lower CD4+/CD8+ cell ratio in smokers vs. non-smokers [19, 20] and an impairment or a true suppression of natural killer cell activity [21] in smokers as a possible result of an enhanced role of macrophages.

The level of interferon γ (INFγ) in the sputum has been reported as being lower in smokers than in non-smokers [22].

Numerous data point to the conclusion that tobacco smoke can increase the risk of onset of TB *via* a reduced immune response, coupled with an impaired non-specific response. It seems that smoking tends to bypass or shorten the steps from infection to disease, resulting in more rapid and severe disease progression.

SUMMARY

Apart from the health problems directly related to tobacco, smoking has little epidemiological impact on the prevalence of TB in countries or regions where the incidence of the disease is low, as in most developed countries. On the other hand, smoking may have a dramatic impact on the prevalence of TB in countries where the rate of latent infection and incidence of active disease is high, as in many developing countries. Considering that smoking prevalence is increasing in developing countries with high incidence rates of TB, and particularly among women, and that a large proportion of the world's population is thought to be infected (one-third according to the World Health Organization), the interaction of smoking on the incidence of TB and reactivation of the disease from the pool of infected subjects should not be underestimated. Furthermore, it also seems clear that smokers frequently belong to social groups with an increased risk of respiratory diseases, particularly TB [23].

REFERENCES

1. WHO – WORLD HEALTH REPORT. Reducing risk and promoting healthy life. Geneva, Switzerland, 2002.
2. Kuemmerer JM, Comstock GW. Sociologic concomitants of tuberculin sensitivity. *Am Rev Respir Dis* 1967; 96:885–892.
3. Altet MN, Alcaide J, Plans P *et al*. Passive smoking and risk of pulmonary tuberculosis in children immediately following infection. A case–control study. *Tuber Lung Dis* 1996; 77:537–544.
4. Jentoft HH, Omenaas E, Eide GE *et al*. Tuberculin reactivity: prevalence and predictors in BCG vaccinated young Norwegian adults. *Respir Med* 2002; 96:1003–1009.
5. Abal AT, Nair PC, Sugathan TN *et al*. Influence of smoking on cutaneous delayed-type hypersensitivity reactions by tuberculin skin test. *Respir Med* 2003; 95:672–675.

6. den Boon S, van Lill SW, Borgdorff MW et al. Association between smoking and tuberculosis infection: a population survey in high tuberculosis incidence area. *Thorax* 2005; 60:555–557.
7. Leung Chi C, Li T, Lam Tai H et al. Smoking and tuberculosis among the elderly in Hong Kong. *Am J Respir Crit Care Med* 2004; 170:1027–1033.
8. Gajalakshmi V, Peto R, Kanaka TS, Jha P. Smoking and mortality from tuberculosis and other diseases in India: retrospective study of 43,000 adult male deaths and 35,000 controls. *Lancet* 2003; 362:507–515.
9. Altet-Gomez MN, Alcaide J, Godoy P et al. Clinical and epidemiological aspects of smoking and tuberculosis: a study of 13,038 cases. *Int J Tuberc Lung Dis* 2005; 9:430–436.
10. Upham JW, Strickland DH, Bilyk N et al. Alveolar macrophages from humans and rodents selectively inhibit T-cell proliferation but permit T-cell activation and cytokine secretion. *Immunology* 1995; 84:142–147.
11. Keane J, Balcewicz-Sablinska MK, Remold HG et al. Infection by mycobacterium tuberculosis promotes human alveolar macrophages apoptosis. *Infect Immun* 1997; 65:298–304.
12. Nouri-Shirazi M, Guinet E. Evidence for the immunosuppressive role of nicotine on human dendritic cell function. *Immunology* 2003; 109:365–373.
13. Rich EA, Ellner JJ. Pathogenesis of tuberculosis. In: Friedman LN (ed). *Tuberculosis: Current Concept and Treatment*. CRC Press, Boca Raton, FL, 1994, pp 27–31.
14. Kluger R. *Asher to Asher: America's Hundred-year Cigarette War, the Public Health, and the Unabashed Triumph of Philip Morris*. Alfred A Knopf, New York, NY, 1996, p 19.
15. Leung CC, Yew WW, Chan CK. Tuberculosis in older people: a retrospective and comparative study from Honk Kong. *J Am Geriatr Soc* 2002; 50:1219–1226.
16. Tollerud DJ, Clark JW, Brown LM et al. The effects of cigarette smoking on T cell subsets: a population based survey of healthy Caucasian. *Am Rev Respir Dis* 1989; 139:1446–1451.
17. Hughes DA, Haslam PL, Townsend PJ, Turner WM. Numerical and functional alterations in circulatory lymphocytes in cigarette smokers. *Clin Exp Immunol* 1985; 61:459–466.
18. Hersey P, Pendergast D, Edwards A. Effects of cigarette smoking on the immune system: follow up studies after cessation of smoking. *Med J Aust* 1983; 2:425–429.
19. Costabel U, Bross KJ, Renter C et al. Alterations in immunoregulatory T cell subsets in cigarette smokers: a phenotypic analysis of bronchoalveolar and blood lymphocytes. *Chest* 1986; 90:39–44.
20. Arcavi L, Benowitz NL. Cigarette smoking and infection. *Arch Intern Med* 2004; 164:2206–2216.
21. Tkeuchi M, Nagai S, Nakajima A et al. Inhibition of lung natural killer cell activity by smoking: the role of alveolar macrophages. *Respiration* 2001; 68:262–267.
22. Geng Y, Savage SM, Razanai-Bouroujerdi S et al. Effects of nicotine on the immune response. II. Chronic treatment induces T cell anergy. *J Immunol* 1996; 156:2384–2390.
23. Bothamley GH. Smoking and tuberculosis: a chance or casual association? *Thorax* 2005; 60:527–528.

18

A 58-year-old woman with COPD and acute fever after visiting relatives in the countryside – farmer's lung

M. Iversen, G. Moscato

BACKGROUND

Allergic alveolitis (farmer's lung) or hypersensitivity pneumonitis [1], which is considered in this case report, is a rare disease. It is a granulomatous inflammation in alveoli and terminal bronchioles caused by inhalation of certain types of organic dust and in most cases fungal spores are involved (farmer's lung). Another important source of disease is exposure to wild birds, racing pigeons or tropical birds (bird fancier's lung).

Allergic alveolitis can occur in any occupational environment with exposure to organic dust and many specific cases have been named in relation to the occupational setting (e.g. cheese-washer's lung – mouldy cheese with *Penicilium casei*). Allergic alveolitis requires sensitization with previous exposures: an initial 'heavy' exposure will not produce allergic alveolitis. During exposure, many subjects will develop precipitating antibodies (usually immunoglobulin [Ig]G) against antigens, but only a very small minority of these will ever experience allergic alveolitis. The inflammation in allergic alveolitis is probably T cell-driven, but humoral factors are also probably involved. The immunological mechanisms are not yet fully understood.

The symptoms and the clinical picture depend on the character of exposure. A short-term, high-level exposure during work produces acute illness within 4–8 h, with high fever, shivering, shortness of breath, myalgia and malaise. Expectoration is frequently found and blood-stained sputum can also occur. Without further exposure, the symptoms will subside after a few days and the patient will be restored to normal health after a few weeks. With repeated low-grade exposure, the symptoms are more insidious, with coughing, shortness of breath and malaise, and the relationship to exposure is less obvious. Clinical studies have shown that patients may be acutely ill, with severe dyspnoea and sometimes cyanosis. Auscultation nearly always reveals fine crepitations in the acute phase. Fever is almost always present.

On an ordinary chest X-ray, acute allergic alveolitis appears as a diffuse haze, in more severe cases with diffusely distributed small nodules and in the most severe cases with confluenting infiltrates. High-resolution computed tomography (HRCT) is the most sensitive radiological method to demonstrate allergic alveolitis with centrilobular nodules and a 'ground glass' appearance (Figure 18.1). The changes are characteristic but not completely specific. Lung function studies show a marked fall in diffusion capacity and a moderate fall in

---

Martin Iversen, Dr Med Sci, Consultant Pulmonologist, Medical Department, Lung Transplantation Unit, Copenhagen University Hospital, Copenhagen, Denmark

Gianna Moscato, MD, Head, Allergy and Immunology Unit, 'Salvatore Maugeri' Foundation IRCCS, Institute of Care and Research, Scientific Institute of Pavia, Pavia, Italy

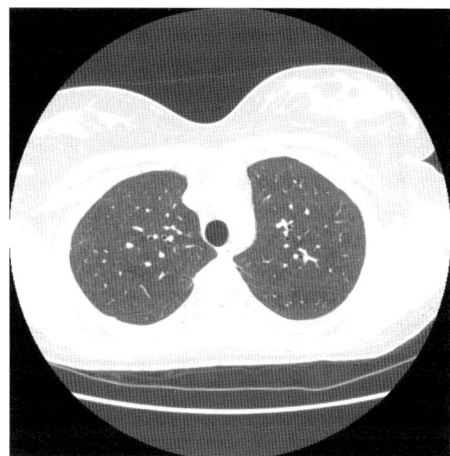

Figure 18.1 HRCT scan of patient with acute allergic alveolitis. Multiple centrilobular small nodules with ground glass pattern.

vital capacity without obstruction. Biochemical tests show a rise in acute-phase reactants without any specific pattern. If bronchial lavage (BAL) is performed, increased cell numbers are shown, with a very high percentage of lymphocytes (>50%), most of these being CD8+. Transbronchial biopsies may, depending on luck and the number of biopsies taken, show patchy inflammation with loose granulomas in the alveoli and terminal bronchioles. Eosinophilia is not a feature of the disorder.

Diagnosis is most often established with a patient history of a known exposure, physical findings and typical radiological and lung function studies. The finding of precipitating antibodies can, at a later stage, corroborate the diagnosis but is not particularly useful in the acute setting. If findings are not typical, a bronchoscopy with BAL and transbronchial biopsies may also be performed.

The most important treatment is the avoidance of further exposure to the precipitant. This must be considered very carefully, because it may have profound socio-economic implications for the patient, and require them to completely change their lifestyle.

In patients with acute allergic alveolitis, the disease will subside without treatment but steroids will accelerate recovery. Chronic forms with long-standing disease will require prolonged treatment with steroids to suppress disease activity. Prednisone at a dosage of 50 mg is continued for 2 weeks and then tapered quickly over the next few weeks to a maintenance dose of 10–15 mg. Patients with isolated episodes of allergic alveolitis will quickly recover their vital capacity and their symptoms will disappear within a few weeks, but diffusing capacity may take several months to return to normal. In patients with long-standing disease and chronic exposure, recovery is slow and incomplete. Although their chest X-ray and vital capacity return to normal, most patients will never have a normal diffusion capacity.

CASE REPORT

A 58-year-old woman living in a small provincial town was visiting her son who ran a small, family-owned farm outside the town. The woman was a former smoker who had stopped smoking 5 years previously, after repeated exacerbations with purulent sputum. At that time, she was found to be moderately obstructive with an forced expiratory volume at the first second (FEV_1) of 55% and forced vital capacity (FVC) of 84%. Now, she experienced on average one exacerbation or pneumonia every winter and chest X-rays suggested the presence of basal bronchiectasis.

A 58-year-old woman with farmer's lung

Previously, for many years, she had worked on the family farm and had on several occasions experienced periods of fever and malaise, some of them related to dust exposure. She had avoided dust exposure for many years.

During the visit, her son cleaned out the large grain silo on the farm. As usual, he was wearing respiratory protection inside the silo because of the amount of dust liberated. After a short while, a cloud of black dust escaped from the opening of the silo and the patient, who feared that a fire had broken out, rushed to the scene where she entered the porthole of the silo. She was immediately overwhelmed by dense black dust and fell to the ground with severe coughing and dyspnoea. She was taken outside by her son and recovered quickly. Two hours later she felt well and returned to her home in the town.

In the evening, 3 h later, she felt unwell with malaise and quickly developed shivering. After 2 h her temperature was 39.7°C. She had coughing, yellow sputum and was short of breath.

The patient at this time considered it to be another episode of pneumonia, took some penicillin tablets that she had left over from last winter, and went to bed. The following morning, the fever was unchanged and the dyspnoea was more severe. The patient went to her family doctor who found crepitation over both lungs and a quick test revealed a moderately elevated C-reactive protein (CRP). The doctor considered it to be pneumonia and advised the patient to continue antibiotics. A chest X-ray performed later the same day did not show any infiltrates. The patient had only very little sputum production.

By the fourth day after exposure, the dyspnoea was still severe and the patient felt ill, but her temperature had declined to 38.2°C. She had now been taking antibiotics for 4 days. The patient again consulted the family doctor who still found rales and a moderately elevated CRP. After a new chest X-ray showed small patchy infiltrates, the doctor considered atypical pneumonia as a possible differential diagnosis and changed the antibiotic treatment to a macrolide.

By the ninth day, the patient had been without fever for several days but the dyspnoea was still present. For the first time, she told her family doctor about the exposure on the farm and previous experience with dust exposure, and a diagnosis of allergic alveolitis was then suspected. After an emergency referral to a pulmonary specialist, an HRCT demonstrated entrilobular nodules with ground glass pattern, predominantly in the upper lobes. Lung function tests showed a mixed obstructive–restrictive pattern with diffusion capacity down to 37%. The PaO_2 was 8.7 kPa and the $PaCO_2$ was 4.5 kPa (Figure 18.2).

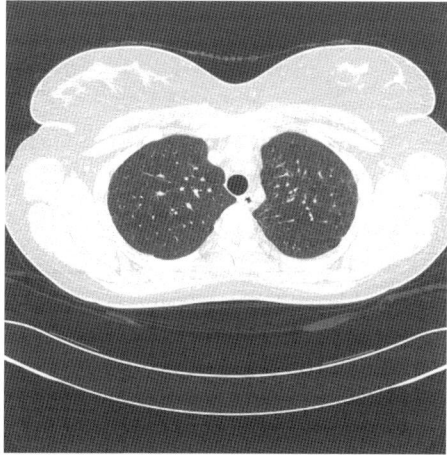

Figure 18.2 HRCT scan of patient with allergic alveolitis after 3 months with prednisolone treatment. Notice the almost complete resolution of infiltrates.

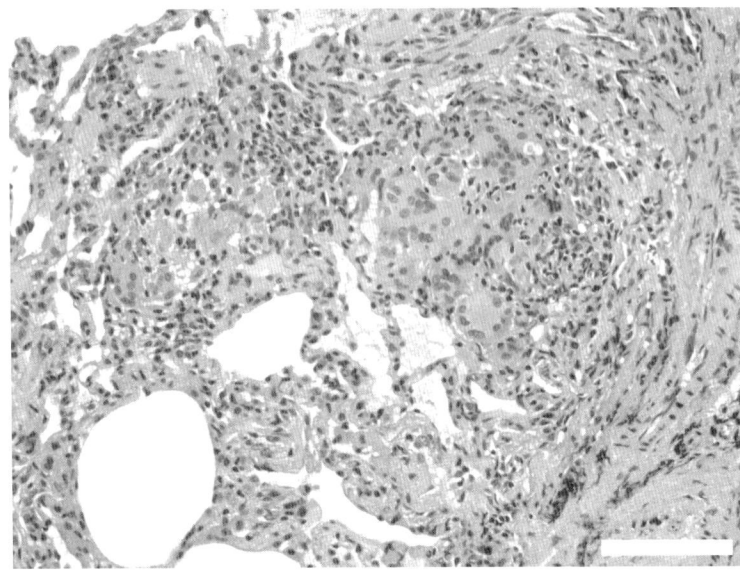

Figure 18.3 Transbronchial biopsy of same patient showing dense cellular infiltration (Scale: white bar = 100 μm).

The patient underwent bronchoscopy with lavage and transbronchial biopsy (Figure 18.3). bronchoalveolar lavage (BAL) fluid showed 70% lymphocytes and biopsies showed interstitial infiltration with small, loose granulomas. Allergic alveolitis was now considered the most probable diagnosis and the patient was started on 40 mg of prednisolone for 2 weeks with tapering of the dosage over the next 2 weeks.

The patient quickly improved, malaise and tiredness disappeared in a few days and the dyspnoea was gone after 2 weeks. A blood sample on day nine later showed a titre 1:32 for thermophilic actinomycetes (*Saccharopolyspora rectivirgula*). At a follow-up visit 2 months after the episode, the titre had declined to 1:8 and the patient's FEV_1/FVC had returned to normal, but the diffusion was still low at 63% predicted. The patient still felt more dyspnoeic on exercise than before the episode. After 4 months, she considered herself to have regained her previous functional level and a measurement of diffusion capacity showed 72% predicted.

DISCUSSION

What was the basic condition of this patient?
This patient had pre-existing chronic obstructive pulmonary disease (COPD) and bronchiectasis. Both previous smoking and previous occupational dust exposure could have played a role in the pathogenesis of COPD. In her previous history, an episode of farmer's lung might have occurred. Due to bronchiectasis, the patient had recurrent infections every winter. Acute reactions to airway irritants can occur in COPD patients [2]. The exposure to a high concentration of grain dust resulted in an onset of acute respiratory symptoms, sputum and fever within 3 h. When mould growth is present, the handling of mouldy material can release a very large number of spores into the air ($>10^9/m^3$). This dust generally contains very high levels of endotoxins or mycotoxins, and this can produce severe acute inflammatory conditions in the airways and lungs. In addition, nitrogen oxides can be

released by the decomposing material in a silo and cause pulmonary oedema some hours after inhalation.

What would be the most probable diagnosis at this time?
Did she have another exacerbation with infection in her bronchiectasis?
Did she develop pneumonia?
Did she experience a toxic response to a very heavy exposure to mouldy dust (organic dust toxic syndrome [ODTS])?
Did she develop an acute attack of allergic alveolitis due to fungal spores?
Did she develop a toxic gas inhalation (NOx) syndrome (silo filler's disease)?

At this time, the characteristics of exposure (high concentration) and the type of dust (grain dust in a silo) suggest an ODTS, whereas a toxic gas inhalation (NOx) reaction seems less likely because of high fever.

The day after the incident, the persistence of fever with very little sputum production and the objective finding of lung crepitation led the family doctor to suspect a new episode of infection/pneumonia similar to those frequently suffered by the patient in her past, and he prescribed antibiotics. A chest X-ray did not show any infiltrate. The patient had only little sputum production.

What was the most probable diagnosis at this time?
Could any of the differential diagnoses be ruled out?

The absence of interstitial infiltrates at chest X-ray should have ruled out the diagnosis of pneumonia, and the absence of sputum an exacerbation of bronchiectasis with infection. NOx syndrome would have provoked more severe pulmonary symptoms without fever. At this time, the history of acute high exposure, consistent symptoms and the absence of pulmonary infiltrates made ODTS the most probable diagnosis, although hypersensitivity pneumonitis was also possible, since in the latter, the pulmonary infiltrates may take some time to become evident on chest X-ray.

ODTS or inhalation fever is an acute reaction to the inhalation of organic dust or aerosol containing fungal spores (mycotoxins) or gram-negative bacteria (endotoxins). The condition has often been named according to the source of the exposure, e.g. grain fever, mill fever, farmer's fever, mycotoxicosis, and humidifier fever. The condition causes high fever, malaise and dyspnoea within a few hours of initial exposure and is usually self-limiting within 48–72 h. Leucocytosis is usually seen, whereas auscultation and chest-X-ray are usually normal [3, 4].

The patchy infiltrates shown by a new chest X-ray in the following days reinforced the diagnosis of pneumonia in the family doctor, who changed the patient's antibiotic prescription. It is worth noting that he clearly did not take any history about the circumstances surrounding the onset of symptoms, nor was he told by the patient herself of the acute exposure to dust until the ninth day. At that time the presence of hypersensitivity pneumonitis was suspected and supported by the results of HRCT, the findings of a mixed obstructive–restrictive pattern during spirometry and the reduction of diffusion capacity. The findings from BAL and biopsy confirmed the diagnosis. The commencement of corticosteroid treatment resulted in a quick improvement of symptoms and objective features.

Even if no bronchoscopy had been performed and the diagnosis of allergic alveolitis was tentative, how many of the differential diagnoses could be ruled out at this time?

The presence of persistent pulmonary infiltrates could rule out the diagnosis of OTDS, which is usually self-limiting within 72 h. The rapid response to corticosteroids would rule out pneumonia as a cause. A diagnosis of allergic alveolitis was also successively supported by the finding of precipitins to *S. rectivirgula* and temporal fluctuation in the titre after the acute illness.

SUMMARY

We have described a case of acute allergic alveolitis after an accidental exposure to a high concentration of grain dust in a woman with pre-existing COPD and bronchiectasis and repeated episodes of pneumonia. Initially, the syndrome was misdiagnosed since both the patient and the family doctor considered the acute respiratory syndrome as another episode of pneumonia similar to those previously suffered by the patient, and antibiotics were therefore administered. When the doctor became aware of the acute environmental exposure, the suspicion of an environmentally related disorder promptly arose. According to the type of exposure and the respiratory and general symptoms, the main possible differential diagnoses could have been allergic alveolitis, ODTS or NOx syndrome. The latter could be excluded due to the presence of high fever. The clinical course of symptoms, physical findings, radiological and lung function studies and the rapid response to corticosteroid therapy eventually led to the diagnosis of allergic alveolitis. Follow-up visits demonstrated a disappearance of symptoms, but lung function and diffusion capacity were still impaired after 4 months.

This case clearly demonstrates that a patient with a pre-existing obstructive respiratory disease may develop another pulmonary disease with a different pathogenesis. A key element for differential diagnosis is the clinical history, which should be carefully taken in any patient, even if already well known for a pre-existing disease. In this case, the family doctor did not ask the patient about the circumstance of onset of her symptoms and, as frequently happens, the patient did not report the acute exposure to dust until several days after the incident.

In the presence of acute respiratory and general symptoms after an accidental exposure to organic dusts, three main syndromes should be considered:

- Allergic alveolitis;
- ODTS;
- NOx.

The main criteria for diagnosis of acute allergic alveolitis are known exposure to offending agents, compatible clinical history and chest radiographs compatible with diffuse bilateral infiltrates, although after the acute exposure the latter may briefly appear normal. In the case described above, another element favouring the diagnosis of allergic alveolitis could have been the previous exposure of the patient to mouldy materials during the period in which she had worked on the family farm. Moreover, during that period, in which it is likely that the sensitization to moulds had occurred, the patient had on several occasions experienced symptoms compatible with allergic alveolitis.

The main medical therapy for acute allergic alveolitis is corticosteroids. The usual starting dose is 0.5–1.0 mg/kg of prednisone per day with tapering of the dose over 4–16 weeks. Such a regimen results in a rapid improvement of symptoms and of lung function. Corticosteroid therapy probably does not change the long-term prognosis of the disease [5].

Avoiding future exposure is an essential element in the management of the disease. Primary prevention measures and the use of personal devices may allow the patient to continue their work in areas of potential high risk, but a close follow-up is essential to ensure that the patient is not showing any 'new' symptoms.

The prognosis for allergic alveolitis is variable. With appropriate treatment and removal from exposure, recovery without lung impairment may occur. Some subjects, however, have progressive fibrosis and disability. The predictive factors for prognosis have not been clearly identified.

REFERENCES

1. Cormier Y. Hypersensitivity pneumonitis. In: Hendrick DJ, Burge PS (eds). *Occupational Disorders of the Lung*. WB Saunders, London, 2002, pp 229–240.
2. Sigurdason ST, Donham J, Kline JN. Acute toxic pneumonitis complicating chronic obstructive pulmonary disease (COPD) in a farmer. *Am J Ind Med* 2004; 46:393–395.
3. Iversen M. Toxic pneumonitis: organic agents. In: Hendrick DJ, Burge PS (eds). *Occupational Disorders of the Lung*. WB Saunders, London, 2002, pp 221–228.
4. Seifert SA, Von Essen S, Jacobitz K et al. Organic dust toxic syndrome: a review. *J Toxicol Clin Toxicol* 2003; 41:185–193.
5. Spurzem JR, Romberger DJ, Von Essen SG. Agricultural lung disease. *Clin Chest Med* 2002; 23:795–810.

19

Higher than expected rest hypoxaemia in a 74-year-old COPD patient with only mild airway obstruction

E. M. Clini, A. M. D'Armini, I. Sampablo

BACKGROUND

Chronic obstructive pulmonary disease (COPD) is a very significant epidemic disease of adulthood [1–3]. For clinical purposes, COPD has a functional definition based on spirometric assessment, and it is defined as a *'syndrome characterized by airflow limitation that is not fully reversible (fixed) (post-bronchodilator $FEV_1/FVC < 70\%$) and progressive'*. However, the updated definition also includes the role of a progressive inflammatory response secondary to inhalation of noxious particles and gases, thus incorporating the most recent insights in pathophysiology [4]. This syndrome generally occurs in subjects with a current or previous history of tobacco smoking presenting with dyspnoea and/or chronic bronchitis [4].

Patients with a fixed airflow limitation (or non-reversible airflow limitation) are often grouped under the general heading of COPD [5]. Although asthmatic patients with fixed airflow limitation are often diagnosed as having COPD, the differential diagnosis between asthma and COPD in patients with fixed airflow limitation must be recognized as the natural history [6], as well as the response to treatment [7], are different, depending on whether fixed airflow limitation is due to COPD or asthma. In fact, although COPD and asthma share two common features (airflow limitation and airway inflammation) they are two distinct chronic respiratory disorders [4, 8].

In this chapter, we will discuss the main factors and mechanisms leading to progressive airway obstruction and hypoxaemia in COPD patients, in reference to the case report presented below.

In COPD, expiratory flow limitation and impaired gas exchange result from varying combinations of obstructive changes in the peripheral conducting airways and destructive changes in the terminal respiratory tracts.

The flow obstruction may be due to many different airway and parenchymal lesions, each of which may be of differing severity and which often occur together but in varying combinations [9]. The known and possible variables related to airflow obstruction involve *bronchi*, *bronchioles* or conducting airways not containing cartilage in their wall, and the *acinus* as the

---

Enrico M. Clini, MD, Associate Professor of Respiratory Medicine, University of Modena, Institute of Respiratory Diseases, Ospedale Policlinico, Modena, Italy

Andrea M. D'Armini, MD, Associate Professor of Cardiac Surgery, University of Pavia, Division of Cardiac Surgery, IRCCS Policlinico San Matteo, Pavia, Italy

Italo Sampablo, MD, Associate Professor of Respiratory Medicine, Universitari Dexeus, Pneumology Service Institute, Barcelona, Spain

© Atlas Medical Publishing Ltd 2007

unit gas-exchanging structure of the lung [10]. The pathological changes of emphysema and narrowing of peripheral airways can be present long before significant disability develops and possibly even before spirometric tests are abnormal. From a pathological point of view, COPD is associated with inflammation of central and peripheral airways (increased number of mononuclear cells, particularly macrophages and T lymphocytes of the CD8+ type, neutrophils, hyperplasia of goblet cells and enlarged mucus glands, metaplasia of airway epithelium that is otherwise well preserved), lung parenchyma (pan-lobular and centrilobular emphysema in various combinations) and pulmonary vessels (loss of vascular bed) [11].

In advanced disease the peripheral airways are the major site of the increase in total airway resistance, but in the early stages of COPD, considerable obstruction can be present in the peripheral airways without causing an increase in total airway resistance or reduction in maximal expiratory flow. The early stages of the disease may also have little effect on overall lung function [12]. Since the pathological changes are distributed irregularly between parallel airways, their effect on lung function can be better detected by tests showing non-uniform behaviour of the lungs, such as the single-breath nitrogen test and closing volume, the frequency dependence of lung compliance and resistance, ventilation scans and the measure of enlarged alveolar–arterial PO_2 difference [13].

At the stage when there are minor changes in the periphery of the lungs, there are few symptoms, no abnormal physical or radiographic signs and exercise capacity is preserved within normal limits [14]. When abnormal breathlessness on exertion develops in COPD, standard tests of overall lung mechanics (i.e. FEV_1) are abnormal and there are increases in static lung volumes and compliance with loss of lung recoil pressure.

Uneven distribution of ventilation, together with destructive changes in the air spaces, leads to inefficiency of the lungs as a gas-exchanging organ. This causes a progressive reduction in arterial oxygenation (PaO_2). It is also notable that, in accordance with the disease progression, secondary changes occur in the chest wall, respiratory muscles, pulmonary circulation, heart and blood flow [15]. The mechanisms impairing the efficiency of pulmonary gas exchange are:

- Imbalance between ventilation and blood flow.
- Impaired diffusion increasing the difference between alveolar (PAO_2) to arterial (PaO_2) oxygen pressure.
- Reduction in PAO_2 due to development of a raised alveolar and arterial PCO_2 (so-called 'alveolar hypoventilation') [13].

The reduction in blood flow may be caused by various mechanisms:

- Local destruction of respiratory vessels by emphysema.
- Active constriction of vessels in the area with hypoxia.
- Passive obstruction by the effects of increased alveolar pressure/distension [13, 16].

The altered distribution of pulmonary blood flow is likely to be mostly accompanied by inequalities within a region [17]. However, the most important contribution to impaired gas exchange in patients with COPD is the mechanism of imbalanced ventilation to blood flow (VA/Q) as suggested by the multiple inert gas elimination technique (MIGET) [18]: combined patterns with units of both abnormally low and high VA/Q ratios are commonly found in COPD as the disease progresses. As progressive impairment of the efficiency of gas exchange develops in COPD, the difference between PAO_2 and PaO_2 widens and PaO_2 falls. Inequality of ventilation also causes reduction in 'accessible' lung volume, so that carbon monoxide transfer factor (DLCO) is reduced.

Several compensations for hypoxaemia are recognized (redistribution of blood flow to vital organs, increase in red blood cell mass, maintenance in cardiac output) so that peripheral oxygen delivery to important organs is maintained. The combination of greatly increased airway resistance together with impaired inspiratory muscle function due to hyperinflation is particularly likely to lead to persisting hypercapnia in the chronic (and most advanced) stable state [19].

CASE REPORT

A 74-year-old man, a mild ex-smoker (21 pack-years) who ceased smoking 5 years ago, affected by mild COPD (FEV_1 = 58% of predicted value; FEV_1/FVC = 61%), chronic respiratory failure (on long-term oxygen therapy [LTOT] since October 2000 and cor pulmonale due to previous pulmonary thromboembolism was admitted to hospital in April 2004, due to progressive severe worsening of his chronic dyspnoea.

He had been stable until 12 days before, when he developed a severe dyspnoea mainly on effort (score 4 on the Medical Research Council [MRC] scale), but also present at rest, needing significantly higher oxygen flow rate (from 2 l/min when stable before, to the current 4 l/min at rest), and initial oedema at the lower extremities. Domiciliary pharmacological treatment consisted of oral anticoagulant, furosemide, and angiotensin-converting enzyme (ACE) inhibitors, with addition of inhaled oxitropium bromide and LTOT for most of the daytime.

Previous medical history was significant for systemic hypertension pharmacologically treated by ACE inhibitors and furosemide for the last 3 years. At the age of 41, the patient had experienced a thrombophlebitis in the right leg (treated by saphenectomy), with a contralateral phlebitis a year later (similarly treated by saphenectomy). A bilateral deep venous thrombosis of the proximal legs was diagnosed 24 years later during an episode of acute pulmonary embolism (PE), treated accordingly with anticoagulants and with the subsequent positioning of a vena cava filter. The patient developed further pulmonary hypertension (PH) leading to the condition of chronic respiratory failure.

At admission, his temperature was 36.5°C, pulse rate 60 bpm, and respiratory rate 18 breaths/min. The systemic arterial blood pressure was 120/80 mmHg.

On physical examination, the patient was alert and cooperative. As the major finding, he presented with severe resting dyspnoea accompanied by cyanosis and bilateral jugular vein enlargement. On examining the thorax a diffuse reduction of pulmonary sounds appeared without any additional signs; normal heart sounds were detected. In a flat and treatable abdomen a mildly liver enlargement was noted. Oedema at the lower extremities was also present.

The electrocardiogram revealed a normally frequent (77 bpm) sinus rhythm, with incomplete right bundle branch block, right axis deviation, and negative T waves at the precordial leads (V_2-V_3).

Blood gas analysis under oxygen (4 l/min) showed severe hypoxaemia (PaO_2 = 51.7 mmHg) with mild hypocapnia ($PaCO_2$ = 32 mmHg) and compensated pH (7.42 with 20 mEq/l bicarbonates): this finding indicated a significant worsening compared with the blood gas analysis recorded at an ambulatory control 7 months earlier with a lower FIO_2 (2 l/min supplement). Lung spirometry did not change consistently when compared with the previous control, showing the presence of a fixed airflow limitation (FEV_1/FVC = 58%), with a moderate reduction in DLCO (59% of predicted).

Laboratory tests resulted only in the presence of mild anaemia (Hb = 12.8 g/dl; RBC = 4.13 × 10^6/ml), the international normalized ratio value of 3.93 being over the recommended value of between 2 and 3 for patients under anticoagulant treatment for chronic thromboembolism. Standard chest X-ray revealed no parenchymal abnormalities; a bilateral hilar enlargement was noted.

The echocardiography indirectly revealed the presence of a high degree of PH (estimated systolic pulmonary artery pressure [sPAP] = 95 mmHg), which represented a value worse than that recorded by the same observer a few months previously.

Based on this evidence, the patient was then addressed to a cardiac surgery centre for further diagnostic assessment and care. At the cardiac surgery centre, laboratory test analyses showed the presence of the following coagulation and immunological abnormalities: elevated serum level of homocysteine, lupus anticoagulant antibodies, anticoagulant C and S protein deficiency, elevated serum level of von Willebrand factor VIII and C677T mutation of *MTHFR* gene (heterozygosis).

The ventilation–perfusion lung scan was suggestive, with a high probability, of pulmonary thromboembolism, as bilateral and numerous segmental perfusion defects were detected in the presence of quite normal ventilation.

Transthoracic echocardiography confirmed the presence of severe PH (sPAP = 100 mmHg), with a dilated and hypertrophic right ventricle, dilatation of the pulmonary trunk and of the right and left main pulmonary arteries.

High-resolution thoracic computed tomography (CT) performed without and with intravenous administration of contrast material showed the presence of a moderate dilatation of the right heart with the right ventricle being 60 mm (short axis) and right ventricle hypertrophy (up to 12 mm), dilatation of the pulmonary trunk (up to 38 mm), anterior and inferior parietal thrombosis of 5 mm on the right main pulmonary artery starting from middle portion and extending to the Boyden truncus causing occlusion of the ventral segmental artery and distal portions of descending branch, and obstruction of proximal mediastinal branch of the left main pulmonary artery (Figure 19.1).

Pulmonary angiography was also performed, showing abnormalities of all left inferior vessels, except the posterior branches, and the occlusion of the right lobar inferior artery.

The right heart catheterization revealed an increase of the pulmonary vascular resistance (PVR) up to 696 dynes/s/cm^5 with a mean pulmonary artery pressure (mPAP) of 43 mmHg; right ventricle ejection fraction (RVEF) was 31% and the cardiac output (CO) was 4.6 l/min.

The echography of the upper abdomen revealed the presence of hepatomegaly, involving both right and left lobes, without signs of portal thrombosis.

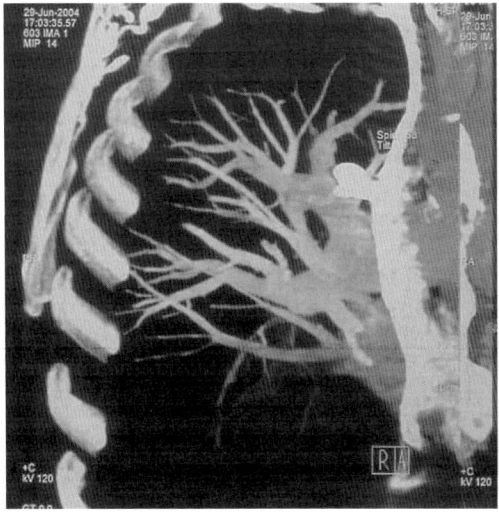 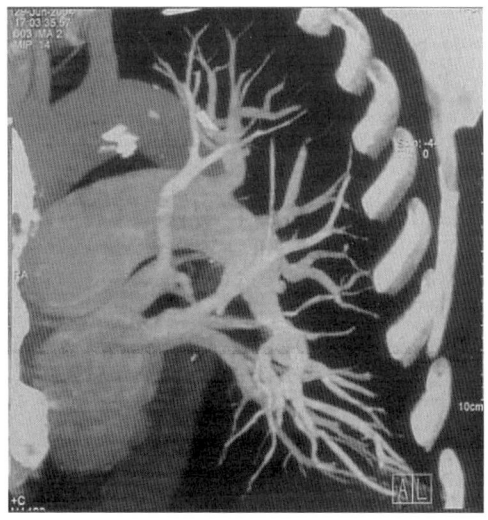

A   *B*

Figure 19.1 High-resolution CT showing segmental artery thrombosis of both right (*A*) and left (*B*) branches (for details see the case report section).

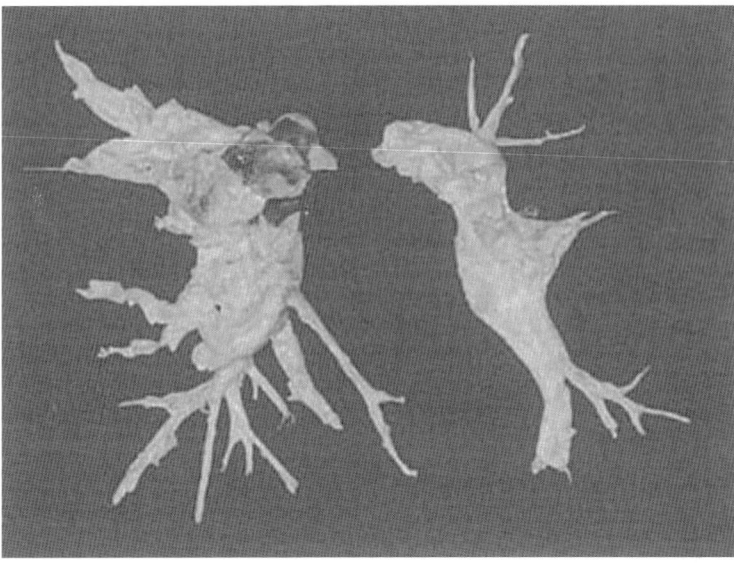

Figure 19.2 The bilateral thrombus surgically removed.

Based on these diagnostic assessments, the diagnosis of chronic thromboembolic PH (CTEPH) was made and the patient underwent a bilateral pulmonary endarterectomy (PEA) a few days later. In Figure 19.2 the bilateral thrombus removed from the arterial pulmonary branches is shown.

DISCUSSION

This patient was certainly affected by a chronic respiratory syndrome, as defined by COPD. Thus, an exacerbation of COPD may be suspected at presentation, based on worsening of respiratory symptoms and gas exchange. Indeed, acute exacerbations of COPD often result from an infectious aetiology [20]. However, in the present situation, some of the typical symptoms like productive cough, rhinitis, or other signs such as fever or leucocytosis were lacking. Similarly, pneumonia was also excluded based on the evidence of absence of a lung parenchyma consolidation or of an interstitial pattern at chest X-ray. Finally, no consistent signs of cardiac decompensation (e.g. oedema) were present.

The requirement for supplemental investigations and the suspicion that a different aetiology was causing the progressive decompensation of this patient was also based on the patient's previous history of pulmonary thromboembolism treated with anticoagulants and with the subsequent positioning of a vena cava filter. In this patient, however, the diagnosis of CTEPH was made very late, since this suspicion had not been investigated previously.

Understanding both the epidemiology and the natural history of CTEPH along with the poor prognosis associated with this disease should enable physicians to screen for incomplete embolic resolution in all patients who have recovered from a documented PE. Screening for PH in every patient with a new-onset or worsening dyspnoea and with a history of previous venous thromboembolism (deep venous thrombosis and/or PE) should be mandatory [21].

From an epidemiological point of view, CTEPH occurs in approximately 0.5–4% [22–25] of patients surviving an acute PE. Moreover, in these subjects, embolism should always be considered as a bilateral disease, as it was found to be unilateral in less than 2% of cases in a series of 1500 consecutive patients [23].

In CTEPH patients, the absence of symptoms during the primary acute event does not preclude evolution into the advanced and more 'dramatic' stage of the disease. Thus, PH should also be considered in the differential diagnosis of dyspnoea whenever there is no clear correlation with an underlying disorder, regardless of whether or not the patient's history seems to suggest several non-thoracic causes. Only a high level of suspicion and the awareness of the extremely wide and non-specific clinical spectrum of CTEPH can allow a timely diagnosis. Recurrences of PE [25, 26], *in situ* thrombosis [26], vascular remodelling, and arteriopathic changes within the small, non-elastic pulmonary arteries [27, 28] are thought to be responsible for the progression of the disease.

The prognosis for medically treated CTEPH patients is poor and it is related to the degree of PH at the time of diagnosis. Indeed, the 5-year mortality is 70% in patients with mPAP > 40 mmHg and it reaches 90% when mPAP is above 50 mmHg [29].

There are three main goals for a physician dealing with a suspected case of CTEPH:

1. To identify the presence of PH.
2. To define the aetiology.
3. To evaluate the most appropriate therapy for the patient.

Each patient with indirect radiological signs of chronic thromboembolic lesions should be assessed for possible surgical therapy. Diagnosis is a step-by-step integrated approach: the purpose of the ventilation–perfusion scan is to identify the ventilation–perfusion mismatched areas caused by the central pulmonary vascular obstruction. This analysis, however, can never be used to assess the extension of the embolic disease as it is known to underestimate the actual degree of vascular occlusion [24]. In patients with intact findings at the perfusion scan examination, right heart catheterization may assist in defining the diagnosis, prognosis and surgical indications [21].

Preventing embolic recurrences and supporting the right ventricle represent the frontline of medical management; however, medical therapy is not able to affect the natural history of the disease and thus is only supportive [30, 31]. PEA must therefore be pursued whenever the surgical indications are met.

Once the need for PEA and the technical feasibility are well established, the next step is to estimate the operative outcome. The principal risk factor for early mortality is the persistence of high PVR after intervention. Postoperative PH leads to acute right ventricular failure, which may worsen mortality rate. The risk-to-benefit ratio of PEA is drawn from a comparative evaluation of both the pulmonary angiography/high-resolution CT scan and observations on right heart catheterization. The status and rate of progression of the underlying disease, as well as the actual operative risk should also be considered when making the final decision [21].

The number of patients who would potentially benefit from PEA is extremely high. Presti *et al.* [32] has found that chronic thromboembolic obstruction of major pulmonary arteries occurred in about 1% of 7753 necropsies performed on subjects with an average age of 67 years. Indeed, in many PEA patients, the disease is only localized to the minor pulmonary arteries, where chronic thrombi are often unnoticed in autopsy studies [33].

On the whole, post-PEA improvement is dramatic and immediate. PVR and PAP usually fall to near-normal levels and cardiac output increases steeply [34]. This is typically evident while the patient is still in the operating room.

In this case study, PEA resulted in a normal pulmonary bilateral revascularization (as revealed by subsequent CT and ventilation–perfusion scans) and an improved cardiac morphology (as revealed by transthoracic echocardiography). Data obtained at 1-year follow-up also confirmed a consistent decrease in mPAP (−35%) and PVR (−49%) as well as an improvement of both RVEF (+32%) and CO (+13). Moreover, a gradual increase in arterial oxygenation has been obtained; at present, the patient does not need oxygen supplementation, presenting with satisfying levels of arterial blood gases while breathing room air (PaO_2 = 80.7 mmHg; $PaCO_2$ = 29.6 mmHg; $SatO_2$ = 96.7 %).

SUMMARY

COPD patients often present with impaired efficiency of pulmonary gas exchange in the advanced stage of their disease [13]. However, the most important contribution to the impaired gas exchange in patients with COPD is the mechanism of imbalanced VA/Q [18]. Although symptoms (even at rest) are commonly associated at this stage, it is clear that acute dyspnoea and/or worsening of symptoms may suggest a different aetiology for the occurrence of decompensation in these severely affected patients.

CTEPH is a very severe potential complication that may occur in subjects with previous thromboembolism, even if it is often misdiagnosed. The natural history of this disease cannot be modified by medical therapy alone. A proper patient selection, an accurate surgical technique and postoperative management are mandatory in order to obtain favourable and (above all) permanent results. Thus, experience and a multidisciplinary approach are required as well as a high turnover of patients. The poor survival rate of medically treated patients, low operative mortality after PEA, and good mid- and long-term outcomes make PEA itself the procedure of choice in the treatment of CTEPH. After a successful procedure, life expectancy is identical to the general age-matched population.

The functional improvement is consequent on the haemodynamic changes immediately after the procedure. Besides, the major cause of immediate postoperative morbidity and mortality is the incomplete dissolution of the obstruction. PEA is a complex procedure and there is undoubtedly a learning curve. This is mainly due to the difficulty in properly recognizing and reversing the embolic lesions. As surgical and clinical experience is gained, the criteria for surgery may be expanded without affecting the outcomes.

Nonetheless, a timely diagnosis of CTEPH and an increasing awareness of the efficacy and safety of PEA among the medical community will enable specialists to provide the optimal treatment to patients. The case reported here clearly indicates the lack of awareness of the problem among the specialists who had this patient in their care.

A careful examination of the patient's history and function and analysis of the data generated by a variety of diagnostic tests may lead physicians to suspect a very serious condition, which underlies but is not caused by the COPD *per se*.

ACKNOWLEDGEMENTS

The authors would like to thank their colleagues Micaela Romagnoli, Matteo Pozzi and Mario Viganò for their help in preparing this chapter.

REFERENCES

1. World Health Organization. World health statistics annual 1995. World Health Organization, Geneva, 1995.
2. Murray CJL, Lopez AD (eds). *The Global Burden of Disease: A Comprehensive Assessment of Mortality and Disability from Diseases, Injuries and Risk Factors in 1990 and Projected to 2020*. Harvard University Press, Cambridge, MA, USA, 1996.
3. Murray CJL, Lopez AD. Evidence-based health policy – lessons from the Global Burden of Disease Study. *Science* 1996; 274:740–743.
4. Global Initiative for Chronic Obstructive Pulmonary Disease (GOLD). Global Strategy for the Diagnosis, Management and Prevention of Chronic Obstructive Pulmonary Disease: NHLBI/WHO workshop report, NIH Publication 2701. April 2001 (Updated 2003): (http://www.goldcopd.com/). US Department of Health and Human Services, Bethesda, USA, 2003.
5. BTS guidelines for the management of chronic obstructive pulmonary disease. The COPD Guidelines Group of the Standards of Care Committee of the BTS. *Thorax* 1997; 52:S1–S28.

6. Burrows B, Bloom JW, Traver GA, Cline MG. The course and prognosis of different forms of chronic airways obstruction in a sample from the general population. *N Engl J Med* 1987; 317:1309–1314.
7. Kerstjens HA, Brand PL, Hughes MD *et al*. A comparison of bronchodilator therapy with or without inhaled corticosteroid therapy for obstructive airways disease. Dutch Chronic Non-Specific Lung Disease Study Group. *N Engl J Med* 1992; 327:1413–1419.
8. Global Strategy for Asthma Management and Prevention. NIH Publication No 02–3659 issued January 1995 (Updated 2002). (www.ginasthma.com). National Institutes of Health, National Heart Lung and Blood Institute, Bethesda, USA, 2003.
9. Hogg JC, Macklem PT, Thurlbeck WM. Site and nature of airway obstruction in chronic obstructive lung disease. *N Engl J Med* 1968; 278:1355–1360.
10. Thurlbeck WM. Chronic Airway Obstruction. In: Petty LT (ed.). *Chronic Obstructive Pulmonary Disease*, 2nd edition. Marcel Dekker Inc., New York, 1985, pp 129–203.
11. Romagnoli M, Clini E, Fabbri LM. Fixed airflow limitation caused by COPD or Asthma: from definition to management. *Med Hypotheses Res* 2004; 1:101–110.
12. Rodriguez-Roisin R, MacNee W. Pathophysiology of chronic obstructive pulmonary disease. *Eur Respir Monogr* 1998; 3:107–126.
13. Pride NB. Chronic Obstructive Pulmonary Disease: Chapter 16.4 Pathophysiology. In: Brewis RAL, Gibson GJ, Geddes DM (eds). *Respiratory Medicine*. Bailliere-Tindall, London, 1990, pp 507–520.
14. Cosio M, Ghezzo H, Hogg JC *et al*. The relations between structural changes in small airways and pulmonary-function tests. *N Engl J Med* 1978; 298:1277–1281.
15. Snider GL, Faling LJ, Rennard SI. Chronic bronchitis and emphysema. In: Murray JF, Nadel JA (eds). *Textbook of Respiratory Medicine*. WB Saunders, Philadelphia, 2000, pp 1187–1246.
16. Wright JL, Lawson L, Pare PD *et al*. The structure and function of the pulmonary vasculature in mild chronic obstructive pulmonary disease. The effect of oxygen and exercise. *Am Rev Respir Dis* 1983; 128:702–707.
17. Riley DJ, Thakker-Varia S, Poiani GJ, Tozzi CA. Vascular remodeling. In: Crystal RG, West JB, Barnes PJ, Weibel ER (eds). *The Lung: Scientific Foundations*. Lippincott-Raven, Philadelphia, 1977, pp 1589–1597.
18. Wagner PD, Dantzker DR, Dueck R *et al*. Ventilation-perfusion inequality in chronic obstructive pulmonary disease. *J Clin Invest* 1977; 59:203–216.
19. American Thoracic Society and European Respiratory Society. Skeletal muscle dysfunction in chronic obstructive pulmonary disease. *Am J Respir Crit Care Med* 1999; 159:S1–S40.
20. Wouters EFM. Management of severe COPD. *Lancet* 2004; 364:883–895.
21. D'Armini A, Zanotti G, Viganò M. Pulmonary endarteriectomy. The treatment of choice for chronic thromboembolic pulmonary hypertension. *Ital Heart J* 2005; 6:861–868.
22. Moser KM, Auger WR, Fedullo PF. Chronic major-vessel thromboembolic pulmonary hypertension. *Circulation* 1990; 81:1735–1743.
23. Jamieson SW, Kapelanki DP. Pulmonary endarterectomy. *Curr Prob Surg* 2000; 37:165–252.
24. Pengo V, Lensing AWA, Prins MH *et al*. Incidence of chronic thromboembolic pulmonary hypertension after pulmonary embolism. *N Engl J Med* 2004; 350:2257–2264.
25. Lewczuc J, Piszko P, Jagas J *et al*. Prognostic factors in medically treated patients with chronic pulmonary embolism. *Chest* 2001; 119:818–823.
26. Fedullo PF, Auger WR, Kerr KM, Rubin LJ. Chronic thromboembolic pulmonary hypertension. *N Engl J Med* 2001; 20:1465–1472.
27. Moser KM, Bloor CM. Pulmonary vascular lesions occurring in patients with chronic major vessel thromboembolic pulmonary hypertension. *Chest* 1993; 103:685–692.
28. Moser KM, Auger WR, Fedullo PF, Jamieson SW. Chronic thromboembolic pulmonary hypertension: clinical picture and surgical treatment. *Eur Respir J* 1992; 5:334–342.
29. Riedel M, Stanek V, Widimsky J *et al*. Long-term follow-up of patients with pulmonary thromboembolism. Late prognosis and evolution of hemodynamic and respiratory data. *Chest* 1982; 81:151–158.
30. Auger WR, Fedullo PF, Moser KM *et al*. Chronic major-vessel thromboembolic pulmonary artery obstruction: appearance at angiography. *Radiology* 1992; 182:393–398.
31. Jamieson SW, Kapelanski DP, Sakakibara N *et al*. Pulmonary endarterectomy: experience and lessons learned in 1500 cases. *Ann Thorac Surg* 2003; 76:1457–1464.
32. Presti B, Berthrong M, Sherwin RM. Chronic thrombosis of major pulmonary arteries. *Hum Pathol* 1990; 21:601–606.

33. Jamieson SW. Pulmonary thromboendarterectomy. *Heart* 1998; 79:118–120.
34. D'Armini A, Cattadori B, Monterosso C *et al*. Pulmonary thromboendarterectomy in patients with chronic thromboembolic pulmonary hypertension: haemodynamic characteristics and changes. *Eur J Cardiothorac Surg* 2000; 18:696–701.

20

A 52-year-old woman with mild COPD and significant oxygen desaturation during exertion

J. Zieliński, T. J. Ringbaek

BACKGROUND

Chronic obstructive pulmonary disease (COPD) is very common in the western world [1]. The natural history of the disease encompasses 40–50 years depending on the rate of annual decline of FEV_1 ranging in the individual patient from 40 to 100 ml per year. The long history of the disease has been divided into four stages according to severity of airflow limitation the patient shows, as assessed by a spirometry test [2] (Table 20.1).

The chronic inflammation of bronchi and destruction of lung parenchyma characterizing COPD lead not only to airflow limitation but also to ventilation–perfusion (V/Q) inequality, hypoventilation and restricted pulmonary circulation. These functional and structural derangements result in abnormal pulmonary gas exchange, heralded by hypoxaemia during exercise and later progressing to respiratory failure, the main cause of death in COPD patients [3]. Pulmonary gas exchange abnormalities develop late in the course of the disease, usually during the third stage, and are typical of the fourth stage of COPD.

Pulse oximetry is an easy, non-invasive method of measurement of arterial blood oxygen saturation (SaO_2) that has made it possible to recognize hypoxaemia (desaturation) of arterial blood at rest or during exercise in a family physician's office. Significant desaturation on exercise is recognized when SaO_2 falls $\geq 4\%$, and below 88% during exercise [4].

Hypoxaemia in COPD reflects high V/Q inequality due to perfusion of hypoventilated or non-ventilated lung regions. This mechanism is rather rare in a patient with mild COPD. Other causes of V/Q inequality should therefore be considered.

Restriction of the pulmonary vascular bed results in ventilation of underperfused or nonperfused lung regions. Closure or narrowing of the large pulmonary artery or severe narrowing of small pulmonary arteries and arterioles both result in hypoxaemia aggravating on exercise [5].

Such abnormalities characterize pulmonary vascular diseases leading to pulmonary hypertension (PH). According to a new classification of PH, the Evian classification, there are four main categories of PH:

1. Pulmonary arterial hypertension (PAH) (idiopathic).
2. Pulmonary venous hypertension.
3. PH associated with disorders of respiratory system or hypoxaemia.
4. PH caused by thrombotic or embolic disease [6].

Jan Zieliński, MD, PhD, FCCP, Professor of Medicine, Department of Respiratory Medicine, Institute of Tuberculosis and Lung Disease, Warsaw, Poland

Thomas J. Ringbaek, MD, DMSc, Consultant in Respiratory Medicine, Department of Cardiology and Respiratory Medicine, University Hospital, Hvidovre, Denmark

Table 20.1 Spirometric classification of COPD*

Stage and severity	FEV_1/FVC	FEV_1 percentage of predicted
Stage I, mild COPD	≤0.7	≥80
Stage II, moderate COPD	≤0.7	50–80
Stage III, severe COPD	≤0.7	30–50
Stage IV, very severe COPD	≤0.7	<30

*Post-bronchodilator values

Our case history illustrates a clinical situation in which a patient with a mild form of a very common pulmonary disease developed a second disease manifested by respiratory symptoms, desaturation and breathlessness.

Oxygen desaturation and shortness of breath are not always linked. The mechanisms responsible for breathlessness during exercise are much more complex and involve ventilatory impairment, dynamic hyperinflation, limitation in pulmonary gas exchange, abnormal cardiac function, neuropsychological impairment, and deconditioning. While supplemental oxygen corrects exercise hypoxaemia, treatment of breathlessness requires the use of bronchodilators, exercise training, modification of breathing pattern (controlled and pursed lips breathing) and anxiolytics. After presenting our case with hypoxaemia of vascular origin, the rationale for supplemental oxygen in COPD patients with exercise-induced dyspnoea and/or oxygen desaturation will be examined using three possible scenarios.

CASE REPORT

A 52-year-old woman, a cook in a factory canteen, reported to her family physician complaining of chronic non-productive cough of 2 years' duration and more recent (6 months) shortness of breath when climbing two flights of stairs. She was an ex-smoker with a history of 20 pack-years of smoking. She had refrained from smoking for the last 5 years. On physical examination no abnormalities were found. Electrocardiogram (ECG) recording was within normal limits. Office spirometry was performed and showed mild airway obstruction: FEV_1 was 81% of predicted, forced vital capacity (FVC) was 96% of predicted and the FEV_1/FVC ratio was 68%. Spirometry was repeated 20 min after inhalation of two puffs of salbutamol (bronchodilating test). No change in measured variables was found.

Chronic cough, exertional dyspnoea and the results of spirometry were compatible with a diagnosis of mild COPD. A short-acting anticholinergic, two puffs every 8 h, was prescribed and the patient was asked to report back in 3 months' time.

Six months later on a follow-up visit of the patient reported that, despite taking the prescribed treatment, her shortness of breath had become worse. Additional tests were ordered. A chest radiograph showed an enlarged heart with a prominent pulmonary artery and dilatation of the central pulmonary vessels. Red cell count was $5.49 \times 10^{12}/l$, haemoglobin of $166 g/l$ and platelet count of $509 \times 10^9/l$. Abnormalities on chest radiograph, polycythaemia and elevated platelet count were not typical for mild COPD. The patient was therefore referred to hospital for further evaluation.

On admission, the patient was in a satisfactory general condition. Her main complaint was exertional dyspnoea – first degree on the Medical Research Council scale. Detailed history revealed two episodes of short retrosternal pain, one 2 years and the other 6 months ago. There was no history of previous illnesses. She was a mother of four children and all pregnancies and deliveries had been normal. She had been in menopause for 3 years. The patient denied any use of hormonal contraceptive treatment or anorexigens in the past. On examination, left parasternal systolic murmur was found. No varicose veins were found.

A 52-year-old woman with mild COPD and oxygen desaturation

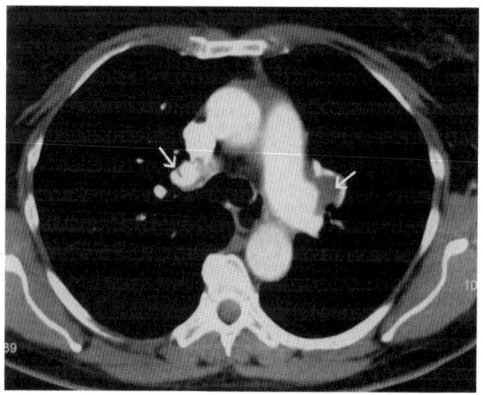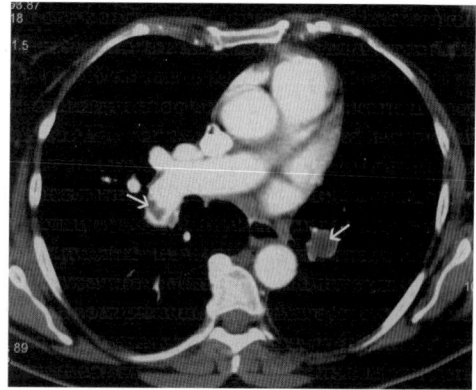

Figure 20.1 Selected HRCT scans of the patient showing multiple bilateral eccentric and central thrombi (arrows) in proximal pulmonary arteries.

A preliminary diagnosis of pulmonary hypertension (PH) in a subject with mild COPD was established.

Differential diagnosis included:

1. Hypoxic PH (HPH).
2. Pulmonary venous hypertension.
3. PAH.
4. PH due to chronic thrombotic or embolic disease.

To confirm the diagnosis, the following tests were performed, in this order:

- Arterial blood gases showed: PaO_2 = 57 mmHg, $PaCO_2$ = 33 mmHg, pH = 7.45.
- Full spirometry confirmed mild airway obstruction.
- Six-minute walking test (6MWD): the test was performed on supplemental oxygen (2 l/min). The patient covered a distance of 580 m. Pulse oximetry recorded during the test showed a significant fall in arterial blood oxygen saturation (SaO_2) from 93% before, to 86% at the end of the test.
- Two-dimensional Doppler echocardiography: the right ventricle was enlarged 30 mm (normal <27 mm) with signs of strain. The pulmonary trunk showed an enlarged diametre of 34 mm (normal <30 mm). The left ventricle showed normal size and contractility. Aortic and mitral valves were normal. Small tricuspid incompetence was found with a high systolic tricuspid gradient of 67 mmHg. Pulmonary artery acceleration time (AcT) was 63 ms (normal >110 ms). ***Conclusion: severe PH.***
- High resolution spiral computed tomography (HRCT): in the main trunk of the pulmonary artery, a linear thrombus penetrating to the left upper and lower lobar arteries and filling their lumen was seen. On the right side, multiple eccentric and central thrombi in the upper lobe, intermediate, and lower lobe pulmonary arteries were visible, along with mosaic perfusion of the lung parenchyma (Figure 20.1).
- Perfusion scintigraphy of the lung: large non-perfused segmental and subsegmental areas, especially in the left lung were seen (Figure 20.2).

The results of the above examinations confirmed severe PH and were compatible with the diagnosis of chronic thromboembolic PH (CTEPH).

HPH could be ruled out. In the majority of COPD patients, HPH develops late in the course of the disease (at stages III and IV). PH in COPD is usually mild and mean

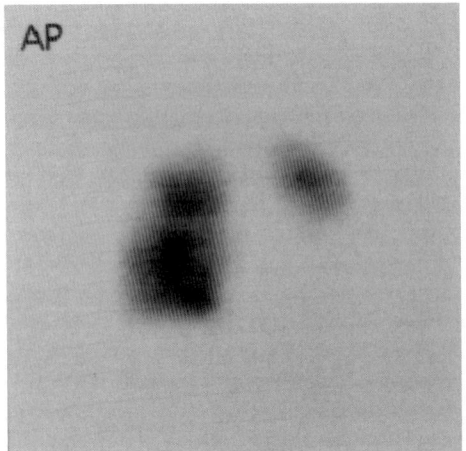 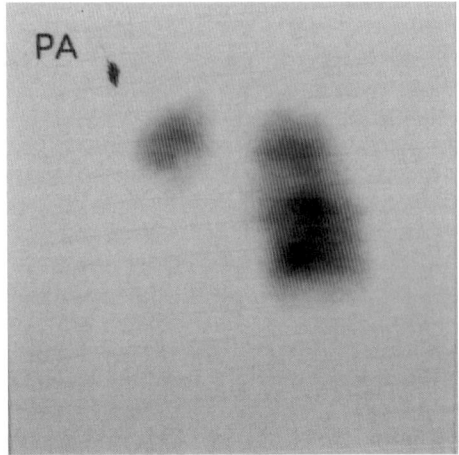

Figure 20.2 Anterior and posterior projections of 99mTc perfusion scintigraphy showing large perfusion defects in both lungs. AP = anterior; PA = posterior.

pulmonary arterial pressure (mPAP) rarely exceeds 40 mmHg. In the largest series of pulmonary haemodynamics studies in COPD, only 27 of 998 patients presented with mPAP ≥40 mmHg [7]. Of those 27 patients, 16 had another disease capable of causing PH. Two of them had CTEPH, and six had severe restrictive pulmonary disease. The remaining eleven with 'pure' COPD presented with moderately/severe airflow obstruction, severe hypoxaemia, and very low diffusion capacity for carbon monoxide (DLCO). Pulmonary fibrosis as a cause of PH could be ruled out by the lack of parenchymal involvement on a chest radiograph and non-restricted lung volumes.

Normal aortic and mitral valves and normal left ventricular function excluded a diagnosis of pulmonary venous hypertension. The results of HRCT and perfusion scintigraphy of the lung allowed the exclusion of idiopathic PAH. Negative history also excluded drug-induced PAH.

Additional examinations were performed to establish the cause of thromboembolic disease. No abnormalities were found on six-point deep vein ultrasonography. Lupus anticoagulant and antiphospholipid antibodies were negative. Antithrombin III level was normal. Finally, bone marrow aspiration showed signs of essential thrombocytosis. This diagnosis could explain a predisposition to thrombus formation.

The history of an episode of acute retrosternal pain of short duration 2 years previously suggested that the disease had started at least 2 years ago. However, recurrent recent embolic episodes could not be ruled out. The patient was started on low molecular weight heparin (LMWH) treatment to prevent further thrombotic episodes and on hydroxycarbamide to control the thrombocytosis, for 3 months. The patient returned to the clinic 7 months later. There was no improvement in breathlessness. The 6MWD was 480 m with a similar severity of desaturation from 92 to 87% (on oxygen supplementation of 2 l/min). Lack of signs of spontaneous resolution of proximal thrombi prompted the decision to opt for surgical treatment.

The patient was referred to the department of cardiac surgery for thrombendarterectomy. The operation was performed in extracorporeal circulation and deep hypothermia was preceded by coronarography, which revealed normal coronary arteries. Thrombendarterectomy of the left and right branches of the pulmonary artery was performed. Pulmonary haemodynamic measurements showed marked reductions in pulmonary arterial pressure and resistance immediately post-procedure. Postoperative recovery was uneventful. At the follow-up visit 6 months after the operation, the patient was in a good general condition. She was no longer short of breath on exertion. Her blood gases improved: $PaO_2 = 75$ mmHg, $PaCO_2 = 36$ mmHg, pH = 7.39, $SaO_2 = 95\%$. 6MWD = 550 m, $SaO_2 = 93\%$ before the test and 92% at the end, with no oxygen supplementation. Cardiac EchoDoppler examination showed no right ventricular hypertrophy or strain. Right ventricle diametre was 25 mm. There was no tricuspid gradient. AcT was 105 ms. Red blood count and haemoglobin levels had returned to normal values but thrombocytosis persisted. The patient continues to take LMWH and hydroxycarbamide.

DISCUSSION

CTEPH seems to be a rare sequelae of acute pulmonary embolism, developing in 0.1–0.3% of survivors of the acute episode [8]. Recent analysis of 223 patients, survivors of an acute pulmonary embolism, showed that at 2 years after the episode, 3.8% of patients presented with PH [9]. Inadequate thrombus resolution seems to be the inciting condition in the development of thromboembolic disease of the proximal pulmonary arteries, leading to severe PH.

The disease has an insidious course. Patients complain of non-productive cough, episodes of acute retrosternal pain probably related to recurrent emboli and exercise-related chest discomfort, frequently leading to an initial diagnosis of coronary artery disease. Sometimes chest pains are of the pleuritic type of a few days' duration from peripherally infarcted lung. Other erroneous diagnoses are: physical deconditioning, psychogenic dyspnoea, late-onset asthma or mild COPD. Exercise-related syncope or presyncope occur late in the course of the disease. The delay from the onset of symptoms to the correct diagnosis ranges between 2 and 3 years [8, 10].

Undiagnosed and untreated CTEPH has a very poor prognosis. Progression of PH leads to right ventricular failure and death. In a historical series of patients with CTEPH followed up before successful surgical treatment was introduced, in patients with mPAP above 50 mmHg, the 10-year survival rate was only 5% [11]. Similarly, a very bad prognosis was found more recently in a group of CTEPH patients treated with anticoagulants only. Poor prognosis was related to mPAP > 30 mmHg, coexisting COPD and low exercise tolerance [12].

Findings on physical examination at the early stages of disease may be limited to the easily-missed accentuated pulmonic component of the second heart sound in the second left intercostal space. In the full-blown disease, right ventricular heave, right ventricular gallop and systolic murmur of tricuspid regurgitation, best heard parasternally in the fourth right intercostal space, are all present. Jugular vein distension, hepatomegaly, ascites, peripheral oedema and cyanosis complete the picture of right ventricle and respiratory failure. Lung auscultation is typically normal. In 30% of cases, a pulmonary flow murmur is heard over the lung fields. This murmur arises from turbulent blood flow through a large branch of the narrowed pulmonary artery. Signs of chronic thrombophlebitis of the lower extremities are frequently present. Chronic thrombophlebitis is the most frequent source of recurrent pulmonary embolization.

Spirometry results are generally normal unless there is a concomitant disease like COPD. At advanced stages of the disease, lung volumes are restricted. A mild-to-moderate reduction of DLCO is usually present. Resting arterial blood gas analysis shows normal or borderline oxygen pressure. CTEPH typically shows an important decline in PaO_2 on exercise. Exercise hypoxaemia reflects the increase in ventilation–perfusion inequalities and a small, inadequate-to-load, increase in cardiac output. The latter is manifested by lowered mixed venous oxygen pressure (< 35 mmHg) and saturation (< 70%) [5].

Chest radiography may be normal at an early stage of the disease. The development of severe PH leads to enlargement of the right ventricle and of the pulmonary outflow tract. Dilatation of the central pulmonary arteries may be erroneously diagnosed as hilar adenopathy.

Right heart catheterization and pulmonary angiography remain a gold standard for defining the extent and proximal localization of organized thromboemboli. Pulmonary angiography also allows an assessment of blood flow dynamics through narrowed vessels [13]. Pulmonary angioscopy allows visualization of the vessel lumen and preoperative assessment of the extent of central thrombi. This procedure is only performed in specialized centres [14].

In patients with a typical clinical picture, invasive diagnostic procedures may be replaced by echocardiography and high-resolution spiral computed tomography [15].

Transthoracic Doppler echocardiography helps to rule out pathology of the left ventricle, valvular disease and intracardiac shunting as possible causes of PH. Pulmonary arterial systolic pressure may be estimated from the transtricuspid systolic pressure gradient and systolic blood velocity in the right ventricle outflow tract (AcT). Right heart chamber enlargement, compression of the left ventricle, paradoxical interventricular septal motion and high pressure in the pulmonary artery are typical findings in CTEPH [16]. HRCT shows dilation of the trunk of the pulmonary artery, irregular reduction of the lumen of the central pulmonary arteries and filling defects in subsequent branches accompanied by mosaic perfusion of lung parenchyma [17]. Normal HRCT does not exclude CTEPH, and patients with a strong suspicion of the disease should undergo pulmonary angiography.

Radioisotopic V/Q scanning plays an important role in distinguishing between CTEPH and idiopathic (or other) forms of PAH. Typical for CTEPH are one or more segmental or larger perfusion defects in regions with normal ventilation. In PAH normal pattern or mottled subsegmental perfusion defects are present [18].

A source of thrombus formation should be established. It may be chronic thrombophlebitis of the lower extremities. Pathological conditions preventing the spontaneous resolution of acute pulmonary embolus should be looked for. Lupus anticoagulant and cardiolipin antibodies may be responsible in 25% of patients [19]. Other pathologies of the coagulation process or fibrinolysis are rare.

Once the diagnosis of CTEPH is established, surgical treatment should be considered. Patients with high pulmonary arterial resistance (>300 dynes/s/cm [5]), severe PH (mPAP > 40 mmHg), and low exercise capacity are suitable candidates [20]. Surgical accessibility of the thrombi is an absolute prerequisite for operational success. Surgical techniques allow the removal of organized thrombi in the main and lobar pulmonary arteries. Dissection of segmental arteries requires great surgical skill and experience. The operation is performed in deep hypothermia and extracorporeal circulation *via* a median sternotomy. Affected pulmonary arteries are longitudinally opened and the organized thrombi are removed, together with intima and part of the medial layer of the arterial wall. Positive haemodynamic effects may be recorded immediately after the procedure. The operation is curative. Haemodynamic improvement has been sustained with recovery of right ventricular function followed by normalization of functional status, improvement in exercise capacity, and quality of life. Mortality in experienced centres averages 4.4% [21]. Patients should continue anticoagulant treatment and, if indicated, other drugs to prevent thrombus formation.

OTHER CLINICAL SCENARIOS

Three clinical scenarios of patients with COPD with different symptoms, oxygen desaturation and effects of supplemental oxygen are shown in Table 20.2 and described below.

Scenario 1: Should transient desaturation during exercise be treated in COPD patients?

American Thoracic Society COPD guidelines recommend that supplemental oxygen during exercise should be considered for patients with a $PaO_2 \leq 55$ mmHg or oxygen saturation of ≤88% during exercise [22]. Patients with normal oxygen tension at rest can show frequent

Table 20.2 Clinical scenarios of exercise dyspnoea, desaturation and effects of supplemental oxygen

Scenario	Dyspnoea and restricted exercise tolerance	Significant desaturation[1]	Effect of supplemental oxygen on	
			Dyspnoea	Exercise tolerance
1	−	+	NA	NA
2	+	±	+	−
3	+	±	+	+

NA: Not applicable.
[1]$SaO_2 < 90\%$ and fall $> 4\%$, as suggested by The British Thoracic Society [4].

and sometimes severe desaturation during activities of daily living [23]. In a study of 5926 patients with moderate COPD (FEV_1 between 1.5 and 2 l) approximately 10% desaturated ≥4% during exercise [24]. In more severe COPD patients (average $FEV_1 = 1.29$ l), Knower et al. [25] found that 26 (32%) of 81 patients desaturated ≥4% and to an SaO_2 of 88% or below. Very little is known about the clinical importance of exercise desaturation. There are no data either on the importance of exercise desaturation or on the effects of oxygen supplementation on hospitalization, pulmonary haemodynamics, quality of life, and survival. Obviously, oxygen desaturation during exercise is poorly correlated to walking distance and breathlessness at exercise [26, 27]. Although supplemental oxygen alleviates the desaturations [28, 29], this intervention cannot be recommended before a beneficial effect is documented.

Scenario 2: What if a patient has exercise dyspnoea, restricted exercise tolerance, and declares that supplemental oxygen relieves dyspnoea?

Several studies have found that oxygen during exercise relieves dyspnoea (reducing the Borg score by 0.5–1.0) and improves performance (5–20%) on a short-term basis [29–38]. However, oxygen supplementation during exercise may pose some problems related to the weight of the device, or the risk of falls and kinking if long tubing is used. According to O'Neil et al. [39], only 19% of patients with oxygen prescribed 'as needed' used it during exercise and 87% used it after exercise. Yet, there is mounting evidence that oxygen given before and after exercise has no effect on dyspnoea or endurance [40–43].

Few studies have looked at the long-term effect of supplemental oxygen. McDonald et al. [32] studied 26 COPD patients. While they found an acute benefit of supplemental oxygen, there was little if any long-term benefit on exercise performance, quality of life or respiratory symptoms after 6 weeks of treatment. Eaton et al. [44] compared ambulatory oxygen 'as needed' with compressed air in a 12-week double-blinded randomized crossover study of 41 COPD patients with resting $PaO_2 > 55$ mmHg, but with exertional arterial oxygen saturation ≤ 88% and dyspnoea. They found that oxygen therapy delivered by a lightweight cylinder (2 kg) improved health-related quality of life as measured by the disease-specific Chronic Respiratory Questionnaire. The improvement was modest though statistically significant in terms of clinical relevance and there was no improvement in generic health-related quality of life [44]. Interestingly, at study completion, 14 of 34 'responders' (41%) did not want to continue oxygen therapy due to poor acceptability.

There are several possible explanations for the disappointing long-term effects of supplemental oxygen during exercise:

1. Many patients are restricted by the weight of portable oxygen cylinders (approximately 3 kg) and sometimes by the available gas delivery time (4–8 h per unit of portable

oxygen). Using an oxygen-conserving device delivering oxygen only during inspiration, the available time with portable oxygen can be increased, but patients often considered it less acceptable than continuous oxygen flow [45].
2. Patients do not wish to wear nasal cannulae (and portable oxygen) in public for cosmetic or emotional reasons [46].

Although most studies have failed to demonstrate any benefits of oxygen supplementation during rehabilitation [34–37], guidelines for pulmonary rehabilitation have recommended providing supplemental oxygen during exercise when clinically significant desaturation ($SaO_2 < 88$–90%) has been found at the training load in the preliminary test [47, 48].

The current evidence does not support the routine use of supplemental oxygen during exercise in symptomatic patients with COPD without resting hypoxaemia.

Scenario 3: What if a patient with mild COPD and desaturation on exercise shows benefits of supplemental oxygen?

The European Respiratory Society has stated that supplemental oxygen may improve performance and reduce breathlessness in subjects with exercise-induced hypoxaemia [49] and, recently, supplemental oxygen has been recommended to patients who desaturate ≥4% and to 90% or below and this improves their exercise capacity on oxygen [33, 50].

Eaton *et al.* [44] in the above mentioned study tested whether this recommendation was able to distinguish patients with improved quality of life after 6 weeks on ambulatory oxygen. The acute response to supplemental oxygen and desaturation during exercise correlated poorly with the 6-week response, either because the daily activity was too different from an exercise test in the laboratory, or because the effect of supplemental oxygen during an exercise test varies, meaning that a patient could be a 'responder' in one test and a 'non-responder' in another test.

Therefore, if supplemental oxygen is prescribed, a 3-month probationary period with evaluation of oxygen use and benefits during activities of daily living is important.

Exercise-induced desaturation seems to correlate with the effect of supplemental oxygen [38]. However, it is important to recognize that patients without exercise desaturation may also benefit from oxygen supplementation [30, 31]. Among 12 COPD patients, four had improved their exercise tolerance for more than 100%, and two of these patients did not desaturate during exercise [31]. In a study of 17 COPD patients, supplemental oxygen increased the exercise tolerance in nine patients. Their oxygen saturation during exercise was not different from the oxygen saturation in patients without the effect of oxygen on exercise tolerance [30].

The modest long-term effect on quality of life does not support a widespread use of supplemental oxygen – even after a positive exercise test. More research is needed to select those patients who could objectively benefit from supplemental oxygen, and to improve the portable oxygen devices.

SUMMARY

- Hypoxaemia is an ominous, life-threatening clinical sign developing in the late stages of COPD. It has been demonstrated that severe hypoxaemia negatively influences survival. Randomized controlled studies have demonstrated beneficial effects of long-term domiciliary oxygen treatment on the survival of patients with COPD and severe resting hypoxaemia.
- Hypoxaemia appearing in a patient with early or moderate COPD is usually caused by another concomitant disease affecting primarily the pulmonary vasculature or interstitium. Appropriate investigations should be undertaken to establish a proper diagnosis and instigate relevant therapy.

- Evidence of benefits of oxygen supplementation in patients who are normoxic at rest but desaturate on exercise is less clear. Oxygen supplementation during exercise has been shown to decrease dyspnoea and increase exercise capacity in an acute experiment. However, long-term effects on daily activities and quality of life are rather small and achieved in only a small proportion of patients. Weight and the obtrusiveness of ambulatory oxygen equipment is an additional confounding factor.
- It seems that the prescription of ambulatory oxygen in this group of patients should be undertaken on an individual basis. More research is needed to select the patients who would derive a benefit from supplemental oxygen. The effects of supplemental oxygen should be objectively measured. Key outcomes of such therapy would include an improvement in quality of life and activities of daily living. Further developments in ambulatory oxygen devices are also needed to enhance patient compliance.

ACKNOWLEDGEMENTS

The authors express their thanks to Professor Adam Torbicki for permission to present the case history of a patient under his care, and to Dr Jakub Ptak for supplying illustrative materials.

REFERENCES

1. Mannino DM. Epidemiology and global impact of chronic obstructive pulmonary disease. *Semin Respir Crit Care Med* 2005; 26:204–210.
2. Celli BR, MacNee W, and committee members. Standards for the diagnosis and treatment of patients with COPD: a summary of the ATS/ERS position paper. *Eur Respir J* 2004; 23:932–946.
3. Zieliński J, MacNee W, Wędzicha J et al. Causes of death in patients with COPD and chronic respiratory failure. *Monaldi Arch Chest Dis* 1997; 52:43–47.
4. BTS Guidelines for the management of chronic obstructive pulmonary disease. *Thorax* 1997; 52:1S–27S.
5. Kapitan KS, Buchbinder M, Wagner PD, Moser KM. Mechanisms of hypoxemia in chronic thromboembolic pulmonary hypertension. *Am Rev Respir Dis* 1989; 139:1149–1154.
6. Simonneau G, Galie N, Rubin LJ et al. Clinical classification of pulmonary hypertension. *J Am Coll Cardiol* 2004; 43:5S–12S.
7. Chaouat A, Bugnet AS, Kadaoul N et al. Severe pulmonary hypertension and chronic obstructive pulmonary disease. *Am J Respir Crit Care Med* 2005; 172:189–194.
8. Fedullo PF, Auger WR, Kerr KM, Kim NH. Chronic thromboembolic pulmonary hypertension. *Semin Respir Crit Care Med* 2003; 24:273–285.
9. Pengo V, Lensing AWA, Prins MH et al. Incidence of chronic thromboembolic pulmonary hypertension after pulmonary embolism. *N Engl J Med* 2004; 350:2257–2264.
10. Simonneau G, Azarian R. Brenot F et al. Surgical management of unresolved pulmonary embolism: a personal series of 72 patients. *Chest* 1995; 107:52S–55S.
11. Riedel M, Stanek V, Widimsky J, Prerovsky I. Longterm follow-up of patients with pulmonary thromboembolism: late prognosis and evolution of hemodynamic and respiratory data. *Chest* 1982; 81:151–158.
12. Lewczuk J, Piszko P, Jagas J et al. Prognostic factors in medically treated patients with chronic pulmonary embolism. *Chest* 2001; 119:818–823.
13. Auger WR, Fedullo PF, Moser KM et al. Chronic major-vessel thromboembolic pulmonary artery obstruction: appearance at angiography. *Radiology* 1992; 182:393–398.
14. Shure D, Gregoratos G, Moser KM. Fiberoptic angioscopy: role in the diagnosis of chronic pulmonary arterial obstruction. *Ann Intern Med* 1985; 103:844–850.
15. Heinrich M, Uder M, Tscholl D et al. CT scan findings in chronic thromboembolic pulmonary hypertension. *Chest* 2005; 127:1606–1613.
16. Dittrich HC, McCann HA, Blanchard DG. Cardiac structure and function in chronic thromboembolic pulmonary hypertension. *Am J Card Imaging* 1994; 8:18–27.
17. Cho SR, Tisnado J, Cockrell CH et al. Angiographic evaluation of patients with unilateral massive perfusion defects on the lung scan. *Radiographics* 1987; 7:729–745.

18. Lisbona R, Kreisman H, Novales-Diaz J, Derbekyan V. Perfusion lung scanning: differentiation of primary from thromboembolic pulmonary hypertension. *AJR Am J Roentgenol* 1985; 144:27–30.
19. Wolf M, Soyer-Neumann C, Parent F *et al*. Thrombotic risk factors in pulmonary hypertension. *Eur Respir J* 2000; 15:395–399.
20. Doyle RL, McCrory D, Channick RN *et al*. Surgical treatments/interventions for pulmonary arterial hypertension. ACCP evidence-based clinical practice guidelines. *Chest* 2004; 126:63S–71S.
21. Jamieson SW, Kapelanski DP, Sakakibara N *et al*. Pulmonary endarterectomy: experience and lessons learned in 1,500 cases. *Ann Thorac Surg* 2003; 76:1457–1464.
22. ATS Statement. Standards for the diagnosis and care of patients with chronic obstructive pulmonary disease. *Am J Respir Crit Care Med* 1995; 152:S77–S120.
23. Soguel Schenkel N, Burdet L, de Muralt B, Fitting JW. Oxygen saturation during daily activities in chronic obstructive pulmonary disease. *Eur Respir J* 1996; 9:2584–2589.
24. Hadeli KO, Siegel EM, Sherrill DL *et al*. Predictors of oxygen desaturation during submaximal exercise in 8,000 patients. *Chest* 2001; 120:88–92.
25. Knower MT, Dunagan DP, Adair NE, Chin R Jr. Baseline oxygen saturation predicts exercise desaturation below prescription threshold in patients with chronic obstructive pulmonary disease. *Arch Intern Med* 2001; 161:732–736.
26. Mak VH, Bugler JR, Roberts CM, Spiro SG. Effect of arterial oxygen desaturation on six minute walk distance, perceived effort, and perceived breathlessness in patients with airflow limitation. *Thorax* 1993; 48:33–38.
27. Baldwin DR, Bates AJ, Evans AH *et al*. Nocturnal oxygen desaturation and exercise-induced desaturation in subjects with chronic obstructive pulmonary disease. *Respir Med* 1995; 89:599–601.
28. O'Donnell DE, D'Arsigny C, Webb KA. Effects of hyperoxia on ventilatory limitation during exercise in advanced chronic obstructive pulmonary disease. *Am J Respir Crit Care Med* 2001; 163:892–898.
29. Jolly EC, Di Boscio V, Aguirre L *et al*. Effects of supplemental oxygen during activity in patients with advanced COPD without severe resting hypoxemia. *Chest* 2001; 120:437–443.
30. Light RW, Mahutte CK, Stansbury DW *et al*. Relationship between improvement in exercise performance with supplemental oxygen and hypoxic ventilatory drive in patients with chronic airflow obstruction. *Chest* 1989; 95:751–756.
31. Dean NC, Brown JK, Himelman RB *et al*. Oxygen may improve dyspnea and endurance in patients with chronic obstructive pulmonary disease and only mild hypoxemia. *Am Rev Respir Dis* 1992; 146:941–945.
32. McDonald CF, Blyth CM, Lazarus MD *et al*. Exertional oxygen of limited benefits in patients with chronic obstructive pulmonary disease and mild hypoxemia. *Am J Respir Crit Care Med* 1995; 152:1616–1619.
33. Snider GL. Enhancement of exercise performance in COPD patients by hyperoxia: a call for research. *Chest* 2002; 122:1830–1836.
34. Garrod R, Paul EA, Wedzicha JA. Supplemental oxygen during pulmonary rehabilitation in patients with COPD with exercise hypoxaemia. *Thorax* 2000; 55:539–543.
35. Emtner M, Porszasz J, Burns M *et al*. Benefits of supplemental oxygen in exercise training in nonhypoxemic chronic obstructive pulmonary disease patients. *Am J Respir Crit Care Med* 2003; 168:1034–1042.
36. Rooyackers JM, Dekhuijzen PN, Van Herwaarden CL, Folgering HT. Training with supplemental oxygen in patients with COPD and hypoxaemia at peak exercise. *Eur Respir J* 1997; 10:1278–1284.
37. Wadell K, Henriksson-Larsen K, Lundgren R. Physical training with and without oxygen in patients with chronic obstructive pulmonary disease and exercise-induced hypoxaemia. *J Rehabil Med* 2001; 33:200–205.
38. Fujimoto K, Matsuzawa Y, Yamaguchi S *et al*. Benefits of oxygen on exercise performance and pulmonary hemodynamics in patients with COPD with mild hypoxemia. *Chest* 2002; 122:457–463.
39. O'Neill B, Bradley JM, Heaney L *et al*. Short burst oxygen therapy in chronic obstructive pulmonary disease: a patient survey and cost analysis. *Int J Clin Pract* 2005; 59:751–753.
40. Killen JWW, Corris PA. A pragmatic assessment of the placement of oxygen when given for exercise induced dyspnoea. *Thorax* 2000; 55:544–546.
41. Lewis CA, Eaton TE, Young P, Kolbe J. Short-burst oxygen immediately before and after exercise is ineffective in nonhypoxic COPD patients. *Eur Respir J* 2003; 22:584–588.
42. McKeon JL, Murree-Allen K, Saunders NA. Effects of breathing supplemental oxygen before progressive exercise in patients with chronic obstructive lung disease. *Thorax* 1988; 43:53–56.

43. Stevenson NJ, Calverley PM. Effect of oxygen on recovery from maximal exercise in patients with chronic obstructive pulmonary disease. *Thorax* 2004; 59:668–672.
44. Eaton T, Garrett JE, Young P *et al*. Ambulatory oxygen improves quality of life of COPD patients: a randomised controlled study. *Eur Respir J* 2002; 20:306–312.
45. Roberts CM, Bell J, Wedzicha JA. Comparison of the efficacy of a demand oxygen delivery system with continuous low flow oxygen in subjects with stable COPD and severe oxygen desaturation on walking. *Thorax* 1996; 51:831–834.
46. Kampelmacher MJ, Kesteren RG, Alsbach GPJ *et al*. Characteristics and complaints of patients prescribed long-term oxygen therapy in the Netherlands. *Respir Med* 1998; 92:70–75.
47. BTS Statement on pulmonary rehabilitation. British Thoracic Society Standards of Care sub-committee on pulmonary rehabilitation. *Thorax* 2001; 56:827–834.
48. Mahler DA. Pulmonary rehabilitation. *Chest* 1998; 113:263S–268S.
49. Siafakas NM, Vermeire P, Pride NB *et al*. Optimal assessment and management of chronic obstructive pulmonary disease (COPD). The European Respiratory Society Task Force. *Eur Respir J* 1995; 8:1398–1420.
50. National Institute for Clinical Excellence (NICE). Chronic obstructive pulmonary disease: national clinical guidelines for management of chronic obstructive pulmonary disease in adults in primary and secondary care. *Thorax* 2004; 59(suppl I):1–232.

21

Hemidiaphragmatic paralysis after cardiac surgery in a 62-year-old COPD patient

S. Zanaboni, L. Appendini, B. Schönhofer

BACKGROUND

The diaphragm is the most important inspiratory muscle with a total surface area [1] of approximately 900 cm^2. Its function (to provide alveolar ventilation) is so critical that it spends more time contracting than any other muscle in the body. In fact, the diaphragm spends 45% of each day contracting, while the soleus muscle spends only 14% [2]. The diaphragm has two components: the non-contractile central tendon and the contractile fibres that radiate circumferentially and insert peripherally into the inner surface of the lower six ribs and costal cartilages anteriorly and into the upper three lumbar vertebral bodies posteriorly. Muscle fibres in the diaphragm can reduce their length by up to 40% between residual volume and total lung capacity [1]. There are many ways in which diaphragm contraction may bring about an increase in lung volume [3]. In upright humans breathing at their functional residual capacity, about 55% of the diaphragm surface area is in the zone of apposition [1, 4] and the first possible mechanism is a pure 'piston-like' action that has the advantage of very efficient conversion of diaphragm muscle fibre shortening into changes in lung volume. The second mechanism is a 'non-piston-like' behaviour in which the zone of apposition remains unchanged but an increase in the tension of the diaphragm domes reduces the curvature, thus expanding the lung. In this situation, the diaphragm behaves like a bubble and Laplace's law dictates the changes in transdiaphragmatic pressure (and lung volume) with changes in diaphragmatic tension. The third mechanism, known as 'piston in an expanding cylinder', incorporates both types of behaviour already described with the expansion of the lower ribcage that occurs with diaphragmatic contraction.

Diaphragmatic dysfunctions occur with a low but not negligible frequency in respiratory medicine. The most common causes of diaphragmatic paralysis are reported in Table 21.1. Diaphragmatic weakness or paralysis can involve either the whole diaphragm (diaphragm paralysis) or only one leaflet (hemidiaphragm paralysis). In motor neuron disease such as amyotrophic lateral sclerosis or Guillain-Barré syndrome, organic destructive processes involving the phrenic nerve such as large tumours, myopathies, muscular dystrophy, systemic lupus erythematosus or an idiopathic aetiology are the most frequent causes of

---

Silvio Zanaboni, MD, Chair of Anaesthesia and Rescuscitation, 'Maggiore della Carita' Hospital, University of Eastern Piedmont, Novara, Italy

Lorenzo Appendini, MD, Consultant in Pneumology and Critical Care Medicine, Division of Pneumology, 'Salvatore Maugeri' Foundation IRCCS, Institute of Care and Research, Scientific Institute of Veruno, Veruno (NO), Italy

Bernd Schönhofer, MD, PhD, Department for Pneumology and Intensive Care Medicine, Hospital Oststadt-Heidehaus, Klinikum Region Hannover, Hannover, Germany

© Atlas Medical Publishing Ltd 2007

Table 21.1 Most common causes of diaphragmatic paralysis

Myopathic causes
Muscle dystrophy
Systemic lupus erythematosus
Amyloidosis
Myasthenia gravis
Organophosphate poisoning
Botulism
Progressive dystrophy (Duchenne)
Neurological causes
Guillaine-Barré syndrome
Amyotrophic lateral sclerosis
Spinal cord disease or trauma
Radiation therapy
Poliomyelitis
Cardiac surgery injury

diaphragm paralysis. In cardiac surgery, paralysis or paresis of the left hemidiaphragm is a common complication [5]. This is not surprising, given the fact that each hemidiaphragm is solely innervated by its ipsilateral phrenic nerve (C3–C5) running near the mediastinum, an anatomical arrangement that predisposes the nerves to damage by topical cooling or surgical procedures. Fortunately, despite the importance of the diaphragm to respiration, hemidiaphragm paralysis usually does not seriously impair ventilation because, depending upon the degree of diaphragmatic compromise, the accessory muscles of respiration assume some or all of the work of breathing and hemidiaphragm paralysis recovers spontaneously in the majority of patients [6]. However, during rapid eye movement (REM) sleep, the contribution of the accessory muscles to breathing is reduced and overt respiratory failure may ensue in patients with isolated bilateral diaphragm paralysis [7], although a recent study demonstrated that these patients recruit extradiaphragmatic muscles in both tonic and phasic REM [8]. Furthermore, in compromised patients, hemidiaphragm paralysis may precipitate the precarious clinical situation into an overt respiratory failure. In these patients, respiratory failure is often ascribed to heart failure, cardiac valve malfunction, over-hydration, obesity, intrinsic lung diseases, pneumonia, or chronic obstructive pulmonary disease (COPD). Diaphragm paralysis-induced respiratory failure can be missed at a first approach. This can be due to many factors. First of all, there is a lack of a specific clinical sign guiding the physician to a correct diagnosis. Second, coexisting problems that often occur in these patients such as infections, malnutrition and reduced inspiratory muscle endurance due to prolonged ventilation [9] can deceive physicians. Third, the assessment of the diaphragmatic activity requires the evaluation of respiratory mechanics, a study in which intensivists are not well versed. For all these reasons, diaphragm disorders are often not recognized and, consequently, their occurrence could be higher than that reported in the literature.

CASE REPORT

A 62-year-old woman with a history of smoking (20 pack-years), COPD and rheumatic heart disease was admitted to a tertiary hospital complaining of acute pulmonary oedema. Mitral valve replacement had been performed 9 years before. Another mitral valve replacement (bioprosthesis) and concurrent tricuspid valve annuloplasty were performed 6 years later. Echocardiography indicated malfunction of the bioprosthetic valve with pressure gradient of 15 mmHg and pulmonary hypertension (pulmonary artery systolic pressure > 50 mmHg). Both the right and left atrium and ventricles were enlarged. The septal wall of the left ventricle was hypokinetic. Serum blood chemistry tests were normal. Chest X-rays showed pulmonary congestion. Bioprosthetic mitral valve replacement and tricuspid valve annuloplasty were again performed. The patient was successfully weaned from mechanical ventilation the day after the surgical procedure and transferred to the ward from the intensive care unit (ICU) on the second day after operation. Nevertheless, one day later, the patient was re-admitted to the ICU because of acute respiratory failure to be intubated and mechanically ventilated. A chest X-ray did not show evidence of pulmonary oedema or pleural effusion. Bilateral basal crepitations, signs of myocardial, valvular or rhythm dysfunction were excluded. Otherwise the patient was in a reasonably stable clinical condition without sepsis, pain, haemodynamic instability, renal or hepatic failure, or altered serum blood chemistry tests.

Several weaning attempts by T-piece failed. Meanwhile, a tracheostomy was performed. After 1 month of mechanical ventilation, the caring physicians classified the patient as difficult-to-wean and transferred her to a chronic ventilatory unit. Here, she was admitted to undergo a programme of progressive discontinuation of mechanical ventilation and to be discharged to a home programme of long-term ventilator assistance as a consequence of weaning failure from mechanical ventilation.

The patient was compliant and in good clinical condition. She was ventilated in the pressure support (PSV) mode set with an inspiratory pressure of 20 cmH$_2$O and a continuous positive airway pressure (CPAP) of 5 cmH$_2$O (total inspiratory pressure of 20 cmH$_2$O) with an oxygen fraction (FIO$_2$) of 30%. With this setting, a tidal volume (V$_T$) of about 700 ml and a respiratory rate (RR) of 12 breaths/min were achieved. Arterial blood gases were acceptable. Further weaning attempts failed again, such that a study of respiratory mechanics during spontaneous breathing was performed after 46 days of mechanical ventilation. Briefly, the study was performed *via* the transnasal placement of two balloon-tipped catheters, one placed at the lower third of the oesophagus to reflect changes in pleural pressure (Ppl) and the other placed in the stomach to reflect changes in abdominal pressure (Pga). Transdiaphragmatic pressure (Pdi) was obtained by subtracting Ppl from Pga. Another catheter and a pneumotachometer were used to sample the pressure (Pao) and the flow (V') at the airway opening. The study performed during spontaneous ventilation showed a tidal volume (V$_T$) = 0.302 l, RR = 19.4 breaths/min, dynamic lung compliance (C$_{L,dyn}$) = 0.066 l/cmH$_2$O (range of normality: 0.08–0.23 l/cmH$_2$O) [10], airways resistance [R$_{aw}$] = 10.1 cmH$_2$O/l/s (range of normality: 1.3–4.4 cmH$_2$O/l/s) [10], dynamic intrinsic positive end-expiratory pressure (PEEPi) = 5 cmH$_2$O (range of normality: 0 cmH$_2$O), maximal inspiratory pressure (PI$_{max}$) = −38.8 cmH$_2$O (normal values: ≤−70.0 cmH$_2$O) [11], maximal expiratory pressure (PE$_{max}$) = 56.6 cmH$_2$O (normal values: ≥90.0 cmH$_2$O) [12], maximal transdiaphragmatic pressure (Pdi$_{max}$) = 32.7 cmH$_2$O (normal value: ≥65.0 cmH$_2$O) [12]. The resulting tension-time index of the diaphragm (TTdi), a predictor of impending diaphragm failure when its value is equal to or exceeds 0.15 [13], was 0.149. Eventually, the patient was discharged home with a mechanical ventilator (PSV + CPAP mode *via* a tracheostomy cannula). Two months later, the clinical situation had improved and the patient was successfully liberated from the mechanical support during the daytime and put on CPAP set at 5 cmH$_2$O during the night. At that time, the respiratory mechanics study was repeated, with the following results: V$_T$ = 0.285 l; RR = 16.3 breaths/min; C$_{L,dyn}$ = 0.062 l/cmH$_2$O; R$_{aw}$ = 9.5 cmH$_2$O/l/s; PEEPi = 4.8 cmH$_2$O; PI$_{max}$ = 43.5 cmH$_2$O; PE$_{max}$ = 140.3 cmH$_2$O; Pdi$_{max}$ = 43.0 cmH$_2$O. The improvement of Pdi$_{max}$ coupled to a substantially unchanged workload resulted in a reduced TTdi that was below the threshold of 0.15 (TTdi = 0.119).

DISCUSSION

Patients with diaphragmatic paralysis report dyspnoea as their main symptom and it is frequently associated with many other clinical conditions in compromised patients and in the postoperative period. Usually, the first diagnostic approach is directed towards cardiac and respiratory failure, common clinical disorders in the ICU setting. However, in this case, good haemodynamic stability and normal PaO_2/FIO_2 ratio during mechanical ventilation excluded cardiac or pulmonary involvement. Because other complications were ruled out, a diaphragm dysfunction was suspected.

Bilateral diaphragmatic paralysis typically presents with dyspnoea that worsens in the supine position [14], paradoxical abdominal wall retraction during inspiration and contraction of the lateral oblique abdominal muscles during expiration. Unfortunately, all of these clinical manifestations are not easily appreciated in patients who experience a dramatic dyspnoea occurring within minutes of removing mechanical respiratory support. Similarly, normal investigations such as chest radiographs are not helpful.

The finding of elevated hemidiaphragms is sometimes difficult to explain because it may be due to other causes such as decreased pulmonary compliance, increased intra-abdominal pressure or pleural adhesion. Although the sniff fluoroscopy test is considered a good tool to show hemidiaphragm paralysis [15], it is impracticable in mechanically ventilated, critically ill patients. The ultrasound technique could be potentially useful to study the diaphragm involvement in respiratory failure, but at present it is not widely used [16].

PI_{max} obtained by voluntary maximal manoeuvres can be used in the ICU to determine muscle weakness (a $PI_{max} > 80\,cmH_2O$ in men and $70\,cmH_2O$ in women excludes clinically important muscle weakness) [11]. Theoretically, respiratory pressures are easier to record in critically ill patients because the majority of them are intubated and thus it is not difficult to achieve a good seal between the patient and the ventilator circuit. In addition, pressure artefacts induced by the compliance of the upper airways are offset by the endotracheal tube. However, this test does not directly reflect the function of the diaphragm, and when a low value of PI_{max} is found, Pdi_{max} measurement is warranted. Finally, it also has to be considered that both Pdi_{max} and PI_{max} can be difficult for critically ill patients to perform. This can limit the usefulness of these tests.

The suggested approach for the diagnosis of respiratory muscle dysfunction in non-cooperative patients is the objective, non-volitional measurement of maximal inspiratory pressure by means of electrical or magnetic stimulation (MS) of the phrenic nerves [12]. The original technique consists of the supramaximal electrical stimulation of the phrenic nerves with surface electrodes positioned on the neck and the concomitant recording of both the diaphragm electromyographic and pressure response to stimulation [17]. This method has the disadvantage that it is poorly tolerated by patients because of pain and discomfort induced by the electrical stimulation itself. Moreover, the localization of the phrenic nerves in the neck can be difficult even by experienced personnel, especially if the patient is obese. More recently, MS of the phrenic nerves has been introduced [18]. MS is technically easier for the operator and causes less discomfort to the patient [12]. Different sites of stimulation are available (cervical, unilateral anterior-lateral, bilateral anterior-lateral). Unilateral anterior-lateral stimulation is more specific than cervical stimulation and gives results comparable to electrical stimulation [12]. Finally, unilateral MS allows the study of hemidiaphragm function, and bilateral MS reliably achieves supramaximal stimulation [12]. In this context, the measurement of transdiaphragmatic pressure during supramaximal MS stimulation (Pdi, tw) provides an index of diaphragm, or hemidiaphragm, strength [12]. The limitations of MS are the cost of the equipment, the need for appropriate skills to perform the tests and the time required to perform the manoeuvre and analyse the data. An accurate cost–benefit analysis seems warranted before implementing such a technique, which in any case should be reserved to a specialized unit [19].

The analysis of respiratory pressures during spontaneous breathing can be of help in the diagnosis and monitoring of diaphragm paralysis. During normal quiet breathing, the diaphragm is the main inspiratory muscle involved in inspiration, its contraction producing a negative change in Pes and a positive change in Pga (Figure 21.1). In the case of complete diaphragmatic paralysis, the inspiratory activity of the accessory inspiratory muscles exerts a suction effect on the flaccid diaphragm, which is pulled upwards. Because the inspiratory

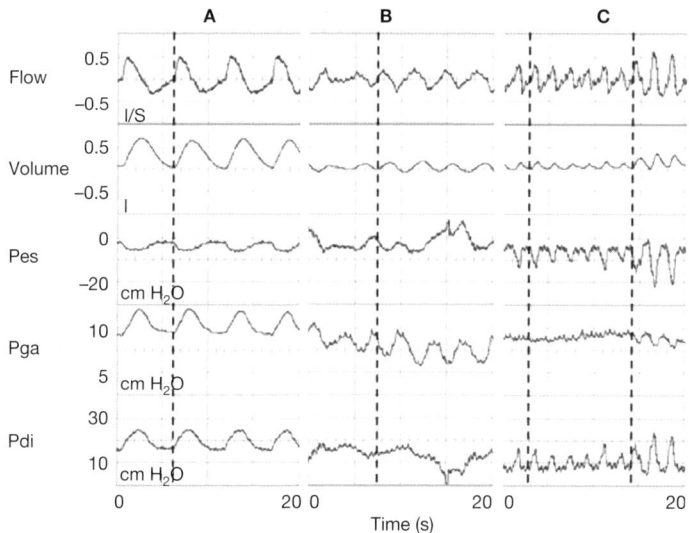

Figure 21.1 Flow, volume and respiratory pressures recorded during spontaneous breathing in a normal subject (A), in a patient affected by bilateral diaphragm paralysis (B), and in a patient with hemidiaphragmatic paralysis (C). Flow = inspiratory (upward) and expiratory (downward) airflow; Volume = tidal volume; Pes = oesophageal pressure; Pga = gastric pressure; Pdi = transdiaphragmatic pressure; vertical dashed lines = beginning of inspiratory pressure. *Note:* (1) the positive inspiratory swing of Pga and Pdi in the normal subject; (2) the negative inspiratory Pab swing associated with the flat Pdi tracing shown by the patient with bilateral diaphragmatic paralysis; (3) the positive inspiratory Pdi swing associated with either a flat or negative Pga swing (due to different levels of respiratory muscle activation) in the patient with hemidiaphragmatic paralysis. See text for further comments.

decrease in Pes is balanced by an equally negative change in Pga, the Pdi (the algebraic difference between Pga and Pes) is nearly nil and the Pdi swings are replaced by a flat trace (Figure 21.1). In the patient presented here, the possibility of obtaining a Pdi_{max}, and the evidence of a positive inspiratory Pdi swing excluded a complete (bilateral) diaphragm paralysis (a representative record of such a condition is represented in Figure 21.1).

The patient history, physical examination and functional evaluations discussed above led to the diagnosis of hemidiaphragm paralysis secondary to intra-operative damage of the ipsilateral phrenic nerve, complicated by a generalized muscle weakness, proven by the low value of PE_{max} and usually observed in critically-ill patients as a result of a generalized sensory-motor neuropathy. To make the situation worse, an increased respiratory workload ($C_{L,dyn}$, R_{aw} and PEEPi) requiring higher respiratory muscle energy expenditure was present due to COPD. The above scenario resulted in the diaphragm's (or better, the intact hemidiaphragm's) incapacity to sustain the effort required to maintain minute ventilation for very long. For this reason, to avoid diaphragm failure, a mechanical respiratory support was provided.

The choice of the particular assisted mode of mechanical ventilation (PSV combined with CPAP) was dictated by the presence of an increased inspiratory workload, mainly due to an increased inspiratory resistance and the presence of PEEPi. A high R_{aw} and PEEPi are causative factors of respiratory failure in COPD patients [20, 21]. In their presence, it has been shown that inspiratory assistance by adequate levels of PSV can support the inspiratory muscles in generating flow and volume, and that the application of CPAP can counterbalance most of the elastic threshold load represented by PEEPi [20]. Moreover, the combination of PSV and CPAP has been demonstrated to be more effective than PSV and CPAP alone in reducing the inspiratory workload and managing the respiratory failure of COPD patients [20, 22].

The clinical status of the patient improved in the following 2 months. Since respiratory mechanics ($C_{L,dyn}$, R_{aw} and PEEPi) due to COPD were substantially unchanged, this improvement was probably due to better muscle performance. As a matter of fact, the increased PE_{max} confirmed the overall muscle function improvement. Moreover, PI_{max} and Pdi_{max} were also increased, but were still below normal values. Notwithstanding this, the Pdi_{max} increase was sufficient to drive TTdi values just below the threshold of diaphragm fatigue. This allowed the patient to breathe spontaneously during most of the day, but the need to maintain some form of home mechanical ventilation during the night (CPAP) remained. The improvement of diaphragmatic function observed in the case report is consistent with data reported in the literature. Curtis et al. [6] reported that recovery from diaphragmatic paralysis secondary to cardiac surgery can occur between 30 days to 2 years. After this period, the lesion can be considered permanent and surgical plication of the paretic hemidiaphragm should be considered in symptomatic patients, since it has been reported to improve the overall respiratory function [23, 24], the latter being maintained over time [25].

The choice of application of CPAP during the night depended on the necessity to counterbalance the presence of moderate levels of intrinsic PEEP, i.e. the amount of isometric contraction required to overcome the inspiratory threshold load throughout inspiration [20]. This choice was based on the reduced need of ventilatory assistance because of the improved inspiratory muscle strength coupled with the evidence that PEEPi can represent up to 40% of the overall respiratory workload in COPD patients with respiratory failure, and that the application of CPAP to counterbalance PEEPi can be as effective as the application of comparable levels of PSV in reducing the inspiratory workload of such patients [20].

The present case report highlights the paramount importance of the concurrence of different pathophysiological mechanisms contributing to the development of overt respiratory failure. In this particular patient both COPD and hemidiaphragm paralysis conspired to generate an imbalance between the force generating capacity (Pdi_{max}) and the inspiratory workload, this imbalance being recognized as the final pathway leading to ventilator dependence [13, 21]. As a matter of fact, neither the reduced maximal inspiratory pressure (more negative than the threshold limit of $-30\,cm\,H_2O$) [26] nor the moderate increase of the mechanical workload of the patient (usually found in stable out-patients with COPD) [27] were sufficient per se to precipitate respiratory failure in the patient at the time of her admission to the chronic ventilatory unit. In this respect, it has to be noted that hemidiaphragm paralysis alone is largely asymptomatic in post-cardiac surgery patients with normal respiratory mechanics [21, 28].

SUMMARY

In summary, hemidiaphragm paralysis is a condition that can precipitate ventilatory failure in post-cardiac surgery patients with impaired respiratory mechanics of whatever origin. Prompt diagnosis should be sought in any of these patients whenever signs of respiratory distress occur. Assessment of respiratory mechanics and the measurement of respiratory muscle force generating capacity are of help in the differential diagnosis of ventilatory failure in this subset of patients.

When hemidiaphragmatic paralysis associated with COPD leads to ventilatory failure, the suggested therapeutic approach is mechanical ventilation in the PSV mode combined with CPAP set at a level close to the PEEPi measured in the patient. The physiological rationale for this combined ventilatory approach is that PSV assists the respiratory muscles in generating inspiratory flow and volume, whereas CPAP counterbalances the elastic threshold load induced by PEEPi itself. The choice of an invasive vs. non-invasive mechanical ventilation interface depends mainly on the severity of ventilatory failure and on the hours spent under mechanical ventilation during the day: full ventilator dependence suggests an invasive approach (tracheostomy), whereas the need for ventilatory assistance only at night shifts the therapeutic choice to the non-invasive approach. Intermediate situations represent the 'grey zone' in which it is hard to give standardized guidelines.

Finally, recovery from ventilator dependence in these patients depends on improvement of respiratory muscle function or of the respiratory workload, or both. Surgical plication of the paretic hemidiaphragm should be considered only as a late therapeutic option.

REFERENCES

1. Gauthier AP, Verbanck S, Estenne M et al. Three-dimensional reconstruction of the in vivo human diaphragm shape at different lung volumes. *J Appl Physiol* 1994; 76:495–506.
2. Sieck GC. Physiological effects of diaphragm muscle denervation and disuse. *Clin Chest Med* 1994; 15:641–659.
3. Petroll WM, Knight H, Rochester DF. A model approach to assess diaphragmatic volume displacement. *J Appl Physiol* 1990; 69:2175–2182.
4. Paiva M, Verbanck S, Estenne M et al. Mechanical implications of in vivo human diaphragm shape. *J Appl Physiol* 1992; 72:1407–1412.
5. Benjamin JJ, Cascade PN, Rubenfire M et al. Left lower lobe atelectasis and consolidation following cardiac surgery: the effect of topical cooling on the phrenic nerve. *Radiology* 1982; 142:11–14.
6. Curtis JJ, Nawarawong W, Walls JT et al. Elevated hemidiaphragm after cardiac operations: incidence, prognosis, and relationship to the use of topical ice slush. *Ann Thorac Surg* 1989; 48:764–768.
7. Millman RP, Knight H, Kline LR et al. Changes in compartmental ventilation in association with eye movement during REM sleep. *J Appl Physiol* 1988; 65:1196–1202.
8. Bennett JR, Dunroy HM, Corfield DR et al. Respiratory muscle activity during REM sleep in patients with diaphragm paralysis. *Neurology* 2004; 13:134–137.
9. Chang AT, Boots RJ, Brown MG et al. Reduced inspiratory muscle endurance following successful weaning from prolonged mechanical ventilation. *Chest* 2005; 128:553–559.
10. Frank NR, Mead J, Ferris BG. The mechanical behaviour of the lungs in healthy elderly persons. *J Clin Invest* 1957; 36:1680–1686.
11. Polkey MJ, Green M, Moxham J. Measurement of respiratory muscle strength. *Thorax* 1995; 50:1131–1135.
12. ATS/ERS. Statement on respiratory muscle testing. *Am J Respir Crit Care Med* 2002; 166:518–624.
13. Moxham J, Goldstone J. Assessment of respiratory muscle strength in the Intensive Care Unit. *Eur Respir J* 1994; 7:2057–2061.
14. Sandham J, Shaw D, Guenter C. Acute supine respiratory failure due to bilateral diaphragmatic paralysis. *Chest* 1977; 72:96–98.
15. Alexander C. Diaphragm movements and the diagnosis of diaphragmatic paralysis. *Clin Radiol* 1966; 17:79–83.
16. Bennett JR, Dunroy HM, Corfield DR et al. Respiratory muscle activity during REM sleep in patients with diaphragm paralysis. *Neurology* 2004; 13:134–137.
17. Newsom Davis J. Phrenic nerve conduction in man. *J Neurol Neurosurg Psychiatr* 1967; 30:420–426.
18. Similowski T, Fleury B, Launois S et al. Cervical magnetic stimulation: a new painless method for bilateral phrenic nerve stimulation in conscious humans. *J Appl Physiol* 1989; 67:1311–1318.
19. Polkey MI, Moxham J. Terminology and testing of respiratory muscle dysfunction. *Monaldi Arch Chest Dis* 1999; 54:514–519.
20. Appendini L, Patessio A, Zanaboni S et al. Physiologic effects of PEEP and mask pressure support during exacerbations of COPD. *Am J Respir Crit Care Med* 1994; 149:1069–1076.
21. Purro A, Appendini L, De Gaetano A et al. Physiologic determinants of ventilatory dependence in long term mechanically ventilated patients. *Am J Respir Crit Care Med* 2000; 161:1115–1123.
22. Appendini L, Purro A, Patessio A et al. Partitioning of inspiratory muscle workload and pressure assistance in ventilator-dependent COPD patients. *Am J Respir Crit Care Med* 1996; 154:1301–1309.

23. Schwartz MZ, Filler RM. Plication of the diaphragm for symptomatic phrenic nerve paralysis. *J Pediatr Surg* 1978; 13:259–263.
24. Schonfeld T, O'Neal MH, Platzker ACG et al. Function of the diaphragm before and after plication. *Thorax* 1980; 35:631–632.
25. Graham DR, Kaplan D, Evans CC et al. Diaphragmatic plication for unilateral diaphragmatic paralysis: 10-year experience. *Ann Thorac Surg* 1990; 49:248–251.
26. Sahn SA, Lakshminarayan S. Bedside criteria for discontinuation of mechanical ventilation. *Chest* 1973; 63:1002–1005.
27. Dal Vecchio L, Polese G, Poggi R et al. 'Intrinsic' positive end-expiratory pressure in stable patients with chronic obstructive pulmonary disease. *Eur Respir J* 1990; 3:74–80.
28. Laroche CM, Carroll N, Moxham J, Green M. Clinical significance of severe isolated diaphragm weakness. *Am Rev Respir Dis* 1988; 138:862–866.

Abbreviations

6MWT	6-minute walk test
ABG	arterial blood gases
ACE	angiotensin-converting enzyme
ACV	assist-controlled ventilatory
ADL	activities of daily living
AECB	acute exacerbation of chronic bronchitis
AMP	adenosine monophosphate
ARF	acute respiratory failure
ATP	adenosine triphosphate
ATS	American Thoracic Society
ATS/ERS	American Thoracic Society and the European Respiratory Society
BAL	bronchoalveolar lavage
BCM	body cellular mass
BHR	bronchial hyperreactivity
BIA	bioelectrical impedance analysis
BMI	body mass index
BNP	brain natriuretic peptide
BODE index	Body mass index, airflow obstruction, dyspnoea, and exercise capacity
CIN	critical illness neuromyopathies
$C_{L,dyn}$	dynamic lung compliance
CO	cardiac output
COPD	chronic obstructive pulmonary disease
CPAP	continuous positive airway pressure
CRP	C-reactive protein
CSA	cross-sectional area
CT	computed tomography
CTEPH	chronic thromboembolic pulmonary hypertension
DEXA	dual-energy X-ray absorptiometry
DLCO	diffusion capacity of the lung for carbon monoxide
DL/VA	DLCO to VA ratio
ECG	electrocardiogram
EELV	end-expiratory lung volume
ERS	European Respiratory Society
ESR	erythrocyte sedimentation rate
ETMV	endotracheal mechanical ventilation
ETS	environmental tobacco smoke
FEV_1	forced expiratory volume during the first second
FFM	fat-free mass
FiO_2	fraction of inspired oxygen
FM	fat mass
FRC	functional residual capacity

FVC	forced vital capacity
GARD	Global Alliance for Respiratory Diseases
GOLD	Global Initiative for chronic Obstructive Lung Disease
GP	general practitioner
HbA1C	glycated haemoblobin
HPH	hypoxic pulmonary hypertension
HRCT	high-resolution computed tomography
HRQoL	Health-Related Quality of Life
IC	inspiratory capacity
ICS	inhaled corticosteroid
ICU	intensive care unit
IFNγ	interferon γ
Ig	immunoglobulin
IMT	inspiratory muscle training
JVP	jugular venous pressure
KCO	carbon monoxide transfer coefficient
LABA	long-acting β_2-agonist
LMWH	low molecular weight heparin
LTB_4	leukotriene B_4
LTOT	long-term oxygen therapy
LV	left ventricular
LVRS	lung volume reduction surgery
M-CSF	macrophage colony-stimulating factor
MEP	maximum expiratory pressure
MIGET	multiple inert gas elimination technique
MIP	maximum inspiratory pressure
MME	macrophage metalloelastase
MMRC	Modified Medical Research Council (scale)
mPAP	mean pulmonary artery pressure
MRC	Medical Research Council
MRI	magnetic resonance imaging
MS	magnetic stimulation
MVV	maximal voluntary ventilation
Nd:YAG	neodymium yttrium-aluminium-garnet [laser]
NETT	National Emphysema Treatment Trial
NHANES	National Health and Nutrition Examination survey
NIV	non-invasive ventilation
NOx	oxides of nitrogen
NPPV	non-invasive positive pressure ventilation
NRT	nicotine replacement therapy
NSCLC	non-small cell lung cancer
ODTS	organic dust toxic syndrome
OR	odds ratio
PA	phase angle
PA-aO_2	alveolar–arterial oxygen difference
PaCO_2	arterial carbon dioxide tension
PAH	pulmonary arterial hypertension
PAO_2	alveolar oxygen pressure
PaO_2	arterial oxygen tension
PAP	positive airway pressure
PAR	population-attributable risk
PC_{20}	provocative concentration of a substance that causes a 20% fall in FEV_1

Abbreviations

PCR	polymerase chain reaction
PD_{20}	provocative dose of a substance that causes a 20% fall in FEV_1
Pdi_{max}	maximal transdiaphragmatic pressure
PE	pulmonary embolism
PEA	pulmonary endarterectomy
PEEP	positive end-expiratory pressure
PEEPe	extrinsic positive end-expiratory pressure
PEEPi	intrinsic positive end-expiratory pressure
PEF	peak expiratory flow
PEFR	peak expiratory flow rate
PE_{max}	maximal expiratory pressure
PET	positron emission tomography
PFT	pulmonary function test
Pga	abdominal pressure
PH	pulmonary hypertension
PI*Z	protease inhibitor phenotype Z
PI_{max}	maximal inspiratory pressure
PI_{max}	maximal static inspiratory pressure
PLB	pursed-lips breathing
PM	particulate matter
Ppl	pleural pressure
PR	pulmonary rehabilitation
PSV	pressure support ventilation
PVR	pulmonary vascular resistance
QoL	quality of life
RANK	receptor activator of nuclear factor κB
R_{aw}	airways resistance
REE	resting energy expenditure
REM	rapid eye movement
rhGH	recombinant human growth hormone
RM	repetition maximum
RR	relative risk
RR	respiratory rate
RV	residual volume
RV	right ventricular
RVEF	right ventricle ejection fraction
SABA	short-acting $β_2$-agonist
SaO_2	oxygen saturation in arterial blood
SB	spontaneous breathing
SBT	SB trial
SC	smoking cessation
SD	standard deviation
SES	socio-economic status
SGRQ	St George's Respiratory Questionnaire
SPAP	systolic pulmonary artery pressure
SpO_2	saturation of oxyhaemoglobin (measured by pulse oximetry)
TB	tuberculosis
TDI	transition dyspnoea index
TLC	total lung capacity
TNFα	tumour necrosis factor alpha
TRISTAM	Trial of Inhaled Steroids and long-acting $β_2$-agonists
TTdi	tension–time index of the diaphragm

V/Q	ventilation–perfusion
VA	alveolar volume
VA/Q	ventilation to perfusion ratio
VATS	video assisted thoracoscopic surgery
VO_2	oxygen uptake
WHO	World Health Organization
WT	walking test

Index

5 As treatment, smoking cessation 30, 31, 32
6-min walking test 51, 52, 54

abdominal obesity 59
ablation, value in atrial fibrillation 140
activity level assessment 52–3
acupuncture, value in dyspnoea 26
acute respiratory failure (ARF) 115–16
   case report 117–18
   management 116–17, 119–21
   non-invasive ventilation 150–1
acute silicosis 138
aerobic capacity, relationship to body mass index 99–100
air leak management, lung volume reduction surgery 2–3, 4, 99
air quality index 33, 34
airflow limitation 169–70
airways resistance, increased 21, 125
allergic alveolitis 161–2, 166
   case report 162–4
   differential diagnosis 165
   effects of grain dust exposure 164–5
allergy to antibiotics, case report 144, 145, 147, 148
α_1 anti-trypsin deficiency 46, 89
   lung volume reduction surgery 4
alveolar hypoventilation 170
ambulatory oxygen 184–6, 187
amoxicillin-clavulanate 144, 147
anabolic steroid therapy 57, 71
anaemia 53
anorexia 20
   association with dyspnoea 37
   case report 38–40
   as side effect of corticosteroids 13
anti-arrhythmic therapy 140
anti-oxidants 12
antibacterial resistance 143–4

antibiotics
   allergy to, case report 144, 145, 147, 148
   choice of agent 146–9
   interaction with methylxanthines 151
   role in management of exacerbations 9, 144, 146
anticholinergics
   effect on exacerbation frequency 9
   use during exacerbations 8, 151
anticoagulation
   in atrial fibrillation 140
   in pulmonary embolism 137
anxiety 11, 79
   and lung volume reduction surgery 4
   role in dyspnoea 22
anxiolytics, value in dyspnoea 23–4
apoptosis, increased in skeletal muscle 66, 102
arrhythmias
   treatment as cause 137
   see also atrial fibrillation
arterial blood gases, monitoring during oxygen therapy 116
aspirin, use in atrial fibrillation 140
assisted ventilation 80
asthma 169
   case study 44
   diagnosis 43
   risk factors 45
   symptoms 46
atrial fibrillation 67
   case report 135–6
   causes 137–9
   management 140
attention strategies in dyspnoea 25, 26

bacterial exacerbations 8, 143
beclomethasone
   risk of osteoporosis 105–6
   value in bronchiectasis 13

benzodiazepines
    effect on ETMV duration 128–32
    value in dyspnoea 23–4
β-1,3-glucan exposure 88
β$_2$-agonists 78
    effect on exacerbation frequency 9
    use during exacerbations 8, 151
    value in dyspnoea 24–5
β-blockers 129
    use in atrial fibrillation 140
bioelectrical impedance analysis (BIA) 37, 67, 68
biopsy appearance, allergic alveolitis 162, 164
bird fancier's lung 161
bisoprolol 129
bisphosphonates 109, 112
blood flow reduction, mechanisms 170
'blue bloaters' 99
BODE index 76
body cellular mass (BCM) 37, 41
body composition assessment 37, 41, 69
body mass index (BMI) 41, 69, 99, 111
    relationship to aerobic capacity 99–100
    relationship to healthcare utilization 100
    relationship to mortality 100–1
bone mass density (BMD) 105
    assessment in glucocorticoid therapy 112
    definition of osteoporosis 108, 109
    relationship to FFM 111
    see also osteoporosis
brain natriuretic peptide (BNP) 139
breathing exercises 59, 79
breathlessness see dyspnoea
bronchial hyperreactivity (BHR) 47
bronchiectasis 8, 13, 164
bronchiolitis obliterans 87
bronchoalveolar lavage, in allergic alveolitis 162, 164
bronchodilator responsiveness 46
bronchodilators 78–9
    effect on exacerbation frequency 9
    use during exacerbations 8, 151
    use in weaning from ETMV 131, 132
bronchoscopic lung volume reduction surgery 5
budesonide
    inhibition of TNF-α release 13
    nebulized 150
    osteoporosis risk 106
    value in bronchiectasis 13

value in dyspnoea 24–5
value in exacerbation prevention 12
byssinosis 87

C-reactive protein 53
    effect on energy expenditure 38
cadmium exposure 86
calcitonin therapy 109
calcium-channel blockers, use in atrial fibrillation 140
calcium supplementation 109, 112
cardiac congestion 51
cardiac surgery, left hemidiaphragm paralysis 192, 195–7
    case report 192–3
cardiopulmonary exercise tests 51, 52
    interpretation 53–4
cardioversion 140
carotid bodies, activity in dyspnoea 21
CD8+ T cells, increase during exacerbations 8
central perception, role in dyspnoea 22, 25–6
cheese-washer's lung 161
chest physiotherapy 79
    use in weaning from ETMV 131, 132
chest X-ray appearances 20
    in emphysema 4
    in mitral stenosis 136, 139
    in tuberculosis 157
    of vertebral fractures 107, 111
children, passive smoking, risk of tuberculosis 158
chronic bronchitis, causative agents 88, 93
chronic obstructive pulmonary disease, definition 169
chronic thromboembolic pulmonary hypertension (CTEPH) 173–5
    case reports 171–3, 180–3
classifications of COPD 75–6
    of exacerbations 80
clinical perspective, smoking cessation 32
coal miners, occupational exposures 86, 87, 88
cognitive behavioural strategies in dyspnoea 25–6
community-based studies, occupational exposures 89
complications, lung volume reduction surgery 4, 5
computed tomography
    in emphysema 2, 4
    of vertebral fractures 111

see also high-resolution computed
    tomography (HRCT)
concrete manufacturing workers,
    occupational exposures 87–8
continuous positive airway pressure (CPAP)
    116, 117, 195–6
corticosteroids, nebulized 150
    see also inhaled corticosteroids; oral
        corticosteroids
cotton dust exposure 87
cough 46
critical illness neuromyopathies (CIN)
    130–1
cuff-leak test 130
cycling
    leg fatigue 54
    role in exercise training 56, 57

D-dimer levels 137
dead space, contribution to ventilatory needs
    54
deconditioning 52
    role in dyspnoea 21, 49, 54
deep venous thrombosis (DVT) 137
delirium tremens 128
depression 11, 79
    and lung volume reduction surgery 4
    role in dyspnoea 22
DEXA examination 108, 109
diabetes mellitus, as cause of muscle
    weakness 40
diagnosis 43
    case studies 43–5, 49–54
    laboratory tests 47
    lung function tests 46–7
    occupationally-related COPD 89–90
    symptoms 46
diaphragm 191
    causes of dysfunction 191–2
    corticosteroid-induced myopathy 56
diaphragm paralysis 193–7
    case report 192–3
digital radiological morphometry 107, 108
digoxin, use in atrial fibrillation 140
distraction strategies in dyspnoea 25–6
domiciliary oxygen therapy, effect on
    exacerbation frequency 9
dynamic hyperinflation 22, 54
    during ETMV 126
dyspnoea 19, 46, 75, 180
    case reports 19–20, 49–54
        cardiac causes 135–6

causes 20–2
    cardiac 135–6
    environmental pollution 31, 33
    differential diagnosis 136–9
    effect on calorie intake 65
    effects of exercise training 57
    effects of supplemental oxygen 185–6
    management 56–9
    protein calorie malnutrition 37
    pulmonary function tests 21
    treatment strategies 22, 26–7
        central perception alteration 25–6
        respiratory muscle function
            improvement 25
        ventilatory demand reduction 23–4
        ventilatory impedance reduction 24–5

echocardiography, diagnosis of pulmonary
    hypertension 140
educational programmes 79
elastase 13, 89
elastic recoil loss 125
emphysema
    α_1 anti-trypsin deficiency 46
    association with malnutrition 99, 100
    lung volume reduction surgery 1–2, 3–5
        case report 2–3
endotoxin exposure 88
endotracheal mechanical ventilation (ETMV)
    125, 126
    weaning 126–7, 129–32
        case reports 127–9, 193, 195–7
endpoints, in trials of antibiotic therapy 144,
    146
energy expenditure 38
energy requirements estimation 67
Enterobacteriaceae infection 147
environmental tobacco smoke (ETS) 31, 33
    risk of tuberculosis infection 158
eosinophilia, diagnostic value 47
Evian classification 179
exacerbations 7–8, 14, 76, 115–16
    antibiotic therapy 144, 146
        choice of agent 146–9
    atrial fibrillation 137
    bronchodilator therapy 151
    case report 10–11
    due to chronic thromboembolic
        pulmonary hypertension 171–5
    indications for hospitalization 80, 149
    infective 143
    management 8–9, 11, 12–13, 80

exacerbations (*continued*)
  mechanical ventilation 80, 116–18, 150–1
  oral corticosteroid therapy 146, 149–50
  prevention 9, 13–14, 80–1
  see also acute respiratory failure (ARF)
exercise, supplemental oxygen 184–6, 187
exercise capacity, effect of nutritional intervention 100
exercise tolerance 53
  relationship to nutritional status 66
  relationship to fat-free mass (FFM) 38
exercise training 56–7, 70–1, 79
  value in dyspnoea 23
exhaled nitric oxide, diagnostic value 47
extubation *see* weaning from ETMV

fans, use in dyspnoea 23
farmers, occupational exposures 88
farmer's lung *see* allergic alveolitis
fat-free mass (FFM) 37, 41, 69, 99
  relationship to exercise tolerance 38
  relationship to osteoporosis 106, 111
fat intake 70
fat mass (FM) 99
fatigue 75
FEV_1 predicted, correlation with bronchiectasis 13
flax dust exposure 87
flow volume loops 54
flunisonide, osteoporosis risk 106
fluoroquinolones 147
  allergic reactions 148
fluticasone
  exacerbation prevention 81
  inhibition of TNFα release 13
  osteoporosis risk 106
  value in bronchiectasis 13
  value in dyspnoea 24–5
formoterol, value in dyspnoea 24–5
fractures 106
free radicals, role in skeletal muscle loss 38

gas exchange impairment, mechanisms 170
gemifloxacin 147
genetic factors 46
Global Alliance for Respiratory Diseases (GARD) 29
GLOBE trial 147
glucocorticoids *see* inhaled corticosteroids; oral corticosteroids
GOLD guidelines
  inhaled corticosteroid use 12
  oral corticosteroid use 11
grain dust exposure 87, 164–5
  case report 162–4
Guillain-Barré syndrome 191

haemoglobin concentration 53
Haemophilus influenzae, antibiotic resistance 147
Haemophilus influenzae colonization 8
hard-rock miners, occupational exposures 87
harm reduction approach, smoking cessation 33
health status assessment 78
healthy worker effect 87
hemidiaphragm, elevated 194
hemidiaphragm paralysis 192, 195–7
  case report 192–3
hemp dust exposure 87
heterogeneity of emphysema 3–4
high-resolution computed tomography (HRCT)
  in allergic alveolitis 161, 162, 163
  in pulmonary arterial thrombosis 172, 181
histone deacetylases, effect of cigarette smoke 14
hormone replacement therapy 112
hospitalization 80, 149
humidification devices, effect on work of breathing 131
hypercapnia 8, 171
  as indication for NIV 119
  oxygen-induced 9, 116
hyperglycaemia, as complication of oral corticosteroids 149
hyperinflation 21–2
  chest X-ray appearance 20
  effect of oxygen therapy 23
hypersensitivity pneumonitis *see* allergic alveolitis
hypnosis, value in dyspnoea 26
hypoxaemia 8, 54, 179–80, 186–7
  carotid body neural discharge 21
  case report 171–3
  in chronic thromboembolic pulmonary hypertension 180–3
  mechanisms 170
  oxygen therapy during exercise 184–6
  role in osteoporosis 110
hypoxic pulmonary hypertension (HPH) 181

ICU admission, indications 149
IgE levels 47

immunomodulator agents 12
immobility, osteoporosis risk 110
immune system
　effects of smoking 159
　response to nutritional supplementation 70
immunodepression 66
incremental exercise tests 51, 52
　interpretation 53–4
industrial workers, occupational exposures 87–8
infective exacerbations 143
　atrial fibrillation 137
　see also exacerbations
inflammation
　during exacerbations 8
　role in skeletal muscle loss 38
　role in weight loss 101–2
　systemic 106, 110
influenza vaccination 9, 12, 80
inhalation fever 165
inhaled corticosteroids
　BMD assessment 112
　exacerbation prevention 9, 12, 81
　risk of osteoporosis 105–6, 110, 112
　value in bronchiectasis 13
　value in dyspnoea 24–5
inhaler technique 56
inspiratory muscle training 25, 55, 57–8, 79
interferon γ levels, effect of smoking 159
international normalized ratio (INR), warfarin therapy 140
intubation 119
　indications 117
ipratropium 78
irritant-induced asthma 87
ISOLDE trial 81

jute dust exposure 87

kyphosis 106, 107, 111

laboratory tests, value in diagnosis 47, 53
lactate accumulation 38, 54
laser procedure, lung volume reduction surgery 1
left ventricular dysfunction, as cause of weaning difficulties 130
leptine 38, 65, 101–2
leukotriene B_4 13
levofloxacin 148
long-acting β_2-agonists 78, 80–1
　see also β_2-agonists

lung cancer 137–8
　case report 98–9
　risk from passive smoking 31
lung function, effect of exacerbations 8
lung function tests 170
　in allergic alveolitis 161–2
　diagnostic value 46–7
Lung Health Study
　effect of smoking cessation 30
　inhaled corticosteroids, osteoporosis risk 106
lung perfusion scans, emphysema 2, 4
lung transplantation, prognostic value of body mass index 100
lung volume reduction surgery (LVRS) 1–5
　association with weight gain 102
　case report 2–3, 98–9
lymphocytes, effects of smoking 159

macrophage metalloelastase (MME) 89
macrophages, effect of smoking 159
magnetic resonance imaging (MRI), of vertebral fractures 111
magnetic stimulation, phrenic nerves 194
malnutrition 37, 65–6
　case reports 38–40, 66–8, 98–9
　differential diagnosis 68
　relationship to healthcare utilization 100
　role in osteoporosis 106
maximum volitional manoeuvres 51
mechanical ventilation 80, 116–17, 150–1
　case report 118
　demonstration of diaphragm paralysis 194
　see also endotracheal mechanical ventilation (ETMV)
metered dose inhalers 151
methylxanthines 151
mid-thigh cross-sectional area 55
mitral stenosis 138–9, 140
Moraxella catarrhalis, antibiotic resistance 147
morphine, value in dyspnoea 24, 27
mortality
　exacerbations as predictor 8
　relationship to BMI 100–1
mortality from COPD 85
MOSAIC trial 147
motor neuron disease 191
moxifloxacin 147
mucociliary clearance, effects of smoking 159
mucolytic agents 12

multiaxial accelerometers 52
muscle hypotrophy 66, 69
muscle strength assessment 51
muscle weakness 13, 37, 38, 41, 55, 99–100
  case reports 38–40, 66–8
  causes 101–2
myopathy, corticosteroid-induced 55, 56
myorelaxant paralysis, role in weaning difficulties 130

nandrolone decanoate therapy 71
narcotics, value in dyspnoea 24, 27
National Emphysema Treatment Trial (NETT) 2, 4
natural killer cells, effects of smoking 159
nebulized bronchodilator therapy 151
nebulized corticosteroids 150
neutrophil elastase 89
neutrophil infiltration, bronchiectasis 13
nicotine, effects on immune system 159
nicotine replacement therapy 30, 32, 33
nitrogen oxides exposure 164–5, 166
nocturnal symptoms 46
nodules, in silicosis 138
non-invasive ventilation 80, 116–17, 119–21, 150–1
  use in weaning from ETMV 129, 130, 131, 132, 193, 195–6
non-small cell lung cancer (NSCLC) 138
NOx syndrome 165, 166
nuisance dust 87
nutritional deficiency, role in dyspnoea 22
nutritional supplementation 25, 70–1
  case report 99

obesity 58–9
occupational exposure
  as cause of lung cancer 138
  contribution to burden of COPD 92
occupationally-related COPD 86–7, 92–3
  case report 85–6
  diagnosis 89–90
  epidemiology 87–9
  management and prevention 90–1
ofloxacin, value during exacerbations 9
opiates, value in dyspnoea 24, 27
oral corticosteroids 12–13, 80
  BMD assessment 112
  GOLD guidelines 11
  side effects 13, 38
    myopathy 55, 56, 66
    osteoporosis 105, 110, 112
  use in allergic alveolitis 162, 164, 166
  use during exacerbations 9, 146, 149–50
organic dust exposure 87
organic dust toxic syndrome (ODTS) 165, 166
osteoporosis 105–6, 110, 150
  vertebral fractures, case report 106–10
osteoprogesterin 110
overweight 58–9
oxygen therapy
  in dyspnoea 23
  during exercise 184–6, 187
  value during exacerbations 9, 80, 116
  value in emphysema 1

particulate matter (PM)
  air quality index 34
  effects 31, 33
passive smoking 31, 33
  risk of tuberculosis infection 158
pathophysiology, COPD 169–71
pedometers 52
PEEPe, application to PSV 130
PEEPi 116, 117, 125, 195, 196, 197
penicillin allergy 144, 147, 148
perfusion scintigraphy, CTEPH 181, 182
pH, indications for NIV 119–21
phase angle (PA) 37, 41
phrenic nerve damage 192
phrenic nerve stimulation 194
physical activity level assessment 52–3
'pink puffers' 99
pneumococcal vaccination 9, 12, 80
pollution
  particulate matter 31, 33
  role in COPD 29
portable oxygen 185–6
positioning, in management of dyspnoea 25
prednisolone
  risk of osteoporosis 105
  use in allergic alveolitis 162, 164, 166
  use during exacerbations 9
pressure support ventilation (PSV) 116–17
  use in weaning from ETMV 129, 130, 131, 132, 193, 195–6
prevention, occupationally-related COPD 90–1
primary care, smoking cessation treatment 31
progression of disease 76
progressive approach, smoking cessation 33
prosthetic heart valves 140

protective equipment, prevention of
  occupational exposure 90, 91
protein intake 70
protein synthesis and turnover 38
Pseudomonas infection 147
psychosocial interventions 79
public health perspective, smoking cessation 32
pulmonary arterial pressure 139–40
pulmonary embolism
  as cause of atrial fibrillation 137
  chronic thromboembolic pulmonary hypertension 171–5, 180–4
pulmonary endarterectomy 173, 174, 182, 184
pulmonary function tests
  changes during exacerbations 7–8
  in dyspnoea 20, 21
  indications for LVRS 2, 3
pulmonary hypertension
  chronic thromboembolic (CTEPH) 172–3, 180–4
  Evian classification 179
  exercise-induced 54
pulmonary rehabilitation 56–7, 79–80
  before lung volume reduction surgery 3
  case report 77–8
  combination with nutritional supplementation 70–1
  effect on exacerbation frequency 9
  role after exacerbations 81
  supplemental oxygen 186
  value in emphysema 1, 2
pulse oximetry 116, 179
pursed-lips breathing (PLB) 24, 59, 79

quadriceps weakness 55
questionnaires, assessment of health status 78

RANK (receptor activator of nuclear factor κB) 110
recombinant human growth hormone (rhGH) therapy 71
reduction-to-stop approach, smoking cessation 33
relapse of exacerbation, risk factors 115–16
relaxation methods, value in dyspnoea 26
REM sleep, respiratory failure in diaphragm paralysis 192
resistance to antibiotics 143–4, 147
resistance training 57
respiratory acidosis, as indication for NIV 119–21

respiratory muscle dysfunction 21–2, 99–100
respiratory muscle function 55
  during weaning from ETMV 127, 130
  improvement 22, 25
respiratory muscle strength assessment 51
respiratory pressure analysis 194–5
respiratory syncytial virus infections, role in exacerbations 8
resting energy expenditure (REE) estimation 67, 69
reversibility 46
rhinovirus infections, role in exacerbations 8, 143
right ventricular function, effect of ETMV 126
risedronate 109
risk factors for COPD 29, 45–6
  passive smoking 31
risk factors for osteoporosis 105, 110
risk factors for weaning/extubation failure 126
risk stratification approach, antibiotic therapy 147, 148
rollators 59

salbutamol 24–5, 151
salmeterol, value in dyspnoea 24–5
sedation, effect on ETMV duration 128–32
self-help associations 80
self-management 56, 79
sex hormones, effects of glucocorticoids 110
short-acting β_2-agonists 78
  see also β_2-agonists
side effects
  of oral corticosteroids 13, 38, 149, 150
    myopathy 55, 56, 66
    osteoporosis 105–6
  of salbutamol 151
  of smoking cessation 30
silicosis 138
silo filler's disease 165
simple nodular silicosis 138
sisal dust exposure 87
skeletal muscle mass loss, case report 38–40
skeletal muscle strength assessment 51
skeletal muscle weakness 13, 37, 38, 41, 55, 99–100
  causes 101–2
sleep apnoea 51
small cell lung cancer 138
'smoker's cough' 14

smoking
    epidemiological studies 87
    gender differences 45–6
    relationship to TB infection 155, 158–9
        case report 155
    role in COPD 29, 85
smoking cessation 9, 12, 14, 29–30, 31–3, 47
    case report 30–1
sniff fluoroscopy test 194
social support, value in dyspnoea 26
socio-economic status (SES), relationship to COPD risk 46
spirometric classification 180
spontaneous breathing trial (SBT) 128, 130, 131
staging, lung cancer 138
staple procedure, lung volume reduction surgery 1
stent placement, emphysema 5
steroids *see* anabolic steroid therapy; inhaled corticosteroids; oral corticosteroids
Streptococcus colonization 8
Streptococcus pneumoniae, antibiotic-resistance 144, 146
stroke risk in atrial fibrillation 140
supplemental oxygen 184–6, 187
surveillance programmes, occupational exposure 91
symptom diaries 26
symptomatic therapy 78–9
symptoms, value in diagnosis 46
systemic symptoms 97
    see also muscle weakness; weight loss

T-piece, use in spontaneous breathing trial 130
testosterone levels 53, 55
testosterone therapy 57
theophylline, value in dyspnoea 24–5
tiotropium 78
    effect on exacerbation frequency 9, 80
    value in dyspnoea 24–5
tracheostomy, use in weaning difficulties 131, 132
triamcinolone, osteoporosis risk 106
TRISTAN (TRial of Inhaled STeroids ANd long-acting β_2-agonists) 12
tuberculosis
    chest X-ray appearances 157
    relationship to smoking 155, 158–9
        case report 155
tumour necrosis factor alpha (TNFα) 13, 106, 110
    effect on protein turnover 66
    role in energy balance 38
tunnel workers, occupational exposures 87

unilateral lung volume reduction surgery 4

ventilation-perfusion (VA/Q) imbalance 170, 179
ventilation-perfusion scans 172, 174, 184
ventilatory capacity, reduced, role in dyspnoea 21
ventilatory demand increase, role in dyspnoea 21
ventilatory demand reduction 22, 23–4
ventilatory impedance reduction 22, 24–5
ventilatory needs, contributory factors 54
vertebral fractures 106
    case report 106–10
    complications 111
    differential diagnosis 108
    management 109–10, 111–12
video assisted thoracoscopic surgery (VATS), lung volume reduction 2
viral infections, role in exacerbations 8, 143
vitamin D intake 109, 112

walking, role in exercise training 56–7
walking aids 59
walking distance, effect of nutritional intervention 100
    see also 6-min walking test
warfarin, use in atrial fibrillation 140
weaning difficulties, ETMV 125, 129–32
    case report 127–9
    due to diaphragm paralysis 193, 195–7
    pathophysiological determinants 126
weaning from ETMV 126–7, 132
weight loss 20, 65–6, 97–8
    assessment 69
    case reports 38–40, 66–8, 98–9
    causes 101–2
        corticosteroids therapy 13
        as complication of vertebral fractures 111
        during exacerbations 8
    management 70–1
weight reduction 58–9
welding fumes exposure 85–6
wheezing 46
women, osteoporosis risk 110–11
World Health Organization, definition of osteoporosis 108, 109

X-ray appearances, vertebral fractures 11, 107